CANCER CARE

THE ROLE OF REPURPOSED DRUGS AND METABOLIC INTERVENTIONS IN TREATING CANCER

2nd Edition

Paul E. Marik, MD, FCCM, FCCP

Published by
Paul Marik Publishing | Norfolk, VA

Publisher's Cataloging-in-Publication Data
Marik, Paul E.

Cancer care : the role of repurposed drugs and metabolic interventions in treating cancer / Paul E. Marik. 2nd edition. - Norfolk, VA : Paul Marik Publishing, 2024.

p. ; cm.

ISBN13: 978-0-9601265-0-7

1. Cancer--Treatment. 2.Cancer--Prevention. 3. Drug resistance. I. Title. II. Marik, Paul E.

RC270.8 M37 2024
616.994--dc23

Printed in the United States of America
28 27 26 25 24 • 5 4 3 2 1

CONTENTS

Disclaimer

This monograph is a review of the published peer-reviewed literature evaluating treatment options for repurposed drugs and lifestyle/dietary changes that can be used as part of a holistic treatment plan for patients with cancer. This monograph is not intended as a stand-alone guide to treating cancer. Nothing in this document should be taken as a basis to initiate treatment without guidance from a medical professional or avoid any treatment prescribed by your treating physician. This information is offered as a basis to assist mutual decision-making between the patient and his/her providers. Cancer care should always be supervised by a healthcare provider. Patients with cancer should ALWAYS consult with their regular oncologist/integrative oncologist as well as an integrative provider, in addition to their primary care provider.

The treatment interventions outlined in this monograph should be used primarily as adjunctive therapy in addition to the treatment provided by an oncologist. The goal is to reduce the toxicity of standard chemotherapy/radiotherapy (and lower the dose of chemotherapy when possible) to prevent severe immunosuppression, organ toxicities, and death from standard chemotherapy and to improve the Quality of Life (QoL). However, the patient may decide to forego conventional chemotherapy and radiotherapy and follow a "holistic" treatment approach based on repurposed drugs and lifestyle interventions; under the principles of true informed consent, patient autonomy and personal decision making the patient has the right to make this choice. It is best that the treatment plan be discussed with the patient's family and the patient's primary health care provider(s) who should supervise the patient's treatment.

Standard chemotherapy targets the rapidly dividing population of cancer cells; these agents commonly adversely affect the tumor microenvironment and may promote the proliferation of cancer stem cells, increasing the potential for metastases. Almost all the interventions listed in this document limit the negative effects on the tumor microenvironment. In addition, many of the agents described herein also target cancer stem cells. This data suggests that these interventions should be used simultaneously with conventional chemotherapy to achieve the best outcomes for our patients.

Note that this document mentions some potential interactions, such as between antioxidants and chemotherapeutic agents, that must be considered.

Target Audience

This information should be of particular interest to patients with cancer, to help guide them through the complicated issue of using repurposed drugs and lifestyle changes for cancer treatment. However, as noted above, it should not be used by patients to self-treat and should be supervised by a qualified healthcare provider. Primary care providers and integrative providers of patients with cancer will find essential information within this document. Furthermore, this document will be of interest to people who would like to reduce their risk of getting cancer. Patients with existing cancers should attempt to discuss the topics of dietary caloric restriction and adjuvant (concurrent) repurposed drugs with their regular oncologist; however, for obvious reasons (vested interests) many oncologists may be unwilling to discuss these topics. In such circumstances patients should engage with an integrative oncologist or integrative primary care provider.

Caution to Patients

This document is based on the highest level of scientific evidence. Patients should review this information, independently validate the reliability of the data, and discuss the treatment options with their family/healthcare advocates. Patients should formulate a treatment plan with their healthcare provider that is compatible with their values and goals. Patients should, however, vigorously avoid unproven and unscientific interventions that only benefit unscrupulous practitioners (see Alternative Medicine).

A repurposed drug is one that is used "off-label," a common basis for prescribing but which means that it has not been reviewed and approved by the U.S. Food and Drug Administration for that indication. Some recommendations may be subject to controversy and differences of opinion among medical authorities. While we believe this monograph offers an accurate view of the current state of science as it is based on solid evidence and pathophysiological principles, public health agencies and regulatory bodies may take contrary positions.

This document represents the author's effort to provide educational material and is not a peer-reviewed publication. The author is not responsible or liable for the use or misuse of the information provided. No guarantees of benefit or the absence of harm can be offered, and reliance on any information provided is solely at your own risk.

Acknowledgments

I would like to thank Dr. Pierre Kory, Dr. 'Justus Hope', Dr. Mobeen Syed, Dr Kathleen Ruddy and Dr. Nathan Goodyear for their valuable contributions to this piece of work. Additionally, I would like to acknowledge the authors of several books on metabolic oncology that were very useful in guiding my thinking. These include Thomas Seyfried (Cancer as a Metabolic Disease), Otto Warburg (The Metabolism of Tumors), Jane McLelland (How to Starve Cancer), Travis Christofferson (Tripping over the Truth), Jeffrey Dach (Cracking the Cancer Toolkit) and Nasha Winter and Jess Higgins Kelley (The Metabolic Approach to Cancer: Integrating deep nutrition, the ketogenic diet, and nontoxic bio-individualized therapies). I am also grateful for groups like Anticancer Fund and the Repurposing Drugs in Oncology (ReDO) group, who provided a framework for this work.

FOREWORD

by Dr. Justus Hope

As a physician and board-certified specialist, I have spent over 30 years caring for patients, mainly those suffering from intractable pain. In January 2020, when my friend contracted Glioblastoma, I began researching to figure out how to help him. What I found annoyed me: my friend could do far better if his doctors would add repurposed drug cocktails to his chemotherapy, radiation, and surgery.

A Harvard professor first stumbled upon repurposed drugs for cancer in the 1990s when he used them to cure his own Glioblastoma. That man is still alive today.

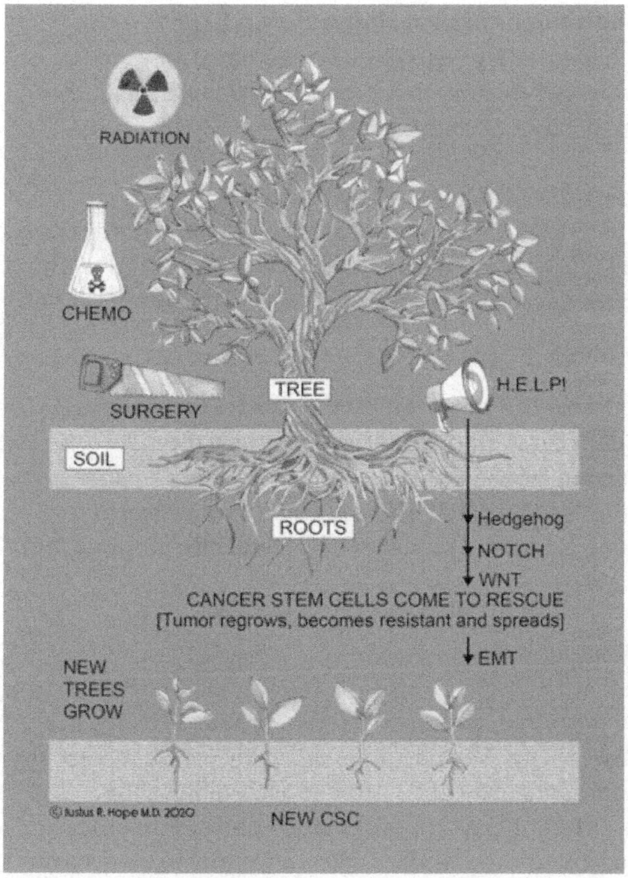

Figure 1: Cancer stem cells are the root of cancer (Source: Dr. Justus Hope)

The most significant problem I see repeatedly is that cancer recurs with resistant metastases. At that point, even with repurposed drugs, it is often a losing battle. This tragedy occurs because the standard treatments of surgery, radiation, and chemotherapy stimulate the growth of cancer stem cells (see Figure 1). Proactively adding repurposed drugs as early as possible can help prevent cancer stem cells from regrowing the tumor into a more resistant and sometimes indestructible form. If we could get all patients and their oncologists to read this document and add a repurposed drug cocktail, along with lifestyle changes, at the onset of a cancer diagnosis (and do this in concert with their treatment plan — whether it be surgery, chemotherapy, and radiation treatment) we would likely see a lot more of these patients not only survive but live better, longer lives.

Justus Hope is a pen name. The author practices medicine under his given name. He has written several books, including *Surviving Cancer, COVID-19, and Disease: The Repurposed Drug Revolution*.

FOREWORD for 2nd EDITION OF CANCER CARE

by Dr. Justus Hope

Dr. Paul Marik, the most published Critical Care Specialist in the United States, has tackled Cancer. Marik reviewed thousands of studies, and in the process, uncovered fundamental truths and busted persistent myths in publishing *Cancer Care 1st Edition*. This 2nd edition expands these and adds propranolol, a relatively unknown anticancer agent. Moreover, Ivermectin is moved up to Tier One based on emerging evidence.

There are numerous practical suggestions, and all are based on PubMed studies so no one can dispute the scientific and evidence basis. Marik gives us some guidance on which three repurposed drugs to take before cancer surgery or biopsy to decrease the risk of spreading the cancer through surgical manipulation. Cutting a tumor has long been known to pose a risk of spreading cancer, yet patients have not been warned of this. Marik notes that studies have shown that these risks can be reduced with the pre-operative use of celecoxib, propranolol, or cimetidine. Better yet, combining all three may have a synergistic effect.

However, my review of Dr. Marik's *Cancer Care 2nd Edition* provided much more, and I am honored to share it here. First, let me start with the root cause of cancer. Dr. Marik notes the Somatic Mutation Theory, the one we are all taught in medical school, is not supported by the growing data. Cancer, as we have been told for decades, is not caused by a series of mutations that result eventually in out-of-control cell division.

Instead, the data provides much more support for the Mitochondrial Dysfunction Model as espoused by Dr. Thomas Seyfried. When cancer cells' mitochondria are transplanted into normal cells, the normal cells become cancerous. However, when cancer cells' nuclei are transplanted into normal cells, the cancer does not transfer. The causative agent is carried in the mitochondria, not in the nucleus. The central issue in cancer is defective mitochondria, not DNA mutations.

Why has this myth that cancer arises from DNA mutations persisted?

Because the Somatic Mutation Theory is the narrative, and the narrative produces expensive and profitable treatments. The results remain lacking. The narrative probably won't change any time soon, however, Dr. Marik notes that addressing cancer treatment according to the Mitochondrial Dysfunction Model produces different therapies and much better outcomes. These treatments, which can be done in addition to the standard of care for most patients, can result in longer survival times - in some cases complete remission. Perhaps more importantly, Marik's recommendations may result in avoiding cancer altogether, a prospect that could demolish the cancer industry's profits.

But I digress.

Let us get to some of the other myths that Marik busts.
"Sunlight is bad for you as it increases your risk of cancer and sunscreen is healthy for you as it decreases your cancer risk."

Wrong. It is quite the opposite. In the 2nd Edition, Dr. Marik convincingly shows, via multiple studies, how sunlight reduces melanoma risk and improves survival and how sunscreen does the opposite.

When my friend and colleague developed Glioblastoma, a serious brain cancer with an average survival of 12.7 months, I dove into the medical literature and found repurposed drugs. After publishing a book in 2020 – *Surviving Cancer COVID-19 and Disease: The Repurposed Drug Revolution* – on my findings including the vast evidence base on Repurposed Drugs for Cancer, my friend added four of these - Atorvastatin, Mebendazole, Metformin, and Doxycycline - to his treatment plan through the US Care Oncology Clinic, and he survived some 46 months - almost 4 times longer than expected.

For this his family was grateful. However, we had all hoped for more. And when he ultimately passed, it was the radiation damage that played the largest role, not the cancer. Dr. Thomas Seyfried has noticed the same issue in his interviews on Glioblastoma. Seyfried explains the brain should never be irradiated.

I only wish we had this information in 2020. We needed Dr. Seyfried's and Dr. Marik's cancer knowledge then. My friend could have done better and lived longer.

Which brings me to propranolol. Dr. Marik ranks this second in evidence support only to Vitamin D3. Why? The book covers all the technical and detailed anti-cancer pathways of propranolol. However, the gist of it is this:
Propranolol is a beta blocker that shields the effect of catecholamines on the body. Catecholamines like norepinephrine and epinephrine are released when we encounter stress, and stress increases the likelihood of developing cancer. Therefore, by blocking the catecholamines, propranolol reduces the risk of developing cancer.
However, the key property of this beta blocker is that it reduces metastatic spread.

This brings me to one of Dr. Marik's favorite parts of his upcoming book. Three repurposed drugs can offer preventative effects against metastatic spread in those undergoing cancer surgery. These include celecoxib, cimetidine, and propranolol. Dr. Marik writes the combination may be synergistic.

Dr. Paul Marik has taken the science of Repurposed Drugs in Cancer to a world-class level. *Cancer Care 1st Edition* is worthy of a PhD thesis with more than 1200 PubMed citations. Marik has earned another PhD with more than 1300 references in this new edition. The most published Critical Care Specialist in the United States has become the most credible scientific voice for repurposed drugs in preventing and treating Cancer.

And on a personal note, talking with Dr. Marik has been a pleasant adventure. Speaking with him is like talking to your best friend albeit with a South African accent and an AI-like knowledge of the subject. He has the most remarkable combination of intellect, compassion, and humility of anyone I know.

Dr. Marik's *Cancer Care 1st and 2nd Editions* will change how the world approaches cancer.

Justus R. Hope, MD
Redding, California
May 2024

PREFACE

By Dr. Paul Marik

"It is more important to know what kind of person has a disease than to know what kind of disease a person has."
Hippocrates (460-370 BC)

"When we have the power to help, we have the duty of doing so."
Mirko Beljanski (1923-1998)

Years ago, when I had more hair and COVID-19 wasn't even a twinkle in anyone's eye, I became known for developing a treatment for one of the most common causes of death in hospitals — medical sepsis, which takes the lives of around 1,000 people each day in this country alone. My 'cocktail' consisted of three safe, inexpensive, easily accessible drugs that could be repurposed for sepsis. Time after time when I gave patients vitamin C, hydrocortisone, and thiamine, their condition turned around within hours. (1)

Repurposing drugs is nothing new. Around 30 percent of all prescriptions in the United States are written for off-label uses. (2) Bringing new drugs to market can take decades and cost billions of dollars while existing licensed drugs can be repositioned to offer safe, affordable, and effective treatments in a short period of time.

We have had great success in using repurposed drugs, as well as vitamins, supplements, and lifestyle changes, to treat COVID, long COVID, and COVID vaccine complications over the past few years. (3) While researching and developing protocols for the above conditions, I began reading huge volumes of information and saw an interesting pattern emerging that led me to investigate the potential role repurposed drugs could play in the treatment of cancer, along with some amazing non-pharmaceutical interventions like intermittent fasting. In doing so, I learned that much of what I once understood about what causes cancer and how it should be treated was wrong or at least misguided.

In putting this document together, I have invested thousands of hours, read more than 1800 peer-reviewed papers, and consulted with dozens of doctors and experts. I want to be clear that I am not suggesting I have found a cure for cancer, nor am I the first to propose using repurposed drugs for cancer. (4-7) What I hope to provide is a well-researched clearinghouse of information that picks up where traditional cancer therapies leave off. I aim to inspire providers caring for cancer patients to broaden their horizons and think creatively about readily available interventions, with science to back up their efficacy, that could improve their patients' outcomes.

While I no longer see patients directly, I will forever be bound by my Hippocratic Oath to 'first do no harm'. I offer this compendium of information as my latest contribution toward that end.

PREFACE to 2nd Edition.

The basic concepts and treatment approach outlined in the first Edition of this monograph have not changed. However, many of the concepts are refined and expanded. A number of additional repurposed drugs have been added to the list. Most importantly, the stratification of the list of preferred repurposed drugs has changed based on newly acquired clinical information. This is a dynamic process, and it is likely that this list will change in future updates.

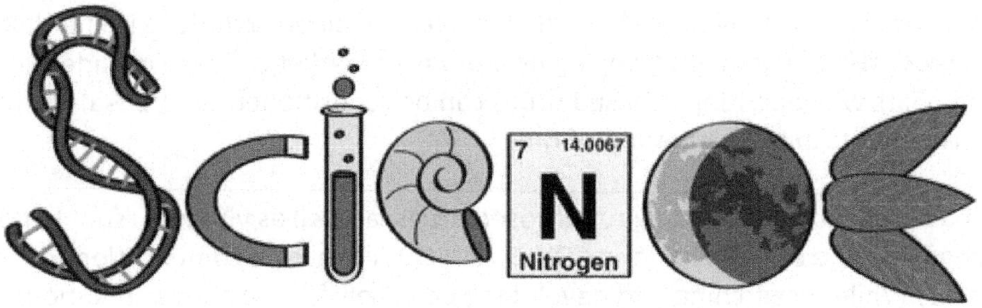

We Need to follow the true science.

Glossary of common abbreviations

AKT: Protein kinase B (PKB or *Akt*)
ALA: alpha-linolenic acid
AMPK: adenosine monophosphate-activated kinase
ARG-1: arginase 1
BRACA1: Breast cancer gene 1
BAX/BAK: members of the Bcl-2 family of apoptotic proteins
CCR6: Chemokine receptor 6
CSC: Cancer stem cells
CI: confidence interval
CGM: continuous glucose monitor
COX: cyclooxygenase
DC: dendritic cell
FOXO1: Forkhead Box O1
EGFR: epidermal growth factor
EGCG: epigallocatechin gallate
ERKs: extracellular-signal-regulated kinases
FGF: fibroblast growth factor
GI: glycemic index
GTCs: Green tea catechins
GDH: glutamate dehydrogenase
HDL: High density lipoprotein
HIF: hypoxia inducible factor
HR: hazard ratio
HK2- Hexokinase-2
HSP: heat shock protein
Hh: Hedgehog pathway
HER2: human epidermal growth factor receptor 2
IGF-1: Insulin-like growth factor 1
IκBα: inhibitor of nuclear factor kappa B
INF: interferon
in vitro: performed in a test tube or culture dish
in vivo: performed in a living organism
GH: growth hormone
IL: interleukin
JAK2: Janus kinase 2
JNK: c-Jun N-terminal kinase
MAPK: mitogen-activated protein kinase
MAMs: metastasis-associated macrophages
MDSC: Myeloid-derived stem cells
MMPs: matrix metalloproteinases
mTOR: mammalian target of rapamycin
NAD: nicotinamide adenine dinucleotide

NF-KB: nuclear factor Kappa beta
NOS: nitric oxide synthase
NK cells: natural killer cells
NSAID: non-steroidal anti-inflammatory drug
Nrf2: nuclear factor E2–related factor 2
OR: odds ratio
PDE5 inhibitor: phosphodiesterase 5 inhibitors
PD-1/PD-1L: Programmed cell death protein 1/ligand
PI3K: phosphoinositide 3-kinase signaling pathway
PGE2: prostaglandin E2
RCT: randomized controlled trial
REM: rapid eye movement
ROS: reactive oxygen species
ReDO: Repurposing Drugs in Oncology
RFS: recurrence-free survival
RR: relative risk
STAT3: signal transducer and activator of transcription 3
TAM: Tumor-associated macrophages
TGF: transforming growth factor
TG: triglyceride
TME: tumor microenvironment
TCR: T cell receptor
TLR: Toll like-receptor
TCGA: The Cancer Genome Atlas Program
TNF: tumor necrosis factor
TRAIL: tumor necrosis factor-related apoptosis-inducing ligand
Tregs: T-regulatory cells
USPSTF: U.S. Preventive Services Taskforce
UV: ultraviolet
VDAC: voltage-dependent anion channel
VCAM1*:* vascular cell adhesion molecule *1*
VEGF: vascular endothelial growth factor
WNT: WNT signaling pathway

CHAPTER 1: INTRODUCTION

We strongly endorse an Integrative approach to the management of patients with cancer. There is much confusion amongst patients (and many health care providers) as to the characteristics of integrative oncology. Furthermore, complementary and alternative medicine (CAM) strategies while outside of the conventional medicine paradigm are quite distinct and should be considered separately. The use of CAM is frequently seen in the oncology setting, with nearly half of cancer patients reporting CAM use following diagnosis and as many as 91% during active chemotherapy and radiation treatment. (8, 9) It is, therefore, imperative that the distinction between complementary and alternative medicine be reviewed with the patient and that oncologists have open non-judgmental discussions with their patients and families and appreciate the potential risks and benefits of CAM to facilitate open and inclusive discussion. This has the potential to allow for the safe integration of complementary (and not alternative) strategies into conventional care and for increased knowledge-sharing between patients and providers. (10)

INTEGRATIVE ONCOLOGY AND OTHER MODELS OF PATIENT CARE

- **Integrative Oncology**. Provision of care by a "true integrative oncologist" is the preferred model of care for the patient with cancer. An integrative oncologist is dual qualified/certified in orthodox medicine (oncology) as well as in integrative medicine (complementary medicine). In many countries — including Israel, Germany, Switzerland, India, and other countries in Asia — by default most oncologists are dually trained and function as integrative oncologists. This is distinct from the United States, Australia, and some European countries, where most oncologists follow the traditional orthodox approach.

  The integrative oncologist has a diverse array of tools (therapeutic options) in his/her toolbox and formulates an individualized and unique treatment plan for each patient. The integrative physician and patient co-design an integrative treatment plan, recruiting the "best of both worlds." This may entail the use of chemotherapeutic agents/radiotherapy together with complementary medicine or complementary medicine alone. Patients participate in their treatment plans in a shared decision-making model. There is open patient-physician communication that is non-judgmental and in keeping with the patient's cultural beliefs.

  Integrative oncology involves a multidisciplinary team with caregivers committed to an integrative care model. The major focus of care is the patient's quality of life with an emphasis on a) relief of symptoms, anxiety, and pain, b) quality of sleep, c) nutrition, d) nutraceutical/herbs and repurposed drugs, and e) lifestyle changes. Integrative oncology complements conventional medicine while keeping within the *boundaries of scientific rigor.* Integrative medicine strives to be based on *rigorous research, conducted in accordance with scientific methodologies*. Integrative oncology focuses on pragmatic research; pragmatic trials test interventions in the full spectrum of everyday clinical settings, in order to maximize applicability and generalizability. Such pragmatic trials allow for a multimodal integrative approach, are individualized, and with patient-centered outcomes. Patients in countries where care is being managed by "orthodox" oncologists should consult with integrative primary care physicians.

- **Complementary medicine.** Complementary medicine involves techniques not considered within the scope of traditional orthodox medicine, but which have a scientific underpinning and are often practiced by non-orthodox practitioners. Examples of complementary approaches include herbal medicine, tai chi, yoga, acupuncture, massage therapy, spinal manipulation, art therapy, music therapy, mindfulness-based stress reduction, and many others. Complementary medicine complements traditional orthodox medicine and when applied by a traditional physician it is known as integrative care.

- **Alternative medicine.** Alternative medicine is used in place of (as an alternative to) conventional medicine. Alternative medicine is ***NOT science-based***. Alternative medicine is any practice that aims to achieve the healing effects of medicine despite lacking biological plausibility, testability, repeatability, or evidence of effectiveness. Unlike orthodox and integrative medicine, which employs the scientific method to test plausible therapies by way of responsible and ethical clinical trials, producing repeatable evidence of either effect or of no effect, *alternative therapies reside outside of medical science* and do not originate from using the scientific method, but instead rely on testimonials, anecdotes, religion, tradition, superstition, belief in supernatural "energies" and pseudoscience. Some alternative practices are based on theories that contradict the established science of how the human body works.

THE SOCIETAL IMPACT OF CANCER

Cancer is a global threat that seriously affects human life, with a prevalence of more than 10 million deaths every year. Nearly 2 million Americans were diagnosed with cancer in 2023, with approximately 609,820 deaths (see Table 1). (11)

Cancer is the second most common cause of death in the United States, exceeded only by heart disease. At least 42% of newly diagnosed cancers in this country are potentially avoidable, including 19% of cancers caused by smoking and at least 18% caused by a combination of excess body weight, alcohol consumption, poor nutrition, and physical inactivity. (11)

Types of Cancer (MALES)	# of cases	% of cases	Types of Cancer (FEMALES)	# of cases	% of cases
Lung & bronchus	61,170	21	Lung & bronchus	59,910	21
Prostate	34,700	11	Breast	43,170	15
Colon & rectum	28,470	9	Colon & rectum	24,080	8
Pancreas	26,620	8	Pancreas	23,930	8
Liver	19,000	6	Ovary	13,270	5
Leukemia	13,900	4	Uterus	13,030	5
ALL SITES	322,080		ALL SITES	287,740	

Table 1: Leading sites of cancer deaths - 2023 estimates (Source: American Cancer Society)

In addition, due to the 'chemicalization' of our society, humans are exposed to numerous carcinogens daily. (12) While these environmental carcinogens have likely contributed to the increasing risk of cancer, the impact is difficult to quantify.

The doctor who goes by the pen name 'Justus Hope' and who wrote a book on cancer and repurposed drugs, says almost everyone who gets cancer shares at least one common risk factor. These include cigarette smoking (40%), insulin resistance (40%), viruses (10%), and hereditary cancers such as familial adenomatous polyposis, BRACA mutations, etc. (10%). (13)

Curiously, it is not being overweight or obese that is most related to cancer; it is the presence of insulin resistance. (13) Furthermore, patients who have insulin resistance and an elevated

TG/HDL ratio (a measure of cholesterol levels) are at an increased risk of not only heart disease and Alzheimer's disease but also cancer. (13, 14)

Current cancer treatments are highly complex and based on multiple modalities (see Figure 2), many of which are extremely expensive and have limited benefit (in terms of quality of life and five-year survival rate), and many of which are also highly toxic. The National Cancer Institute estimated that in 2020 cancer-related medical costs in the U.S. were $208.9 billion, which is likely a gross underestimate due to the increasing costs of individual medications. (11)

In 2000, only two oncology drugs garnered more than $1 billion in sales. Just 10 years later, the top 10 oncology drugs each exceeded $1 billion in revenue. By 2010, there were three oncology drug sales representatives for every 10 oncologists in the United States. Cancer, you see, is big business. (15) Patients and their families frequently face extreme financial burdens and distress as a result of cancer treatment — this is known as "financial toxicity." (16)

Despite the vast spending on treating common cancers like lung, breast, colorectal, prostate, and pancreas, age-adjusted death rates have remained remarkably stable or have even increased since 1930. (11) Compared to the improvements in preventing and treating heart disease, cancer mortality has remained relatively unchanged over the past 30 years. (17)

Based on data collected between 1992 and 1997 for the 22 most common malignancies, Morgan et al estimated the overall contribution of curative and adjuvant cytotoxic chemotherapy to 5-year survival in adults was estimated to be 2.3% in Australia and 2.1 % in the U.S. (18) More recent data from the U.S. indicate that the 5-year cancer survival rate has only increased from 63% to 68% over the last 25 years (1995 to 2018).). Ladanie et al. showed that over the past fifteen years, the improvement in overall survival by new cancer therapies is a meager 2.4 months.(19) The study by Del Paggio et al reports an improvement of 3.4 months over the last thirty years. (20)

This data suggests that despite the billions of dollars spent on cancer therapy, the "traditional" approach has largely failed; alternative, less expensive, less toxic, and more effective therapies are urgently required.

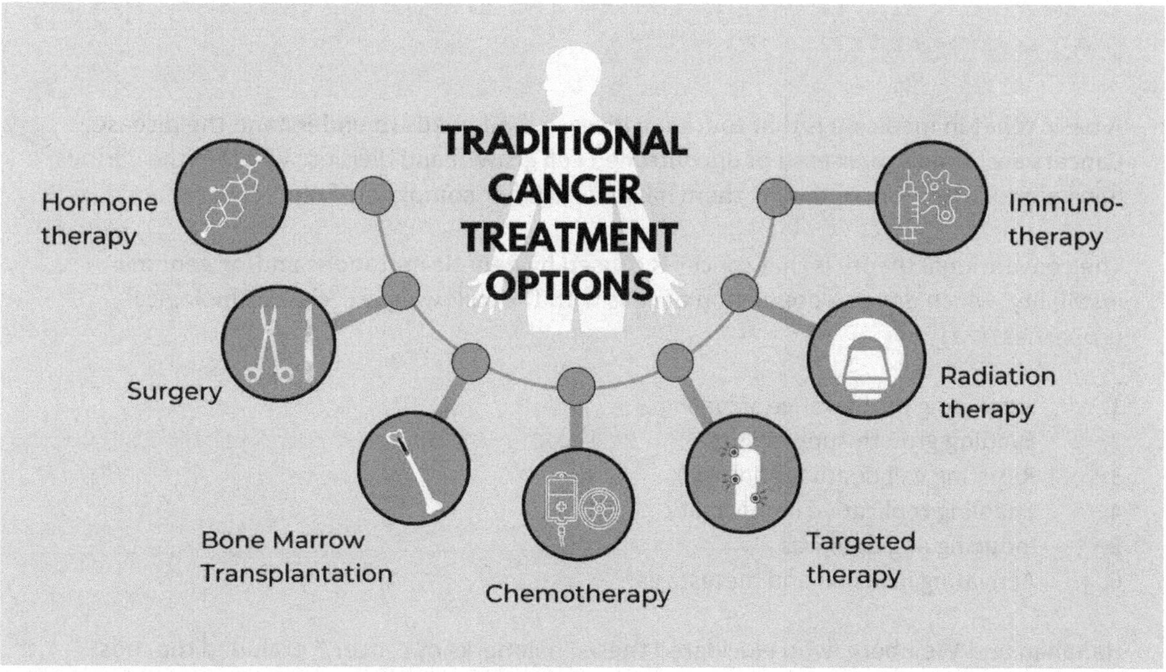

Figure 2: "Modern" cancer treatments are expensive and have limited benefit (Source: FLCCC)

CHAPTER 2: WHAT IS CANCER: UNDERSTANDING ITS PATHOGENETIC CAUSES

A basic tenet in medicine is that to treat a disease, one needs to understand the disease. Cancers are, simply, a disease of uncontrolled cell growth and division, wherein the various natural processes for containing them have partially or completely failed.

The conventional theory is that cancer is caused by genetic mutations and/or genomic instability, which drives a population of cells with the following six "classic" biological properties: (21)

1. Sustaining proliferative signaling
2. Evading growth suppressors
3. Resisting cell death (apoptosis)
4. Enabling replicative immortality
5. Inducing angiogenesis
6. Activating invasion and metastasis

Hanahan and Weinberg, who elucidated these "hallmarks of cancer," excluded the most important and universal finding in all cancer cells, (22) namely the metabolic reprogramming of cancer cells, with aerobic glycolysis — the so-called "Warburg effect" that we will explore below. (23, 24)

Conventional thinking suggests cancer arises from a single cell due to specific mutations in that cell, which are then characteristic of the patient's "cancer genome." The loss of genomic "caretakers" or "guardians," involved in sensing and repairing DNA damage, has been proposed to explain the increased mutability of tumor cells. The loss of these caretaker systems allows genomic instability, thus enabling pre-malignant cells to reach the six essential hallmarks of cancer.

The Cancer Genome Atlas Program (TCGA), modeled after the human genome project, was an attempt to determine the characteristic mutations of common cancers. (25) The TCGA assessed mutational signatures using 84,729,690 somatic mutations from 4,645 whole-genome and 19,184 exome sequences that encompassed most types of cancer. (26, 27) The finding of this massive project raises serious doubts concerning the mutation theory of cancer.

The TCGA identified 49 single-base-substitution, 11 double-base-substitution, 4 clustered-base-substitution, and 17 small insertion-and-deletion signatures. However, no specific mutation was characteristic of any particular cancer (except CML and the Philadelphia chromosome). In many tumors no mutation was found, and there was marked heterogeneity of mutations between tumors of the same cell type (intertumoral heterogeneity) and within the same tumor (intratumoral heterogeneity). (7) In pediatric tumors such as medulloblastoma, the number of driver genes was low (zero to two). In common adult tumors, such as pancreatic, colorectal, breast, and brain cancers, the number of mutated driver genes was frequently between three to six, but several tumors had only one or two driver mutations. The notion that cancer is caused solely by mutations to key genes is becoming harder to maintain. (7) The inconsistencies are too numerous and pronounced.

AN ALTERNATE THEORY: CANCER IS A METABOLIC DISEASE

Travis Christofferson, in his book entitled "Tripping over the Truth", articulated the following:

"No researcher can point to any single mutation or combination of mutations and say with confidence that it is alone the cause of cancer. Nor can researchers point to a series of cellular systems rendered dysfunctional by mutations and make the same claims with confidence." (7)

In a 2009 op-ed for The New York Times, James Watson, a Nobel Prize winner known as the "father of DNA," suggested that *"we may have to turn our main research focus away from decoding the genetic instructions behind cancer and toward understanding the chemical reactions within cancer cells."* (28)

Although very specific processes underlie malignant transformation, many non-specific influences can initiate diseases — including radiation, chemicals, viruses, inflammation, etc. Indeed, it appears that prolonged exposure to almost any provocative agent in the environment can potentially cause cancer. (29) That a very specific process could be initiated in very unspecific ways was considered "the oncogenic paradox" by Szent-Gyorgyi. (29) This paradox remains largely unresolved. (30)

Still, the concept of genetic mutations and genetic instability underpins most conventional cancer treatments. Big Pharma and the medical establishment have propagated this concept to promote the use of very expensive and toxic chemotherapeutic drugs; as mentioned above, cancer is profitable for the pharmaceutical industry. Curing cancer is not the goal.

There is considerable evidence that the genetic mutation theory may not be entirely correct. Dr. Thomas Seyfried provides a compelling argument that cancer is primarily a metabolic rather than a genetic disease. (30, 31) His underlying hypothesis is that cancer is a mitochondrial disorder with impaired oxidative phosphorylation and energy production; the genomic abnormalities are likely secondary to disordered energy production and cellular metabolism. Dr. Seyfried has clearly demonstrated that disordered mitochondrial function and energy production are common to all cancers. (30, 31) The view of cancer as primarily a metabolic disease will dramatically impact the approach to cancer management and prevention. However, it is clear that a very complex and bi-directional relationship exists between genetic instability and mitochondrial dysfunction.

The idea that cancer is a metabolic disease was first noted by Otto Warburg in 1927, who was awarded the Nobel Prize in Medicine and Physiology in 1931 for his discoveries. (23, 24) Dr. Warburg, reported that cancer cells are dependent on aerobic glycolysis (breakdown of glucose to lactate) with impaired oxidative phosphorylation (pyruvate does not enter the Krebs cycle in the mitochondria). (23, 24) In simple terms, this means cancer feeds on glucose.

In contrast to normal differentiated cells, which rely primarily on mitochondrial oxidative phosphorylation to generate the energy needed for cellular processes, most cancer cells instead rely on aerobic glycolysis, a phenomenon termed “the Warburg effect.” (32) Dr. Warburg proposed that irreversible damage to respiration was the prime cause of cancer. Aerobic glycolysis in cancer cells involves elevated glucose uptake with lactic acid production in the presence of oxygen. (30)

Following his extensive research on tumor metabolism, Dr. Warburg stated: “Cancer, above all other diseases, has countless secondary causes. But, even for cancer, there is one prime cause. Summarized in a few words, the prime cause of cancer is the replacement of the respiration of oxygen in the normal body cell by fermentation of sugar.” (23, 24)

This metabolic phenotype is the basis for tumor imaging using labeled glucose analogs and has become an important diagnostic tool for cancer detection and management. Genes for glycolysis are overexpressed in the majority of cancers examined. (30) Numerous studies show that tumor mitochondria are structurally and functionally abnormal and incapable of generating normal levels of energy. (33-38) In addition, there is compelling evidence that mitochondrial dysfunction, operating largely through the RTG response (mitochondrial stress signaling), underlies the mutator phenotype of tumor cells. (39-43) Impaired mitochondrial function can induce abnormalities in tumor suppressor genes and oncogenes.

It is well documented that tumorigenicity can be suppressed when cytoplasm from enucleated normal cells is fused with tumor cells to form cybrids, suggesting that normal mitochondria can suppress the tumorigenic phenotype. (44, 45) Singh and co-workers provided additional evidence for the role of mitochondria in the suppression of tumorigenicity by showing that exogenous transfer of wild-type mitochondria to cells with depleted mitochondria (rho0 cells) could reverse the altered expression of the APE1 multifunctional protein and the tumorigenic phenotype. (46) It is also well documented that nuclei from cancer cells can be reprogrammed to form normal tissues when transplanted into normal cytoplasm, despite the continued presence of the tumor-associated genomic defects in the cells of the derived tissues. (47, 48)

Viruses have long been recognized as the cause of some cancers. It is interesting that several cancer-associated viruses localize to, or accumulate in, the mitochondria. Viral alteration of mitochondrial function could potentially disrupt energy metabolism, thus altering expression of tumor suppressor genes and oncogenes over time. Viruses that can affect mitochondrial function include the Epstein-Barr virus (EBV), Kaposi’s sarcoma-associated herpes virus (KSHV), human papillomavirus (HPV), hepatitis B virus (HBV), hepatitis C virus (HCV), and human T-cell leukemia virus type 1 (HTLV-1) as well as SARS-CoV-2. (49-51)

A cell’s first line of defense against becoming cancerous is apoptosis. The apoptotic pathway is kept in check by anti-apoptotic factors; these two systems function in balance, and when one or the other becomes dominant, the cell either apoptoses, or it resists apoptotic signals. *The metabolic approach to cancer treatment promotes apoptotic pathways.*

In addition to the ultrastructural abnormalities in mitochondria and mitochondrial-associated membranes, no cancer cell has been found with a normal content or composition of cardiolipin, the cristae-enriched phospholipid that contributes to oxidative phosphorylation (OxPhos). Cardiolipin is recognized as essential for the proper function of the electron transport chain (ETC) super complex structures, which are linked directly to cristae ultrastructure. (52) Apart from these documented abnormalities in mitochondria structure and function, genetic abnormalities that alter mitochondrial function have also been recognized in many cancers. The p53 mutation, which is found in many cancers, can disrupt mitochondrial OxPhos. The retinoblastoma tumor suppressor protein, Rb, has been linked to abnormalities in mitochondrial mass and OxPhos function. (52) It appears that few, if any, cancer types are free of mitochondrial abnormalities, whether structural or functional, making OxPhos inefficiency the signature metabolic hallmark of cancer. As tumor cells require a significant ATP/ADP ratio for invasion, an alternative system for ATP synthesis must be in place to compensate for OxPhos inefficiency. A reliance on cytoplasmic (glycolysis) and mitochondrial substrate level phosphorylation (SLP) can provide both the necessary ATP and the metabolic building blocks needed for tumor cell proliferation and invasion in either aerobic or anaerobic growth environments. (52)

Cells using oxygen consumption for ATP synthesis will die quickly under hypoxia or when treated with cyanide. As many cancer cells can survive when treated with cyanide or in hypoxia, ATP synthesis in these cells must come from sources other than OxPhos. (52) The genomic instability and random somatic mutations seen in most cancers arise largely as downstream epiphenomenon of ROS production and OxPhos dysfunction.

Since the 1950s, it has been recognized that tumors require large amounts of glutamine for growth and survival (hence the inclusion of glutamine in most culture media). The high-affinity glutamine transporter Slc1a5 (ASCT2) is upregulated in multiple types of cancer including glioblastoma multiforme (GBM) and has been implicated in mediating net glutamine uptake. (53) Several decades later, it was recognized that glutamine is a major energy source in tumor cells including GBM. (30, 31, 52-55) The interconversion of glutamine and glutamate is bidirectional in normal cells, with glutamine synthetase catalyzing glutamine formation. In tumors, however, overexpression of glutaminases and suppression of glutamine synthetase favor the forward reaction toward glutamate. Glutaminase activity correlates well with tumor growth rates in vivo. Glutamine not only provides nitrogen for synthesis of nucleotides and NEAAs but also provides a-ketoglutarate to serve as a precursor for ATP synthesis through substrate-level phosphorylation in the citric acid cycle.

Abnormalities in the cancer cell mitochondrial network would reduce OxPhos efficiency, thus forcing the cell to rely more heavily on SLP for ATP synthesis. The succinate-CoA ligase (SUCL) is a mitochondrial matrix enzyme that catalyzes the conversion of succinyl-CoA and ADP to CoA-SH, succinate, and ATP. Notably, when the SUCL proceeds toward ATP formation it is termed "mitochondrial substrate-level phosphorylation" (mSLP), a process that can yield high-energy phosphates in the absence of oxygen. Energy generation through mSLP is critically important in several metabolic pathways and could compensate for inefficient energy production through Ox-Phos in cancer cells. The glutaminolysis pathway would support production of high-energy phosphates through the sequential metabolism of glutamine → glutamate → α-ketoglutarate → succinyl CoA → succinate. (30, 31, 52-55) Glutamine has long been considered an essential metabolite for tumor cell growth. (56) Glutaminase is an enzyme that catalyzes the production of glutamate from the amino acid glutamine, which then feeds into the TCA cycle.

Chen et al. showed that glutamine utilization is a common feature of cells with partial defects in OxPhos, irrespective of the specific OxPhos complex affected. (57) OxPhos inefficiency could account in large part for the glutamine addiction of cancers. Glutamine-supported mSLP can compensate for OxPhos deficiency in either hypoxic or normoxic growth environments.

It is well recognized that most, if not all, tumor cells are dependent on glucose and glutamine for growth. Although amino acids other than glutamine can also provide energy through mSLP, glutamine is the only amino acid not requiring expenditure of energy for the metabolic interconversions necessary to produce succinyl-CoA. (52)

Mitochondrial substrate level phosphorylation (mSLP) in the glutamine-driven glutaminolysis pathway, substantiated by the succinate-CoA ligase reaction in the TCA cycle, can partially compensate for reduced ATP synthesis through both Ox- Phos and glycolysis. A protracted insufficiency of OxPhos coupled with elevated glycolysis and an auxiliary, fully operational mSLP, would cause a cell to enter its default state of unbridled proliferation with consequent dedifferentiation and apoptotic resistance, i.e., cancer. (52) The simultaneous restriction of glucose and glutamine offers a therapeutic strategy for managing cancer.

Insulin and cancer

Insulin, insulin-growth factor-1 (IGF-1), phosphoinositide 3-kinase (PI3K) and mTOR are nutrient sensors and cellular growth factor associated with initiation and propagation of cancer.(58) Established risk factors for cancers include obesity, sedentary lifestyle and type 2 diabetes mellitus which are characterized by hyperinsulinemia and insulin resistance. (59) Higher circulating insulin and C-peptide (a marker of insulin resistance and long-term insulin secretion) have also been associated with an increased risk of cancer. The association between hyperinsulinemia and cancer suggests that a diet inducing an elevated insulin response may contribute to tumour growth. A recent study showed that higher dietary glycemic load was associated with an increased risk of recurrence and death in stage III colon cancer patients. (60) Yuan et al determined the association of post-diagnosis dietary insulin scores with survival among 2006 patients from two large prospective cohorts who were diagnosed with colorectal cancer.(59) The insulin score was developed to quantify postprandial insulin response for various food items. In the study by Yuan et al the adjusted HRs for colorectal cancer specific mortality comparing the highest to the lowest quintiles of the dietary insulin load was 1.82 (95% CI: 1.20–2.75, p=0.006).

Carcinogens

Carcinogens and other environmental factors are strongly associated with the development of cancer. These factors are likely due to chronic cellular injury and mitochondrial damage. See Table 3.

COVID-19, SPIKE PROTEIN, AND "TURBO CANCERS"

Published case reports and social media reports have reported that exposure to the spike protein, particularly following mRNA vaccination for COVID-19, is associated with "turbo cancers."(61-63) These include new cancers that are highly malignant, often in young patients and rare cell types/locations, as well as tumor recurrences in patients after remission. It has also been proposed that long COVID-19 can predispose recovered patients to develop cancer and accelerate cancer progression. (64) The U.S. Department of Defense Medical Epidemiology Database (DMED) (65) reported a 664% increase in malignant neoplasms following the deployment of COVID-19 mRNA vaccination in the military (until this data was erroneously removed). This information is now supported by an analysis of the VAERS database which has demonstrated a strong "safety signal" for many cancers but particularly for breast, colon, liver lung and kidney cancer. (66) Death trends for cancers in the USA (ICD codes C00-D48) for individuals aged 15-44 demonstrated a rise which started in 2020 (1.7%) and accelerated substantially in 2021 (5.6%) and 2022 (7.9%). (67) A similar trend has been reported in the UK.(68) It is likely that this trend has continued into 2023 and 2024. It should be noted that cancer is largely a disease of the aged and the increase in cancers deaths in this young cohort of patients is alarming. A recent Japanese study demonstrated a significant increase in age-adjusted mortality rates from cancer as a whole, as well as some specific types of cancer, namely leukemia, as well as ovarian, prostate, oropharyngeal, pancreatic, and breast cancers.(69) In this study some excess cancer mortalities was observed in 2021 after mass vaccination with the first and second vaccine doses, and significant excess mortalities were observed for all cancers after mass vaccination with the third dose in 2022. The increasing risk of cancer with the increasing number of "shots" may be related to increasing immuno-suppression likely caused by immunological imprinting (antigenic sin).(70, 71) In addition, the systemic toxicity of spike protein (spikopathy) increases with the number of vaccines.(72)

It has been suggested that SARS-CoV-2 converts normal cells into cancer cells by modulating central metabolic pathways or hampering genomic integrity mechanisms, consequently inhibiting the apoptotic machinery and/or enhancing cell proliferation. (64, 73) It is likely that decreased CD8+ cells with impaired immune surveillance plays a major role in turbo cancers. This may explain the explosion of turbo cancers after repeated "boosters" rather than the primary vaccine series. Angues and Bustos have suggested a multi-hit hypothesis to explain the increased risk of cancer associated with COVID mRNA vaccination.(74) The specific pathogenic mechanisms by which SARS-CoV-2 and/or the spike protein leads to increased tumorigenesis have not been well studied, however, several possible mechanisms exist. The spike protein damages mitochondria and alters mitochondrial function; this may play a central role in cancer cell development and propagation. (75-78) SARS-CoV-2 results in dysregulated innate and adaptive immunity. Depletion of CD8+ and natural killer cells reduces immune surveillance and alters the tumor microenvironment to promote tumor proliferation and metastases. (79) The retinoblastoma protein (pRB) is a tumor suppressor protein that prevents excessive cell growth by inhibiting cell cycle until a cell is ready to divide. The non-structural protein 15 (Nsp15) of coronaviruses induces the nuclear export and ubiquitination of pRB leading to its degradation via proteasomes. (80) A second potential oncogenic mechanism has been hypothesized for SARS-CoV-2 consisting of the degradation of the tumor suppressor protein p53 mediated by NSP 2 and Nsp3. (81) The open reading frame 8 (ORF8) protein of SARS-CoV-2 interacts with p62, the main autophagic cargo receptor, thereby inhibiting autophagy. (82) Jiang et al reported that spike protein localizes in the nucleus and inhibits DNA damage repair by impeding key DNA repair protein BRCA1 and 53BP1 recruitment to the damage site. (83) Spike protein impairs type I IFN signaling increasing the risk of cancer as type I IFN signaling suppresses proliferation of cancer cells by arresting the cell cycle, in part through upregulation of p53 and various cyclin-dependent kinase inhibitors. (84, 85) Metabolic reprogramming is a distinctive feature of SARS-CoV-2, and this may play a role in tumorigenesis. Metabolic reprogramming includes amino acid and lipid metabolism, carbohydrate, and energy metabolism, and immune-related pathways. (64) More recently Simian Virus 40 (SV40) DNA plasmids have been isolated in the vials of the COVID-19 vaccines (social media reports). SV40 is a known oncogenic virus. (86) IgG4 Antibodies are induced by repeated COVID-19 vaccination.(87, 88) IgG4 plays an essential role in cancer immune evasion. (89, 90)

In a patient with cancer, it may be difficult to establish a causal role with SARS-CoV-2/spike protein. However, the tumor can be stained for spike protein, establishing this causal association. As these “turbo” cancers are frequently highly malignant, an aggressive treatment is suggested including the guidance offered in this monograph.

Table 3. Exposure to 'carcinogens" and environmental factors and impact on cancer.

Factor	Trend	Impact on cancer in isolation	Exposure level
Smoking	Global decrease of 28% for men and 38% for women between 1990 and 2019 (92)	RR=46 for small cell lung cancer (SCLC) for male current smokers compared to men who have never smoked. RR=22 for SCLC for female current smokers compared to women who have never smoked (93)	11.5% of US adults smoke (2021) (94)
Pesticide exposure-occupational	Increase in pesticide use 7% between 1996 and 2011 (95)	Non-Hodgkins Lymphoma associated with glyphosate exposure: RR=1.3 (96) RR=2.02 (97)	2.4 million farmworkers in USA (2013) (98) 0.6% of USA farming acreage is organic
Glyphosate use	Glyphosate tonnage grew by 17% on average annually between 1990 and 2014 (99)	Organic food consumption associated with a decreased risk (RR=0.79) of non-Hodgkin Lymphoma (100)	On average 1.0kg per hectare of farmland applied in USA (99) 59% of corn and soy samples test positive for glyphosate and glufosinate residues
Beauty products	Global annual growth rate of 4.5% over the last 20 years Decrease of 13% in North America from 1998 to 2007	Breast cancer hazard ratio 1.15 for frequent white female users of beauty products relative to infrequent users (101)	85% of adolescent girls use body products on a daily basis (102)
Fire retardants in furniture	Production of chlorinated organophosphate flame retardants increases from 14,000 tons per year (mid-1980's) to 38,000 tons per year (2012) (103)	Flame retardants decabromodiphenyl ether and tris(2-chloroethyl) phosphate associated with greater risk (RR=2.3) of papillary thyroid cancer (104)	Ubiquitous in furniture owing to flame-retardant requirements of furniture (105, 106)
Radon exposure	Should be stable, Radon's source primarily geological (107)	Every 100 Bq/m^3 increase in Radon concentrated estimated to increase relative risk for lung cancer by 8-16% (108)	Second biggest cause of non-occupational lung cancer behind smoking (108)

Azo dyes	Azo dyes banned in EU (109)	Unknown	Azo dyes comprise majority of industrial dyes (110)
Antibiotics	Drop in recent years in USA. 5% decrease in number of prescriptions between 2011 and 2016. 25% drop between 2016 and 2020 Global increase from 9.8 defined daily doses (DDD) per 1000 per day in 2000 to 14.3 DDD per 1000 per day in 2018 (111)	RR=1.37 between lowest and highest exposure group for cancer (112)	In USA, 613 antibiotic prescriptions per 1000 persons in 2020
EMF exposure	Increasing (113)	Increased RR=2.0 for childhood leukemia for exposures of ≥0.4 μT compared to <0.1 μT (114)	Ubiquitous
Sedentary lifestyle	Increase in 39% in rates of meeting physical activity guidelines between 1998 and 2013. (115)	Combined healthy lifestyle reduced risk of cancer (RR=0.29 compared to those reporting no physical exercise or positive health behaviors) (116)	2/3 of adults do not meet physical activity guidelines (150 min per week of moderate to vigorous physical activity) (115)
Sleep deprivation	Relatively stable sleep duration in adults (117, 118) but decreases in sleep quality (119)	Increased risk of colorectal cancer (RR=1.08) and lung cancer (RR=1.11) in poor sleep category (120)	More than 1/3 of US adults sleep fewer than 7 hours per night (2014) (121)
Stress	Work stress has been on the rise in Europe (122)	Association between work stress and risk of colorectal (RR=1.36), lung (RR=1.24) and esophageal (RR=2.12) cancers (123)	71% of employees typically feel tense or stressed out during the workday (2019)

Caesarean birth	Increase in rate of caesarean section from 30% in 2003 to 37% in 2010 (124, 125)	Increased rate of childhood kidney cancer (RR=1.25) (126)	Approximately one-third of North American births in 2010 (127)
Family size	Decrease from 3.33 in 1960 to 2.50 in 2022	Hodgkin's Lymphoma risk lower for increased number of older siblings: RR=0.72 for three or more older siblings compared to none (128) RR=0.41 for five or more older siblings compared to none (129) acute monocytic leukemia RR=0.35 for three or more older siblings compared to none (129) acute lymphoblastic leukemia RR=0.69 for three or more older siblings compared to none (129)	Average family size of 2.50 in 2022
Mother's age at first birth	Increasing (130)	RR~1/3 for women giving birth before age 18 compared to those giving birth after 35 (131, 132)	Average age in USA is 27.1 years (2020)
Febrile illness	No trend in presentation rates to emergency department (133)	Lower rates on non-breast cancers for adults experiencing childhood febrile illness (134)	2.8 million children <2 years with fever present to emergency departments annually in USA (133)
Hormonal birth control	In the UK, hormonal birth control prescription proportion dropped 45% between 2000 and 2018. (135) Between 1995 and 2010, approximately 82% of sexually experienced women use the pill, staying relatively constant (136)	RR=1.20 for breast cancer for users compared to non-users (137)	one in four US women aged 15-44 using oral contraceptives (2013) (138)

Breastfeeding (mother)	Increase in proportion of mothers breastfeeding from 75% in 2010 to 81.1% in 2016	Decrease in 2% breast cancer risk for every 5 months breastfeeding. (139) Decreased risk of premenopausal breast cancer (RR=0.88) (140) RR=0.76 for invasive epithelial ovarian cancer (141)	81.1% of mothers breastfeed at birth (2016)
Breastfeeding (child)	See above box	No association (140)	83.2% of infants are ever breastfed (Born 2019)

CANCER SIGNAL PATHWAYS

Signaling pathways are a core system in which cells regulate various physiological processes and respond to external stimuli. Normally, cells have a complete set of regulatory mechanisms for initiating and/or inhibiting signal reception, cascade transmission, and ultimately gene expression, but in cancer cells, the signaling pathway is usually overactivated, and the balance is broken. Almost all the nutraceutical and repurposed drugs listed in this document have anticarcinogenic effects by promoting and/or inhibiting signal transmission through the targeted regulation of multiple links in important signal pathways. The most relevant pathways include the following:

Hexokinase-2 (HK2) pathway. In 1977, Pete Pedersen isolated the metabolic defect responsible for the Warburg effect: the hijacking of normal hexokinase by hexokinase II (HK2), followed by its massive overproduction. (7, 142) Hexokinase is the first step in glycolysis in the cytoplasm. Cancer cells have switched to an embryonic form of hexokinase (HK2), which then translocates from the cytoplasm to the outer mitochondrial membrane, where it is attached to the voltage-dependent anion channel (VDAC). (143-145) The VDAC is a pore-like opening in the outer membrane involved in shuttling nutrients and signaling molecules in and out of the mitochondria. HK2 is the major bound hexokinase isoform expressed in cancer cells that exhibit the Warburg effect. By stationing itself on the outer mitochondrial membrane, HK2 helps immortalize cancer cells, escapes product inhibition, and gains preferential access to newly synthesized ATP for phosphorylating glucose. (146) The attachment of HK2 to the VDAC on the outer mitochondrial membrane creates a state of apoptosis resistance and shunts ATP out of the mitochondria to the cytoplasm to support glycolysis. When bound to HK2, the VDAC gate is "locked", preventing the release of cytochrome c, thereby preventing apoptosis, and effectively immortalizing the cell. Several drugs target HK2, separating the enzyme from the outer mitochondrial membrane; these include 3-bromopyruvate, curcumin, resveratrol, and its derivatives pterostilbene and quercetin.

The p53 pathway (the tumor suppressor pathway). (147) The p53 pathway is activated by sensor kinases which monitor the cell's DNA for damage or errors. Upon detection of damage, they phosphorylate the nuclear localization factor of the p53 tumor suppressor protein, allowing it to translocate to the cell nucleus and begin expressing p21, p16, p15, and p19; this activates the cell cycle arrest pathway, initiating DNA repair, and preventing cell division. If the repair is deemed to have failed, BAX, BAK, and/or PUMA are expressed, among others, initiating the mitochondrial caspase cascade, which initiates apoptosis.

The TGF-β pathway. The TGF-β pathway plays a crucial role in regulating cell growth, differentiation, and apoptosis. (148) Upon binding to its cell surface receptors, TGF-β activates SMAD transcription factors, leading to the repression of anti-apoptotic genes and the activation of pro-apoptotic genes. This pathway acts as a tumor suppressor by promoting apoptosis in abnormal cells and inhibiting the growth of precancerous cells. Defects in this pathway can lead to uncontrolled cell growth and the development of cancer.

The Wnt signaling pathway. The Wnt/beta-catenin pathway is a family of proteins that is implicated in many vital cellular functions such as stem cell regeneration and organogenesis. The Wnt signaling pathway plays a crucial role in the regulation of cell proliferation and differentiation. (149) In normal conditions, Wnt signaling maintains the balance between cell proliferation and apoptosis to ensure healthy tissue growth. However, when the pathway is activated excessively or inappropriately, it can lead to the development of cancer. Wnt activation has been observed in breast, lung, and hematopoietic malignancies and contributes to tumor recurrence.(150) The Wnt pathway cross talks with the Notch and Sonic Hedgehog pathways, which has implications for therapeutic interventions in cancers.

The Notch signaling pathway. The Notch signaling pathway is a signaling mechanism that plays a role in cell differentiation, proliferation, and apoptosis. (151) Disruptions in the Notch pathway, such as mutations in Notch receptors or ligands, can lead to the dysregulation of cell proliferation and differentiation, contributing to the development of cancer. Notch signaling plays a crucial role in the development of colon cancer; targeting the Notch pathway may sensitize colon cancers to various adjuvant agents.(152)

The PI3K/AKT signaling pathway. The phosphoinositide 3-kinase (PI3K) signaling pathway is linked to both growth control and glucose metabolism. The activation of the PI3K/AKT signaling pathway occurs when growth factor receptors on the cell surface bind to their ligands, triggering the activation of PI3K. (153) Once activated, AKT phosphorylates and inhibits the activity of pro-apoptotic proteins, such as BAD and FOXO. AKT also activates mTORC1, which regulates cellular metabolism and promotes cell survival by stimulating the expression of anti-apoptotic genes Bcl-2 and Bcl-xL.

The Hedgehog Pathway. Hedgehog (Hh) is one of the few signaling pathways that is frequently used during development for intercellular communication. (154) Hh is important for the organogenesis of almost all organs in mammals, as well as in regeneration and homeostasis. Further, Hh signaling is disrupted in diverse types of cancer. Mebendazole decreases the activity of the Hedgehog pathway, which is common in gliomas, melanomas, lung cancers, ovarian cancers, and colorectal cancer. (155)

The insulin growth factor-1 (IGF-1) pathway. Insulin-like growth factor 1 (IGF-1) is produced primarily by the liver as an endocrine hormone, as well as in target tissues in a paracrine/autocrine manner. IGF-1 signaling is mainly mediated by binding to its specific receptor, the insulin-like growth factor 1 receptor (IGF-1R) leading to the activation of the AKT signaling pathway resulting in cell growth, proliferation, and inhibition of programmed cell death. An elevated level of circulating IGF-1 is an established risk factor for many cancer types, whereas a decrease in IGF-1 levels is associated with lower cancer incidence.

CANCER IMMUNITY

Inflammation is an essential pillar of immune defense. However, chronic inflammation is considered a hallmark of cancer initiation and progression. Chronic inflammation demonstrates a potential to induce complex changes at molecular, cellular, and organ level and thereby alter the tumor microenvironment (TME). Cancer cells frequently secrete several growth factors that stimulate myelopoiesis and recruit myeloid cells to TME (see Figure 3). (156, 157) Therefore, the TMEs of various cancers are characterized by the high infiltration of monocytes, macrophages, granulocytes, and dendritic cells. Most myeloid cells within TMEs are present in an immature form; however, cancer-derived growth factors modify these myeloid cells into cells that support carcinogenesis by enhancing proliferation, migration, and metastasis and enabling cancer cell survival and immune evasion. Therefore, in addition to abnormalities in apoptosis, patients with cancer have derangements in immunity with the immune system failing to recognize the cancer cell as foreign. The following cells play a major role in altering the TME and promoting carcinogenesis.

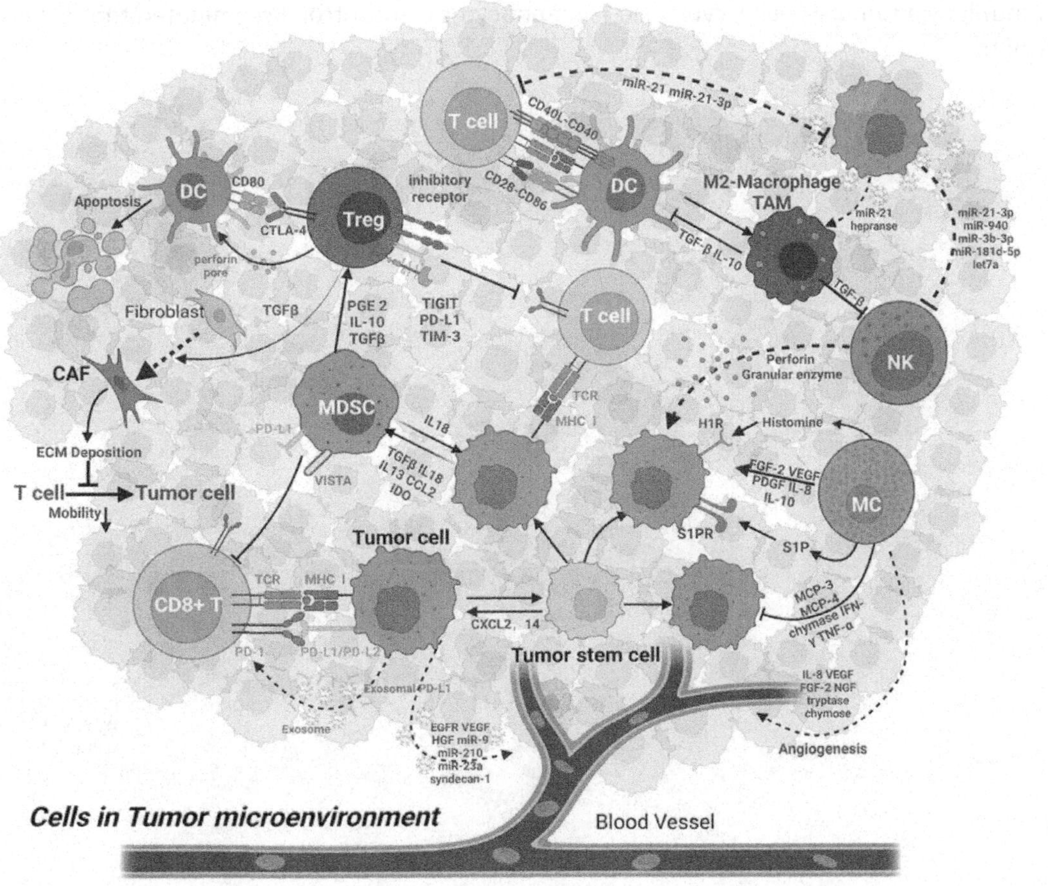

Figure 3. The cellular and structural components in the tumor microenvironment (source: Wang et al. Reproduced under Creative Commons Attribution International license) (157)

Myeloid-derived stem cells (MDSC). The establishment of primary tumor cells in distant organs, termed metastasis, is the principal cause of cancer mortality. Despite "curative" resection of the primary tumor, many patients have disseminated tumor cells at the time of diagnosis. Tumor cells can be found in the bone marrow of cancer patients at the time of their primary tumor resection. (158) These patients may then develop overt metastases months, years, or even decades later. This latency period, during which cancer cells do not grow and remain in a quiescent or equilibrium state, is known as "cancer dormancy." The timeline of metastatic dormancy is regulated by interactions between the tumor, its microenvironment, angiogenesis, and tumor antigen-specific T-cell responses. One such mediator of dormancy is myeloid-derived suppressor cells (MDSCs), whose number in infiltrating tumors has been associated with cancer stage, grade, patient survival, and metastasis in a broad range of tumor pathologies (see Figure 4). (159, 160)

Extensive studies have revealed a role for MDSCs in tumor escape from adaptive and innate immune responses, facilitating tumor progression and metastasis. (159, 161-165) Host immunity via tumor-specific cytotoxic T-lymphocytes can control disseminated tumor cell growth,

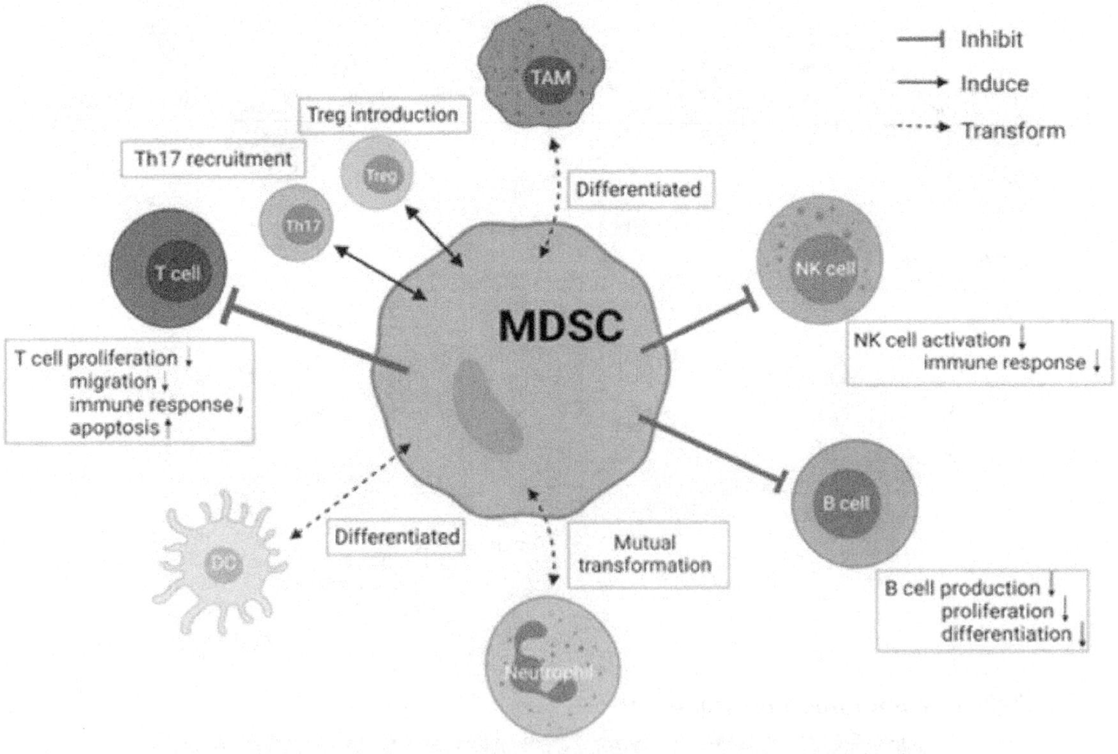

Figure 4. Crosstalk between MDSCs and other immune cells. Up arrows mean increased, and down arrows mean decreased. (Source Ma et al. Reproduced under Creative Commons Attribution International License) (160)

resulting in a dormant lesion that can be held in stasis for years or decades until released from dormancy in association with an increase in MDSCs reversing host T-cell responses. MDSCs contribute to immune evasion by inducing T-cell dysfunction through the production of reactive oxygen species, arginase-1 (ARG1), and nitric oxide synthase (NOS). ARG1 hydrolyzes extracellular L-arginine into urea and ornithine. L-arginine is required for T-cell proliferation, cytokine production, and expression of the T-cell receptor. (166)

MDSCs can not only inhibit clonal expansion of activated effector T cells, but also induce tumor-specific Treg lymphocytes to further establish and maintain T-cell tolerance in the tumor-bearing host. (164, 167, 168) In addition, by downregulating interferon, overexpressing inflammatory cytokines, and creating leaky vasculature by overexpressing matrix metalloproteinase 9 and other remodeling factors which compromise the integrity of the extracellular matrix and the basal membrane, MDSCs promote cancer cell invasion. (163)

T-regulatory cells (Tregs). Tregs universally labeled by CD4+CD25+Foxp3+CD127low/− are differentiated from traditional T lymphocytes. (169-172) To maintain immune homeostasis, Treg cells inhibit abnormal or excessive immune reactions to self- and non-self-antigens. By stifling the anti-tumor immune response of effector T cells, NK cells, and dendritic cells, Treg cells contribute to the growth and spread of tumors in the TME. (170, 172, 173) An unfavorable prognosis is associated with high Treg cell infiltration in the TME in patients with diverse cancer types. (173-179) Treg cells cause immune suppression by the production of immunosuppressive cytokines, the consumption of interleukin-2 and IL 2 receptors, modulation of CD80 and CD86 expression by dendritic cells, and direct killing of effector T cells. (173) Tregs also contribute significantly to angiogenesis via the VEGF/VEGFR pathway.

Natural Killer Cells (NK cells). Natural killer (NK) cells are the most relevant cancer-fighting cells of the innate immune system. NK cells play a vital role in recognizing and responding to abnormal cells, including cancerous and infected cells, in the immune system. T-cells possess T-cell receptors (TCRs) that allow them to bind MHC-I-peptide complexes on the cell surface, which determines whether an immune response will be initiated. Failures occur in the expression of the transporter associated with antigen processing (TAP) complex, and β2-microglobulin; these cause a loss of MHC-I self-antigen transport and surface presentation capacity, which causes the failure of the NK cell to destroy the cancerous cell.

Tumor-associated macrophages. Macrophages recruited from circulating monocytes to tumors and influenced by the presence of cancer to promote tumor malignancy and progression are often referred to as tumor-associated macrophages (TAMs) (see Figure 5). (180-182) Macrophages are divided into the M1 and M2 subgroups based on morphological, phenotypic, and functional variability. M2 macrophages have been shown to have protumor characteristics and to promote tumor development and metastasis, whereas M1 macrophages play a critical role in antitumor immunity and largely mediate proinflammatory activities in the tumor microenvironment (TME). (182-184) In metastatic tumors, macrophages have different phenotypes and functions from primary tumors and are often called metastasis-associated macrophages (MAMs).

TAMs mostly arise from bone-marrow-derived monocytes with the chemokine CCL2 produced by tumor cells being the major recruitment factor. Bone-marrow-derived monocytes include both classical monocytes and monocytic MDSCs (M-MDSCs), (185) and are crucial for the negative regulation of immune responses. (186, 187)

The immune system is skewed toward a tumor-promoting response because of the release of IL-10 by MDSCs, which inhibits the secretion of IL-12 by macrophages. Macrophages also cause MDSCs to produce more IL-10, which raises levels of IL-6 and TNF- in macrophages. (186) MDSC IL-6 was reported to be elevated by tumor cells, and vice versa. (186) The ratio of tumor cells to MDSC and macrophages controls inflammation within solid tumors, and interactions between these cells have the potential to drastically change the inflammatory environment within the tumor microenvironment. (183, 186) A high infiltration of macrophages in human solid tumors is associated with poor clinical outcomes. (182-184, 186-195) Similarly, the expression of macrophage growth factors or their chemoattractants, such as CSF1 and CCL2, in tumors or in the circulation is often associated with poor prognosis. (180)

TAMs are the crucial and dominant immune cells in the TME and significantly contribute to tumor progression by promoting angiogenesis, mediating tumor immunosuppression by inhibiting T cell function, they secrete chemokines which contribute to the recruitment of T regulatory cells in the tumor microenvironment and promote tumor cell intravasation via VEGF expression (see Figure 5). TAMs are activated by mediators secreted from tumor-infiltrating lymphocytes such as Th2, Treg cells, IL-10, TGF-β. (196) By reducing antitumor immunity, Foxp3+ regulatory T (Treg) cells and tumor-associated macrophages (TAMs) both aid in the growth of tumors. Researchers identified TAMs and Tregs as responsible for direct tumor immune evasion. (197) TAMs and Tregs combine to form a cellular network that is partially redundant and contributes to the robustness of tumor immunosuppression as well as resistance to immunotherapy. (183, 197)

TAMs play a major role in tumor metastases. (198) Cancer-associated fibroblast are produced because of the mesenchymal transition of endothelial cells during the growth of tumors, and they secrete Heat shock protein-90 alpha (*Hsp90α)*, which promotes M2 polarization and maintains an immunosuppressive milieu. (199) By secreting different mediators that alter the tumor promoting TME, TAMs can accelerate the growth of tumors. Proangiogenic growth factors, such as vascular endothelial growth factor (VEGF), platelet-derived growth factor (PDGF), fibroblast growth factor (FGF), and transforming growth factor- (TGF-), NF-kB-mediated factors that prevent apoptosis, and proangiogenic growth factors (190) that promote cancer cell migration and metastasis. (183) TAMs can also increase the tumor stemness, which upregulates the release of immunosuppressive cytokines such as IL-1ra. (183, 200) By releasing growth factors like the epidermal growth factor receptor (EGFR), which encourages the proliferation of cancer cells, TAMs may directly drive the proliferation of cancer cells. (201) In hepatocellular carcinoma, active Wnt/-catenin signaling induced by a greater number of invading macrophages can promote the proliferation of tumor progenitor cells, and targeted macrophage reduction can diminish Wnt and slow tumor growth. (202)

By controlling the PI3k/Akt pathways in cancer cells, TAMs may block proapoptotic cytokines such tumor necrosis factor-related apoptosis-inducing ligand (TRAIL). (203) By introducing miRNAs into cancer cells, such as colorectal cancer and pancreatic ductal adenocarcinoma cells, exosomes produced by M2 macrophages spread malignancy. (204) Metastatic cells use the Cysteine-cysteine motif chemokine ligand 20 (CCL20), also known as macrophage inflammatory protein-3α, MIP*3α*) - Chemokine receptor 6 (CCR6) axis/pathway to attract monocytes and differentiate them into metastasis-associated macrophages (MAMs) that support tumor cell survival and metastasis by suppressing T cells. (183, 189) Additionally, TAMs release several enzymes, such as matrix metalloproteinases (MMPs) and cyclooxygenase type-2 (COX-2), which all work to promote angiogenesis by destroying the matrix and enabling endothelial cells to invade. (205) Despite TAMs having pro-tumorigenic characteristics, they can ingest tumor cells, and cause tumor apoptosis by releasing NO, ROS, and IL-12, which encourage anti-tumor responses and limit tumor growth in specific situations. (206) This suggests that immunosuppressive and immunostimulatory TAM can coexist in the same tumor. (183, 186, 207)

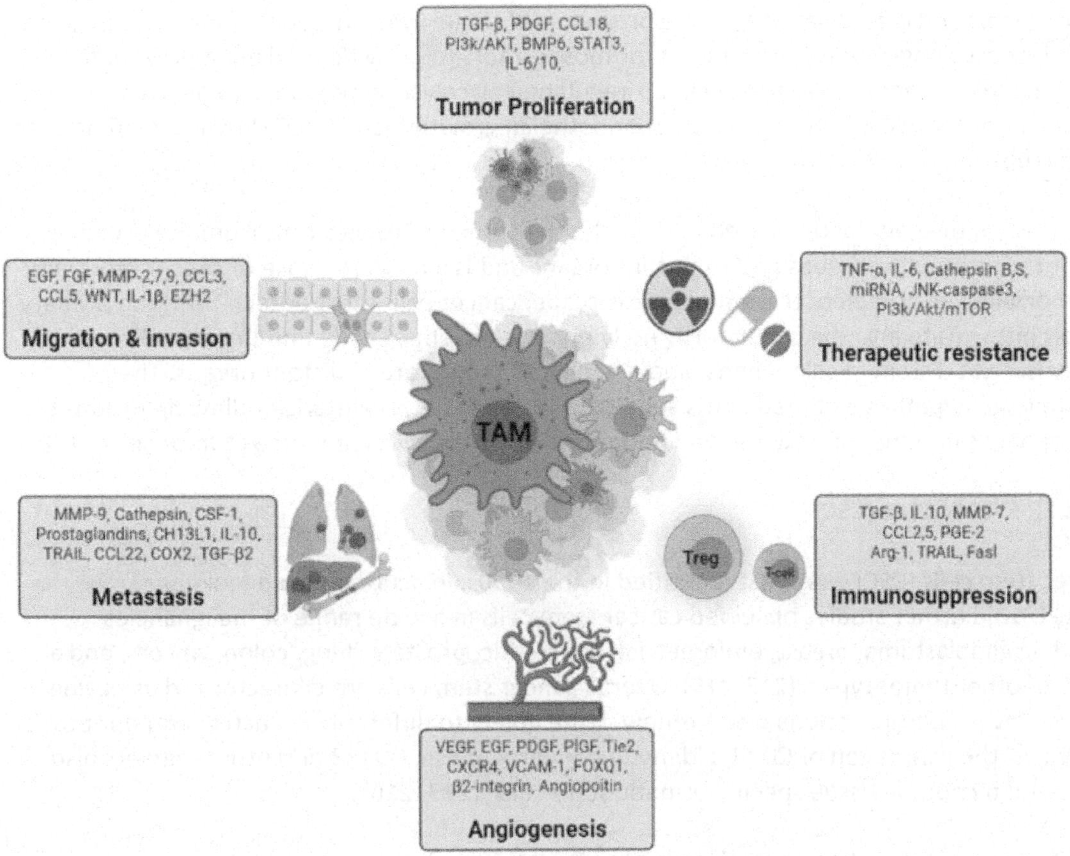

Figure 5. The role of tumor associated macrophages in cancer. (Source: Reproduced from Kumari et al under Creative Commons Attribution 4.0 International License). (182)

PLATELETS AND CANCER

Platelets have been implicated in enabling successful metastasis and worsening the prognosis of patients with cancer by guarding tumor cells from immune elimination and promoting arrest and extravasation of tumor cells. (208-210) Direct signaling between platelets and cancer cells induces an epithelial-mesenchymal-like transition and promotes metastasis. Platelet-derived TGFβ and direct platelet-tumor cell contacts synergistically activate the TGFβ/Smad and NF-κB pathways in cancer cells, resulting in their transition to an invasive mesenchymal-like phenotype and enhanced metastasis in vivo. (208) In a symbiotic manner, tumor-derived bioactive molecules have been shown to prompt an increase in platelet activation and production. (211, 212)

ANGIOGENESIS AND METASTASIS

Angiogenesis involves neovascularization or the formation of new capillaries from existing blood vessels and is associated with the processes of tissue inflammation, wound healing, and tumorigenesis. Angiogenesis is required for most tumors to grow beyond an approximate size of 0.2-2.0 mm. In addition to its role in up-regulating glycolysis in response to hypoxia, HIF-1α is the main transcription factor for vascular endothelial growth factor (VEGF), which stimulates angiogenesis.

Metastasis is the general term used to describe the spread of cancer cells from the primary tumor to surrounding tissues and to distant organs and is a primary cause of cancer morbidity and mortality. To complete the metastatic cascade, cancer cells must detach from the primary tumor, intravasate into the circulatory and lymphatic systems, evade immune attack, extravasate at distant capillary beds, and invade and proliferate in distant organs. The macrophage hypothesis of metastasis suggests that metastatic cells arise following fusions of macrophages or bone marrow-derived hematopoietic cells with committed tumor cells. (198)

CANCER STEM CELLS (CSC)

Cancer stem cells (CSC) were first identified in the 1990s, in acute myeloid leukemia (AML).(213) Further studies observed cancer stem cells in a wide range of malignancies including glioblastoma, breast, endometrial, pancreatic, prostate, lung, colon cancers, and a range of other tumor types. (213-215) Overall cancer stem cells are characterized as having distinct key properties including self-renewal, the ability to differentiate, active anti-apoptotic pathways, the expression of CD44, aldehyde dehydrogenase, CD133 and other markers also expressed by normal tissue specific somatic stem cells. (213, 216)

Despite arising initially from a single cell, almost all tumors become very heterogeneous, expressing different markers, and containing proliferative and more differentiated cells. Tumor heterogeneity may be responsible for tumor progression, metastasis, resistance to therapy, and relapse. (217) Fast-growing cancer cells make up the bulk of a tumor with a smaller population of cancer stem cells (CSC). CSCs are a cell population similar to stem cells with characteristics of self-renewal and differentiation potential in tumor tissue. (218) Although CSCs are similar to stem cells in terms of function, because of the lack of a negative feedback regulation mechanism for stem cell self-renewal, their powerful proliferation and multidirectional differentiation abilities are unrestricted, which allows CSCs to maintain certain activities during chemotherapy and radiotherapy. When the external environment is suitable, CSCs will rapidly proliferate to reactivate the formation and growth of tumors. (216)

CSCs are defined by their functional properties and can self-renew and propagate the tumor over an extended period and recapitulate the different cell lineages found in the primary tumors. CSCs reside in particular tumor microenvironment niches that play an important role in regulating their proliferation, renewal, differentiation, and stemness. (217) Inflammation and hypoxia promote the acquisition of a CSC phenotype and its maintenance. (217) Chemotherapy induces changes in the tumor microenvironment that support CSC survival and tumor relapse.

The CSC colony is slow-growing and resembles normal cells in many respects. Chemotherapy and radiation all attempt to kill the fast-dividing cancer cells; however, they also kill fast-dividing normal cells, including the hair, lining of the gastrointestinal tract, and bone marrow.(13) However, like normal cells, chemotherapy spares CSC. Furthermore, both chemotherapy and radiation treatment have a stimulating effect on the CSC population, causing them to grow resistant new tumor cells and replace the bulk of what was removed (See Figure 1). (13, 217, 219) Dr. Hope considers this like the effect of "pruning a tree thereby stimulating new growth" (see Foreword). The tumors of patients with breast cancer brain metastasis were reported to be highly cancer stem-like cell-enriched, suggesting that brain metastases probably arise by the seeding of cancer cells with stem features. (220) In bladder cancer, the resistance of tumor cells to chemotherapy was caused by slow-cycling CSCs that were stimulated to proliferate in between cycles of chemotherapy. (221) The proliferative response of CSCs was promoted by prostaglandin E2 (PGE2) release by cancer cells that were killed by the chemotherapy. Targeting PGE2 by monoclonal blocking antibody or by the administration of cyclooxygenase-2 inhibitor attenuated chemoresistance and suggested that targeting this pathway in between cycles of chemotherapy may enhance the therapeutic response in bladder cancer.

The successful elimination of a cancer requires an anticancer therapy that will affect both differentiated cancer cells and CSC. At present, conventional therapy that includes radio-, chemo-, and immunotherapy kills rapidly proliferating and differentiated cells. These treatments may cause the tumor to shrink but will not prevent it from recurring. Thus, a combination of treatments that target both rapidly-proliferating cancer cells and the quiescent or slow-proliferating cancer stem cells is required. (146)

Adding repurposed drugs to attack CSC should be a priority and should be done at the time of initiation of chemotherapy and radiation therapy. (13) Common repurposed drugs that can attack CSC include green tea extract, melatonin, vitamin D3, metformin, curcumin, statins (atorvastatin), berberine, mebendazole, doxycycline, ivermectin, resveratrol, aspirin, diclofenac phosphodiesterase 5-inhibitors, and omega-3 fatty acids. (13, 222-225)

HOW CHEMOTHERAPY ACTIVATES CANCER AGGRESSIVITY

Another problem with chemotherapy is that the drugs make cancer more aggressive by activating massive inflammation in the body. Chemotherapy activates the inflammatory master controller, NF-KB, which produces the inflammatory cytokine IL-6. (226) This massive, chemotherapy-induced increase in inflammation has the following consequences: (146)

- Stimulates more rapid cancer growth (proliferation).
- More resistance to apoptosis (programmed cell death).
- More invasive and metastatic behavior of the cancer.
- Stimulates angiogenesis.
- Creates a chemo-resistant cancer cell population.

These findings suggest that patients should receive anti-inflammatory therapies concomitant with chemotherapeutic agents. In addition, almost all the repurposed anticancer drugs listed in this monograph potentiate the effects of standard chemotherapy agents, allowing a dose reduction of these agents.

CHAPTER 3: PREVENTING CANCER

As previously mentioned, at least 42% of newly diagnosed cancers in the United States could potentially be avoided. (11, 227) The most important interventions to reduce the risk of cancer include: quitting smoking, limiting (or stopping) alcohol consumption, improving nutrition, adopting time-restricted eating, treating metabolic syndrome/insulin resistance, engaging in moderate physical exercise, and supplementation with vitamin D3. (11) Smoked and processed meats should be avoided as they are related to several cancers, most notably gastric cancer. (228, 229) In addition, the topical application, consumption, and inhalation of carcinogenic substances should be limited as much as possible. (12) The World Cancer Research Fund (WCRF)/American Institute for Cancer Research (AICR) published ten Cancer Prevention Recommendations, updated in 2018, that encourage a healthy lifestyle pattern, including eating a healthy diet, maintaining a healthy body weight, and undertaking adequate physical activity.(230) Greater adherence to these recommendations was associated with a reduced risk of all cancers combined and of breast, colorectal, kidney, oesophageal, ovarian, liver, and gallbladder cancers. (227)

The DO-HEALTH trial was a three-year, multicenter, 2 × 2 × 2 factorial design double-blind, randomized controlled trial to test the individual and combined benefit of supplemental vitamin D3 (2000 IU/day), and/or 1 g per day of marine Omega-3s, and/or a simple home strength exercise program. These were compared to placebo and control exercise. (231, 232) While each intervention individually reduced the risk of cancer, the combination was synergistically highly effective in reducing the risk of cancer (the adjusted hazard ratio of adjusted HR was 0.39). Although reported as a negative study, the Vitamin D and Omega-3 Trial (VITAL) funded by the NIH further corroborated the protective effect of vitamin D on cancer mortality, reporting lower rates of death caused by cancer among participants randomized to vitamin D3 vs placebo (HR, 0.72 [95% CI, 0.52-1.00]). (233) In addition, many other nutraceuticals appear to be highly effective in preventing cancer. Published peer-reviewed studies strongly support the use of green tea catechins in reducing the risk of numerous cancers. (234, 235) In addition, melatonin has numerous health benefits including increasing health span and decreasing the risk of neurodegenerative diseases; it is likely that this natural product may be highly effective in preventing cancer.

Metformin suppresses tumor initiation, growth, and spread and is recognized as an effective anticancer drug even for non-diabetics. Diabetics taking metformin had a lower all-cause mortality than normal non-diabetics not taking it. (236) Metformin has been demonstrated to reduce the risk of prostate cancer in men with type 2 diabetes. (237) Meta-analyses have examined the role of metformin in the primary prevention of cancer, where it was found to significantly reduce overall cancer incidence. (238, 239) Metformin should be considered as an add on in those patients at high risk of developing cancer. i.e., strong family history, previous cancer, increased genetic risk, etc.

Based on this data we suggest the following interventions for all individuals to reduce their risk of cancer:

- Quit smoking.
- Reduce or limit the use of alcohol.
- Lose weight: adopt a healthy diet, manage insulin resistance, and follow a time-restricted eating plan.
- Avoid processed food and processed vegetable oils. (240)
- Avoid sugary beverages and pure fruit juices. (241, 242)
- Limit consumption of red meat to no more than 3 portions/week. (230)
- Vitamin D3: 5000 u/day and adjusted according to vitamin D3 level (see Table 3). Target a Vit D level of 50-70 ng/ml.
- Omega 3 fatty acids: 2-4 g/day.
- Green tea catechins: 500-1000 mg/day. (234, 243) Green tea extract should be taken during/after a meal, rather than on an empty stomach. (244) See precautions in the section labeled 'Green Tea'.
- Melatonin: 0.75–5 mg (extended/slow release) at night. (222, 245)
- Metformin: Metformin should be considered in anyone at high risk of cancer, whether their risk extends from diabetes, prediabetes, insulin resistance, chronic viral infection, smoking, or genetics. Requires doctor's evaluation, approval, and prescription. (Suggested dose ranges from 250-2000 mg daily.) (13)
- Regular aerobic exercise and resistance training 30 minutes/day (walking, home strength training, etc.).
- Reduce stress (meditation, yoga, mindfulness exercises, etc.). (246-248)
- Get at least 8 hours of high-quality sleep (ensure adequate sleep hygiene). (248-251)
- Avoid known carcinogens. (12)

Familial adenomatous polyposis (FAP) is a hereditary condition that causes colon cancer at a young age. Many patients choose to have a total colectomy before the age of 20 rather than risk fatal cancer development. In a mouse model of FAP, the combination of mebendazole and sulindac (an NSAID) reduced the number of polyps by 90%. (252) (152) In an experimental adenomatous polyposis coli model, ashwagandha was associated with a 59% reduction of tumor and polyp initiation and progression. (253)

These preclinical findings support the consideration of clinical trials for patients with FAP as well as other high-risk cancer patients. The use of phosphodiesterase-5 inhibitors (e.g., sildenafil) is associated with a lower risk of colorectal cancer in men with benign colorectal neoplasms. (254)

Female patients with the BRACA 1 and 2 mutations are at an approximately 70% lifetime risk of developing breast cancer and a 20-40% risk of developing ovarian cancer. (255) However, it should be noted that the risk of these patients developing a malignancy has doubled over the last four decades, suggesting that environmental and lifestyle factors may increase the risk of cancers in this population. The management of these patients is complex and needs to be individualized. Oral selenium is a good candidate for chemoprevention in women who carry a mutation in the BRCA1 gene.(256) The guidance as provided in the monograph should be considered even in those patients that elect to undergo prophylactic surgery.

CHAPTER 4: THE METABOLIC APPROACH TO TREATING CANCER

Although mitochondrial replacement therapy could, in principle, restore a more normal energy metabolism and differentiated state to tumor cells, it is unlikely that this therapeutic approach would be available in the foreseeable future. (30, 31) However, if cancer is primarily a disease of energy metabolism, then rational approaches to cancer management can be found in therapies that specifically target energy metabolism.

The goal of metabolic adjunctive treatments is to "starve the cancer cell" by modulating energy pathways that are important to the survival of cancer cells and thereby reduce cancer growth and cancer metastases (the cause of death in over 90% of cancer patients). An approach to cancer treatment is emerging with research showing impressive results from the use of metabolically targeted drug cocktails alongside conventional chemotherapy. The metabolic protocol is designed to work primarily by restricting the overall ability of cancer cells to take up and use (i.e., 'metabolize') energy. By starving cancer cells of energy substrates, metabolic interventions may reduce the capacity of cancer cells to defend themselves against chemotherapy and radiation. The metabolic protocol may also act on the many dysregulated signaling pathways within cancer cells helping to enable apoptosis, or "programmed cell death," allowing chemotherapy and radiation to kill cancer cells more effectively.

The most important and central approach to the metabolic treatment of cancers is dietary calorie (glucose) restriction. This is supplemented with pharmacologic and nutraceutical compounds that target specific cancer pathways and interventions that restore "normal" anticancer immunity and prevent metastases.

It is important to emphasize that there is no single "magic bullet" and that multiple interventions act synergistically and simultaneously to promote cancer cell death. The combination of dietary interventions together with multiple repurposed drugs/nutraceuticals which act synergistically is strongly recommended. This approach is similar to that of the Care Oncology Clinic, which uses the patented *Metabolic Oncology COC Protocol™* consisting of a combination of conventional pharmaceuticals (metformin, atorvastatin, mebendazole, doxycycline, and an NSAID) that theoretically work together to restrict the overall ability of cancer cells to take up and use energy. (257) However, similar to the work of Jane McLelland, (4) we suggest a more extensive and targeted list of pharmacologic and nutraceutical compounds combined with glucose restriction and a ketogenic diet. (Please note that the Care Oncology Clinic has now been dissolved in the United States and our mention of it herein is in no way an endorsement or recommendation.)

The metabolic approach to cancer should be considered as adjunctive to more "traditional" approaches to cancer treatment. The metabolic treatments will likely act synergistically with the more traditional approaches, thereby increasing tumor response rate, limiting the toxicities of standard chemotherapy, limiting the risk of metastasis, and leading to an improvement in overall quality of life. This combined approach will allow for reduced dosages of standard chemotherapeutic agents, drastically reducing their toxicity (see metronomic dosing, Chapter 12).

DIETARY CALORIC RESTRICTION, THE KETOGENIC DIET, AND "REAL" FOOD

Numerous studies show that dietary energy restriction is a general metabolic therapy that naturally lowers circulating glucose levels and significantly reduces the growth and progression of numerous tumor types, including cancers of the breast, brain, colon, pancreas, lung, and prostate. (258-264) An impressive body of evidence indicates that dietary energy restriction can retard the growth rate of many tumors regardless of the specific genetic defects expressed within the tumor. (258-264) Hyperglycemia with high insulin levels is associated with tumor recurrence. (60, 265) Sugar sweetened beverages are associated with an increased risk of cancer. (266-268) Both experimental and clinical data suggest that fructose, particularly fructose-corn syrup, to be more carcinogenic than glucose. (242, 269, 270)

As demonstrated by Dr. Otto Warburg, almost all cancer cells are dependent on glucose as a metabolic fuel via aerobic glycolysis, (23, 24) with hyperglycemia being a potent promotor of tumor cell proliferation and associated with poor survival. (271) Although the mechanisms responsible for the caloric-restriction-mediated reduction in tumorigenesis have not been unequivocally identified, they may involve caloric-restriction-induced epigenetic changes as well as changes in growth signals and in the sirtuin pathway. (272)

Insulin resistance plays a major role in the initiation and propagation of cancer. (273) Reversing insulin resistance is therefore a major goal in patients with cancer. Dietary energy restriction specifically targets the IGF-1/PI3K/Akt/HIF-1α signaling pathway, which underlies several cancer hallmarks including cell proliferation, evasion of apoptosis, and angiogenesis. IGF-1 production is stimulated by growth hormone (GH) and can be inhibited by calorie restriction, suggesting it could play a central role in the protective effect of calorie restriction. In this regard, humans with mutations in the GH receptor (known as Laron syndrome) have low serum IGF-1 levels, and have a remarkably low risk of developing cancer. (272) Glucose reduction not only reduces insulin but also reduces circulating levels of IGF-1, which is necessary for driving tumor cell metabolism and growth. In diabetics, those on insulin or insulin secretagogues were demonstrated to be more likely to develop solid cancers than those on metformin. (274)

Dietary energy restriction targets inflammation and the signaling pathways involved with driving tumor angiogenesis. Indeed, calorie restriction is considered a simple and effective therapy for targeting tumor angiogenesis and inflammation. Calorie restriction results in the downregulation of multiple genes and metabolic pathways regulating glycolysis. Besides lowering circulating glucose levels, dietary energy restriction elevates circulating levels of fatty acids and ketone bodies (β-hydroxybutyrate and acetoacetate). Fats, and especially ketones, can replace glucose as a primary metabolic fuel under calorie restriction. This is a conserved physiological adaptation that evolved to spare protein during periods of starvation. Many tumors, however, have abnormalities in the genes and enzymes needed to metabolize ketone bodies for energy. Elevation in ketone bodies is well known to be able to suppress blood glucose levels and glycolysis, which are major drivers of tumor growth. A transition from carbohydrates to ketones for energy is a simple way to target energy metabolism in glycolysis-dependent tumor cells while enhancing the metabolic efficiency of normal cells. Metabolism of ketone bodies and fatty acids for energy requires inner mitochondrial membrane integrity and efficient respiration, which tumor cells largely lack. Under fasting conditions, ketone bodies are produced in the liver from fatty acids as the main source of brain energy. Ketone bodies bypass the glycolytic pathway in the cytoplasm and are metabolized directly to acetyl CoA in the mitochondria.

The ketogenic diet is a high-fat, low-carbohydrate diet with adequate protein and calories originally developed in the 1920s as a treatment for intractable epilepsy.(275) The traditional ketogenic diet is a 4:1 formulation of fat content to carbohydrate plus protein. (275) A classic 4:1 ketogenic diet delivers 90% of its calories from fat, 8% from protein and only 2% from carbohydrate. Ketogenic diets of the 1920s and 1930s were extremely bland and restrictive diets and, therefore, prone to noncompliance. In recent years, alternative keto-genic protocols have emerged, making adherence to the diet much easier.(276) Alternatives to the traditional keto-genic diet include a medium-chain triglyceride (MCT)-based ketogenic diet and the Atkins diet. Compared to long-chain triglycerides, MCTs are more rapidly absorbed into the bloodstream and oxidized for energy because of their ability to passively diffuse through membranes. Another characteristic of MCTs is their unique ability to promote ketone body synthesis in the liver. Thus, adding MCTs to a ketogenic diet would allow significantly more carbohydrates to be included. (276)

A ketogenic diet KD has tumor growth-limiting effects, protects healthy cells from damage by chemotherapy or radiation, accelerates chemotherapeutic toxicity toward cancer cells, and lowers inflammation. (276) Altered availability of glucose and induction of ketosis influence all the classically defined hallmarks of cancer.(277) Weber et al demonstrated that ketogenic diets slow melanoma growth in vivo regardless of tumor genetics and metabolic plasticity. (278) Moreover, ketogenic diets simultaneously affected multiple metabolic pathways to create an unfavorable environment for melanoma cell proliferation. In glioma cancer models a ketogenic diet has been shown to reduce angiogenesis, inflammation, peri-tumoral edema, migration and invasion. (279) Similarly, a ketogenic diet altered the hypoxic response and affects expression of proteins associated with angiogenesis, invasive potential and vascular permeability in a mouse glioma model. (280) The ketogenic diet may work in part as an immune adjuvant, boosting tumor-reactive immune responses in the microenvironment by alleviating immune suppression.(281) A meta-analysis on the use of ketogenic diet in animal models demonstrated significantly prolonged survival time and reduced tumor weight and tumor volume. (282) The ketogenic diet was effective across a broad range of cancers. The ketogenic diet is an effective adjuvant to radiation therapy for the treatment of malignant glioma.(283)

Ketone bodies have been shown to inhibit histone deacetylases and may decrease tumor growth. In addition, the ketone body β -hydroxybutyrate acts as an endogenous histone deacetylase inhibitor, resulting in downstream signaling that protects against oxidative stress.

(284-287) Calorie restriction, which lowers blood glucose and elevates blood beta-hydroxybutyrate, reduces nuclear expression of phosphorylated NF-kB (p65), cytosolic expression of phosphorylated IkB, total IkB, and DNA promoter binding activity of activated NF-kB. (288) NF-kB is a major driver of inflammation in the tumor microenvironment.
The randomized controlled trial by Chi et al describes how adhering to a caloric-restricted diet for 6 months can have therapeutic benefits in slowing the growth of prostate cancer. (289) The men in the control group were instructed to avoid any dietary changes, whereas the men in the calorie-restricted group were coached by a dietician to restrict dietary carbohydrates to <20 grams/day. The authors found that elevated levels of serum ketone bodies (3- hydroxy-2-methylbutyric acid) at both 3 and 6 months were associated with significantly longer prostate cancer antigen doubling time ($p < 0.0001$), which is a marker of prostate cancer growth rate. Similarly, in a post hoc exploratory analysis of the CAPS2 randomized study the PSA doubling time was significantly longer in the low carbohydrate diet versus control diet (28 vs. 13 months, $P = 0.021$) arms.(290) These findings support the concept that elevations in ketone bodies are associated with reduced tumor growth. In a randomized trial in women with endometrial or ovarian a ketogenic diet was associated with a significant improvement in physical function scores with less fatigue.(291) In this study the ketogenic diet resulted in the selective loss of fat mass, retention of lean mass with lower fasting serum insulin levels. (292) In a randomized controlled trial Khodabakshi et al determined the feasibility, safety, and beneficial effects of an MCT-based Ketogenic diet in patients with locally advanced or metastatic breast cancer and planned chemotherapy. (293) Compared to the control group, fasting blood glucose, BMI, body weight, and fat% were significantly decreased in intervention group ($P < 0.001$). Overall survival in neoadjuvant patients was higher in the ketogenic group compared to the control ($P = 0.04$).

A ketogenic diet following completed courses of chemotherapy and radiotherapy was further reported to be associated with long-term survival in a patient with metastatic non-small cell lung cancer. (294) “Long-term” survival has been reported in patients with glioblastoma on a ketogenic diet. (294, 295) Furthermore, evidence shows that therapeutic ketosis can act synergistically with conventional chemotherapeutic drugs, irradiation, and surgery to enhance cancer management, thus improving both progression-free and overall survival. (295) In addition, it is highly likely that therapeutic ketosis acts synergistically with the repurposed anticancer drugs reviewed in this document. Therapeutic ketosis requires a blood glucose < 90 mg/dl and a blood ketone > 2 mmol/l, aiming for a Glucose-Ketone Index < 2. (296) See the Glucose-Ketone Index Calculator in the section on caloric restriction. There are no known drugs that can simultaneously target as many tumor-associated signaling pathways as can calorie restriction. Hence, energy restriction can be a cost-effective adjuvant therapy to traditional chemo- or radiation therapies, which are more toxic, costly, and generally less focused in their therapeutic action than dietary energy restriction. It should be noted that the medium-chain fatty acids that are present during the consumption of a ketogenic diet directly inhibit glutamate receptors. (297) Shukla et al observed reduced glycolytic flux in tumor cells upon treatment with ketone bodies. Ketone bodies also diminished glutamine uptake, overall ATP content, and survival in multiple pancreatic cancer cell lines, while inducing apoptosis. (298) According to Dr. Seyfried: “Most human metastatic cancers have multiple characteristics of macrophages. We found that neoplastic cells with macrophage characteristics are heavily dependent on glutamine for growth. We have not yet found any tumor cell that can survive for very long under prolonged restriction of glucose and glutamine. Furthermore, we have not yet found any fatty acid or ketone body that can replace either glucose or glutamine as a growth metabolite. It, therefore, becomes essential to simultaneously restrict both glucose and glutamine while placing the person in nutritional ketosis for successful cancer management."

Although dietary energy restriction and anti-glycolytic cancer drugs will have therapeutic efficacy against many tumors that depend largely on glycolysis and glucose for growth, these therapeutic approaches could be less effective against those tumor cells that depend more heavily on glutamine than on glucose for energy. Glutamine is a major energy metabolite for many tumor cells and especially for cells of hematopoietic or myeloid lineage. Green tea polyphenol (EGCG) targets glutamine metabolism by inhibiting glutamate dehydrogenase activity under low glucose conditions (see section below). (234, 299-303) In addition, mebendazole, curcumin and resveratrol inhibit glutaminolysis. (13, 304) Glioblastoma, breast cancer, pancreatic cancer, lung cancer, prostate cancer, and lymphoma may depend on glutamine as a source of energy. (13)

REAL FOOD: THE BANTING DIET

Patients are strongly recommended to eat "real food" and not processed food. If it looks like food, it is likely food. If it comes in a box or carton, has a food label, and/or a long list of chemicals and additives with long and complex names it is not food. A high proportion of the population (60-80%) eating a Western diet are addicted to processed food. (305) Processed food addiction is a recognized "substance use disorder" (SUD) and should be treated as such.(305) Animal experiments demonstrate that sugar and fructose are more addictive than cocaine and heroin and that carbohydrate addicts demonstrated many of the behaviors of those with an SUD. (305) Results from the NutriNet-Santé prospective cohort study demonstrated that a 10% increase in the proportion of ultra-processed foods in the diet was associated with a significant increase of greater than 10% in risks of overall and breast cancer.(240) The EPIC Cohort study investigated the association between dietary intake according to amount of food processing and risk of cancer at 25 anatomical sites using data from the European Prospective Investigation into Cancer and Nutrition (EPIC) study. (306) In this study, in a multivariate model, substitution of 10% of processed foods with an equal amount of minimally processed foods was associated with reduced risk of overall cancer (hazard ratio 0·96, 95% CI 0·95-0·97), head and neck cancers (0·80, 0·75-0·85), oesophageal squamous cell carcinoma (0·57, 0·51-0·64), colon cancer (0·88, 0·85-0·92), rectal cancer (0·90, 0·85-0·94), hepatocellular carcinoma (0·77, 0·68-0·87), and postmenopausal breast cancer (0·93, 0·90-0·97).

A low carbohydrate-high fat (LCHF) dietary pattern is especially important for patients with cancer. As already discussed, a low carbohydrate ketogenic diet is essential to control blood glucose levels. Furthermore, a real food diet high in both soluble and insoluble fiber and fermented foods is critical to normalize the microbiome. Alterations in the microbiome play an important role in both tumorigenesis and tumor propagation. Altered gut microbiota is associated with resistance to chemotherapeutic drugs while restoration of a normal microbiome improves the response to the anticancer drugs. (307-310) Antibiotics cause severe dysbiosis; this is associated with an increased risk of cancer and reduced response to chemotherapy. (311, 312)

The Banting Diet comes close to meeting the criteria of the ideal real-food diet. (313-315) William Banting (1796-1878), a Victorian undertaker, is regarded as the father of the low-carbohydrate diet. In 1863, Banting wrote a booklet called *Letter on Corpulence, Address to the Public,* which contained the particular plan for the diet he followed. (313, 315) It was written as an open letter in the form of a personal testimonial. Banting accounted for all his unsuccessful fasts, diets, spas, and exercise regimens in his past. His previously unsuccessful attempts had been on the advice of various medical experts. He then described the dietary change that finally had worked for him, following the advice of another medical expert. "My kind and valued medical adviser is not a doctor for obesity, but stands on the pinnacle of fame in the treatment of another malady, which, as he well knows, is frequently induced by [corpulence]." His own diet consisted of meat, greens, fruits, and dry wine. The emphasis was on avoiding sugar, saccharine matter, starch, beer, and milk. Banting's pamphlet was popular for years to come and would be used as a model for modern diets.

The Banting diet consists mainly of animal protein (including poultry, eggs, and fish), saturated animal fats (including lard, duck fat, and butter), coconut oil, olive oil, and macadamia oil, some cheeses and dairy products, some nuts and seeds, fresh vegetables grown mainly above the ground and a few berries. (314) The Banting diet excludes all processed “food”, pre-packed, boxed, and “food” in wrappers as well as “fast food”. It excludes all foods with sugar, fructose, and maltose as well as grain products (wheat, barley, oats, rye) and soy products. (314) Soy products are genetically modified, toxic non-foods. (314) Replace all seed oils (canola, sunflower, safflower, cottonseed, soy) with healthy saturated fats; extra virgin olive oil and virgin coconut oil are freely encouraged. High-fat dairy products are suggested and not skimmed or fat-free dairy.

MANAGEMENT OF CANCER CACHEXIA

A high percentage of patients with cancer are nutritionally impaired and at risk for malnutrition.(316) Cancer-associated cachexia is a disorder characterized by loss of body weight with specific losses of skeletal muscle and adipose tissue. (317, 318) It is characterized by a negative protein and energy balance. Cancer cachexia is driven by a variable combination of reduced food intake and metabolic changes, including elevated energy expenditure, excess catabolism, and inflammation. (317) Cancer cachexia is defined as weight loss greater than 5%, or BMI <20 and any degree of weight loss >2%; or skeletal muscle index consistent with sarcopenia (males <7·26 kg/m²; females <5·45 kg/m²). (319) Cancer cachexia is associated with reduced physical function, reduced tolerance to anticancer therapy, and reduced survival. (317, 318) Cancer cachexia is common in patients with advanced cancer.

The therapeutic strategy is to address coexisting treatable factors. The treatment of cancer cachexia should be chosen in a way that can be continued according to the patient's condition and lifestyle. Patients with advanced cancer who can complete an exercise program show improvements in physical function and quality of life (see exercise [intervention 2] in section on lifestyle interventions for the treatment of cancer). In RCTs in patients with advanced cancer, nutritional therapy alone has not demonstrated consistent efficacy on weight, quality of life, and survival. (320, 321) Nevertheless, we suggest three nutrient-dense meals a day (following the Banting Diet). Intermittent fasting/time-restricted feeding should be avoided (except during chemotherapy); however, patients should avoid snacking between meals and should avoid eating within 3-4 hours before going to sleep (to promote autophagy while sleeping).

Shukla et al demonstrated that ketone body-induced intracellular metabolomic reprogramming in pancreatic cancer cells leads to a significantly diminished cachexia in cell line models. The cachectic phenotype is in part due to metabolic alterations in tumor cells, which can be reverted by a ketogenic diet, causing reduced tumor growth and inhibition of muscle and body weight loss. (298) In addition, we suggest a complete nutritional "shake" containing superfoods such as plant protein, super green, omega-3 fatty acids, vitamins, adaptogenic herbs, probiotics, fiber, mushrooms, and berries (e.g., Ka'Chava ™ https://www.kachava.com/ and 310 Shakes™ https://310nutrition.com/). These "superfood shakes" are preferred over regular protein shakes. Tube feeding should be avoided as this may negatively impact quality of life. Pharmacological therapies for cachexia have limited efficacy and are difficult to improve the severely reduced muscle mass in patients with cachexia. (318) Anamorelin, a ghrelin receptor agonist, is currently the only drug available for the indication of cancer cachexia in a limited number of countries. (322) However, it has been reported that anamorelin elevates IGF-1 which promotes tumor growth. (323)

INTERMITTENT FASTING, AUTOPHAGY, AND CANCER

Fasting has a profound effect on promoting immune system homeostasis, improving mitochondrial health, and increasing stem cell production. (324-328) Fasting stimulates the clearing of damaged mitochondria (mitophagy), misfolded and foreign proteins, and damaged cells (autophagy). Intermittent fasting/time-restricted eating is the single most effective method to activate autophagy. However, the role of intermittent fasting and autophagy in cancer is complex (see below).

The 2016 Nobel Prize in Physiology or Medicine was awarded to Yoshinori Ohsumi for his initial elucidation of the morphological and molecular mechanisms of autophagy in the 1990s. (329, 330) Macroautophagy (herein referred to as autophagy) is a conserved lysosomal degradation pathway for the intracellular recycling of macromolecules and clearance of damaged organelles and misfolded proteins to ensure cellular homeostasis. (331) Dysfunctional autophagy contributes to many diseases, including cancer. However, theoretically autophagy can suppress or promote tumors depending on their developmental stage and type. Modulating autophagy for cancer treatment is a therapeutic approach currently under intense investigation.

During autophagy, cytoplasmic constituents (damaged proteins, misfolded proteins, foreign proteins) are engulfed within double-membrane vesicles called autophagosomes, which subsequently fuse with lysosomes to form autolysosomes, where the cargo is degraded or recycled (see Figure 6). Autophagy occurs at basal levels under physiological conditions and can be upregulated in response to stressful stimuli such as hypoxia, nutritional deprivation, DNA damage, and cytotoxic agents. (331) The molecular machinery that mediates the autophagic process is evolutionarily conserved in higher eukaryotes and regulated by specific genes (ATG genes), which were initially characterized in yeast. The process of macroautophagy can also lead to cell death or "autophagic cell death," as a result of the accumulation of autophagosomes and autolysosomes in the cytoplasm. The effects of fasting, autophagy and cancer are still under study, but many researchers propose that intermittent fasting could help with the treatment and eradication of tumors and cancer cells.(332)

Intermittent fasting/time-restricted eating is the most effective therapy for the treatment of insulin resistance, metabolic syndrome, and type II diabetes. Intermittent fasting has additional benefits in prolonging health span, alleviating the symptoms/curing many chronic diseases, as well as preventing cardiovascular disease, Alzheimers disease and cancer. (333, 334) To gain the maximum benefits of intermittent fasting, it is thought that feeding times should be scheduled to align with circadian rhythms and activities so that timely nutrient metabolism favors healthy physiology.

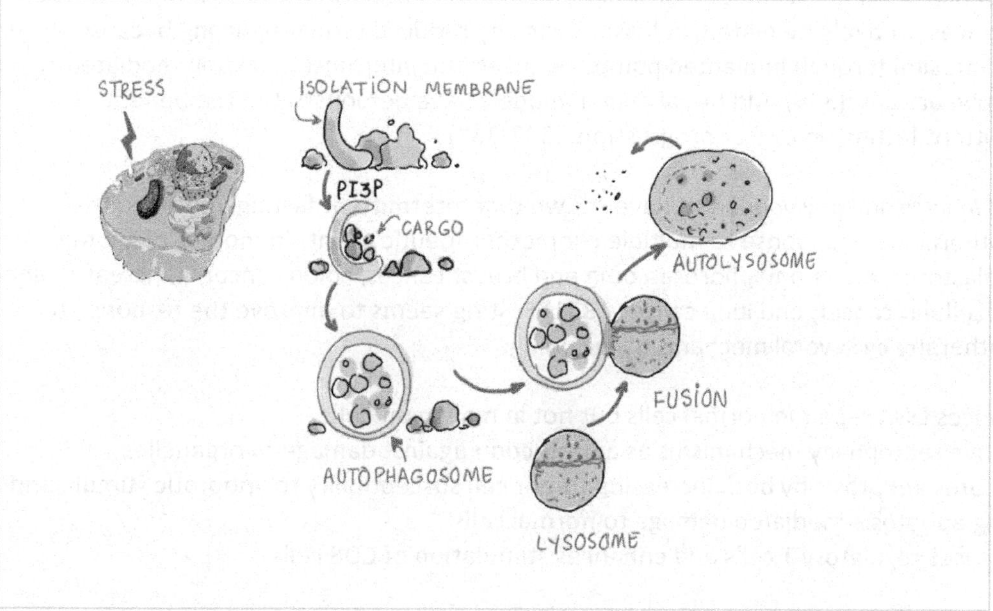

Figure 6. Autophagy pathway (Source: Dr. Mobeen Syed)

The metabolic effects of intermittent fasting are numerous and include increasing insulin sensitivity, decreasing blood glucose levels, decreasing insulin levels, decreasing insulin-like growth factor, activating the sirtuin pathway, and activating autophagy. Intermittent fasting is the most effective means of activating autophagy and accounts for many of its beneficial effects. These effects likely explain the benefits of intermittent fasting in patients with cancer.

There has been some concern that while autophagy may play an important role in preventing the development of cancer, it may paradoxically promote cancer cell proliferation. Once a tumor is established, the main function of autophagy is to provide a means to cope with cellular stressors, including hypoxia, nutritional and growth factor deprivation, and damaging stimuli, thus allowing tumor adaptation, proliferation, survival, and dissemination. Autophagy, by degrading macromolecules and defective organelles, supplies metabolites and upregulates mitochondrial function, supporting tumor cell viability. While autophagy may theoretically promote cancer cell proliferation multiple studies have demonstrated that autophagy leads to cancer cell death. (335) Almost all the repurposed drugs listed in this monograph have been demonstrated to enhance tumor cell death by activating the autophagy pathway.

Limited rodent studies and human studies have evaluated the independent effects of intermittent fasting/time restricted eating in modulating cancer progression. In a study of a high-fat driven, postmenopausal breast cancer mouse model, intermittent fasting markedly inhibited tumor initiation, progression, and metastasis compared with mice fed *ad libitum* in the absence of calorie restriction or weight loss. (336) This beneficial effect of intermittent feeding was probably mediated, at least in part, by reduced insulin signaling because systemic insulin infusion through implanted pumps reversed the intermittent fasting-mediated cancer-protective actions. (336) Additional animal models have demonstrated the benefit of intermittent fasting on cancer progression. (337-339)

Recent *in vitro* and *in vivo* models have shown that intermittent fasting improved the chemotherapeutic response to multiple chemotherapeutic agents in models of glioma, neuroblastoma, melanoma, fibrosarcoma and breast cancer, colon cancer, pancreatic cancer, hepatocellular cancer, and lung cancer. (331) Fasting seems to improve the response to chemotherapy by several mechanisms including:

- Enhances DNA repair in normal cells but not in malignant cells
- Improves autophagy mechanisms as a protection against damage to organelles
- Promotes apoptosis by both increasing tumor cell susceptibility to apoptotic stimuli, and averting apoptosis-mediated damage to normal cells
- Decreases regulatory T cells and enhances stimulation of CD8 cells

Interestingly, fasting in combination with cytotoxic agents elicited differential responses in normal and cancer cells, a phenomenon known as differential stress resistance (DSR). For DSR, normal cells prioritize maintenance pathways and inactivate growth factor signaling when nutrients are absent. In contrast, cancer cells, due to oncogene activation, do not inhibit stress resistance pathways, thus becoming vulnerable to cytotoxic treatment. In a colon cancer model, intermittent fasting inhibited tumor growth without causing permanent weight loss and decreased M2 polarization of tumor-associated macrophages in mice. (340) When intermittent fasting cycles were combined with chemotherapy, tumor growth was slowed and overall survival was prolonged in breast cancer, melanoma, and neuroblastoma animal models. (341)

The role of intermittent fasting and the enhancement of autophagy in patients with cancer is complex. While animal models demonstrate a benefit of intermittent fasting in several tumor models, clinical data in humans is limited. While time-restricted feeding (intermittent fasting) may theoretically promote cancer cell proliferation, this concept has not been observed in patients with cancer. Furthermore, more prolonged fasting of 24-96 hours has been well tolerated in patients with cancer and appears to improve quality of life and disease symptoms.(12) This data suggests that the approach to intermittent fasting should be individualized in patients with cancer according to each patient's response.

Data from small trials in humans suggest that many types of intermittent fasting regimens positively affect risk factors for poor breast cancer outcomes, such as glucoregulation, inflammation, obesity, and sleep. Experimental animal models and human data support the hypothesis that a prolonged nightly fasting interval (time restricted eating) could reduce cancer risk and improve cancer outcomes. Marinac et al investigated whether the duration of nightly fasting predicted recurrence and mortality among women with early-stage breast cancer. (342) Data were collected from 2413 women with breast cancer but without diabetes mellitus who were aged 27 to 70 years at diagnosis and participated in the prospective Women's Healthy Eating and Living study. Nightly fasting duration was estimated from 24-hour dietary recalls collected at baseline, year 1, and year 4. The mean fasting duration was 12.5 ± 1.7 hours per night. In repeated-measures Cox proportional hazards regression models, fasting less than 13 hours per night was associated with an increase in the risk of breast cancer recurrence compared with fasting 13 or more hours per night (HR 1.36; 95% CI, 1.05-1.76).

INSULIN POTENTIATION THERAPY FOR CANCER?

In vitro studies suggest that insulin may potentiate the effects of chemotherapeutic drugs.(343) However, there are no clinical studies to support this concept. Furthermore, such treatment may be hazardous (causing severe hypoglycemia) and is counterintuitive, as it may likely promote tumor cell proliferation. Insulin is responsible for cellular glucose uptake and mitogenic signaling cascades in cancer cells and can promote cell proliferation, survival, invasiveness, angiogenesis, immunomodulation, and chemoresistance (as reviewed in this document). (344) Tumor cells express significantly more insulin receptors on their cell surface as compared to normal effects. (12) Insulin will promote further glycolysis and provide metabolic fuel for the cancer cell!

Some medical practitioners claim that the combined use of insulin and glucose (insulin potentiation therapy) can improve the outcomes of patients with cancer and facilitate cancer therapy de-escalation? (146, 345) Supporters of insulin potentiation therapy (IPT) and IPT with low-dose chemotherapy (IPTLD) for patients with cancer claim that insulin increases cancer cells' permeability to chemotherapeutics relative to surrounding healthy tissues, because of the high expression of insulin receptors on these cells. (344) Other supporters suggest anticancer drugs enter cells through the same mechanism as that of glucose, conflating glucose transport with multidrug uptake transport.

There are only two published clinical trials assessing insulin potentiation therapy. Damyanov et al enrolled 16 patients with castration-resistant prostate cancer to receive insulin (0.4 U/kg) and docetaxel or a non-standard drug combination. (344) Those patients who received insulin and chemotherapy had a worse outcome (median survival of 11 months compared with 18.9 months). The second prospective study examined methotrexate response and toxicity in 30 patients with metastatic breast cancer. (346) Stable disease was reported to be more frequent in the group receiving methotrexate plus insulin compared with those receiving methotrexate alone; however, patient-centered outcomes were not provided.

Practitioners of IPT are convinced by the efficacy of this technique despite the lack of convincing scientific evidence. The role of this treatment modality therefore remains uncertain.

CHAPTER 5: METABOLIC AND LIFESTYLE INTERVENTIONS FOR CANCER TREATMENT

1. Glucose Management and Ketogenic Diet

A carbohydrate-restricted diet (less than 25 g of carbs per day) that is high in saturated fat and Omega-3 fatty acids (ketogenic diet) is suggested. Avoid all processed food. (240) Contrary to current dogma, saturated fatty acids are "healthy," but you should avoid processed Omega-6 vegetable oils (see below). (347, 348) Avoid foods that are high on the glycemic index and follow the "hacks" to flatten the blood glucose curve (see below). (349)

A continuous glucose monitor (CGM) is essential to track changes in blood glucose levels. Patients must keep accurate records to identify (and avoid) any food that might spike blood glucose. Target a baseline blood glucose of 60-80 mg/dl (3.3 – 4.4 mmol/l) and a postprandial (after a meal) glucose of less than 120 mg/dl (6.6 mmol/l). The ideal is a flat blood glucose curve; the blood glucose should not increase by more than 20 mg/dl after a meal. In addition, a blood ketone meter (blood level of beta-hydroxybutyrate) is recommended to confirm that the patient has entered ketosis (normal level < 0.5 mmol/l). Ideally, the blood ketone level should be over 2 mmol/l. The optimal therapeutic range is between 3 and 5 mmol/l. It is important to track changes in blood glucose and ketones with both fasting and exercise. Therapeutic ketosis requires a blood glucose < 90 mg/dl and a blood ketone > 2 mmol/l, aiming for a Glucose-Ketone Index (GKI) of < 2. (296)

The GKI can be calculated at: https://keto-mojo.com/glucose-ketone-index-gki/ and https://perfectketo.com/glucose-ketone-index-calculator/

The Glycemic Index

The glycemic index is a value assigned to foods based on how quickly those foods cause increases in blood glucose levels and how high they spike. The glycemic index ranks food on a scale from 0 to 100. Pure glucose is arbitrarily given a value of 100, which represents the relative rise in the blood glucose level after two hours (see Figure 7). The glycemic index of a specific food depends primarily on the quantity and type of carbohydrate it contains (see Table 4). Foods that are low on the glycemic index (GI) scale tend to release glucose slowly and steadily. Foods that are high on the glycemic index release glucose rapidly. It should be noted that the glycemic index varies between individuals. (350, 351) A CGM allows for the individual assessment of the glucose excursion (glycemic index) of various foods.

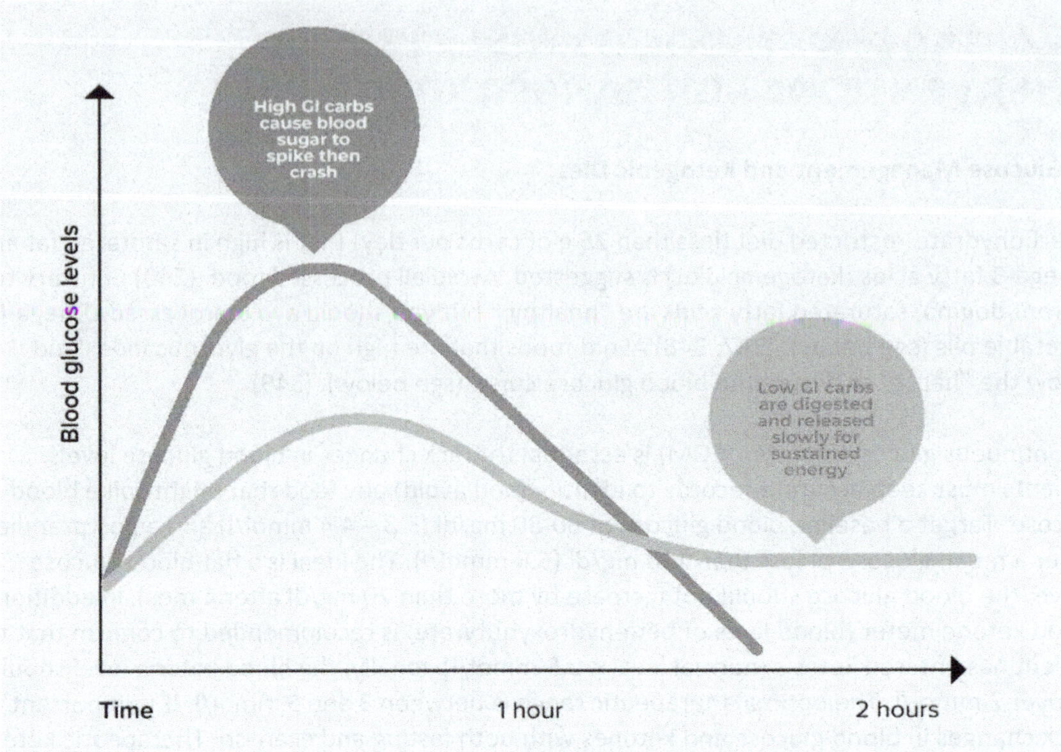

Figure 7: The blood glucose profile of high and low glycemic index foods (Source: adapted from Glycemic Index Foundation)

What to eat and what not to eat

The most important intervention to reduce obesity, metabolic syndrome, type II diabetes, cancer, cardiac disease, neurodegenerative diseases, autoimmune diseases etc., is to eat real food and not processed food. (240, 305, 352) Telling the difference is quite simple. If it looks like food, it is real. If it comes in a box or has a food label, it's likely processed. The more ingredients listed on a product's label and the more chemicals you see with strange and unpronounceable names, the more processing the product has undergone. Recent evidence suggests that processed foods in themselves can cause insulin resistance. (353)

Healthy foods include:

- All vegetables (especially avocados, and cruciferous and leafy vegetables)
- Nuts (almonds, brazil nuts, cashews, and pistachios)
- Peanut butter (but avoid the white bread and grape jelly!) and chia seeds
- Fish (wild fresh fish especially Alaskan/Pacific salmon and sardines)
- Chicken breast (free range, no hormones, no antibiotics)
- Eggs (they've been giving a bad rap!); free range "organic" eggs are suggested

- Meat (grass-fed, no hormones, avoid processed meats)
- Blueberries (limit volume if insulin resistant)
- Coffee with heavy cream or coconut oil; choose Stevia (without erythritol) over sugar or artificial sweeteners.

Table 4: Glycemic index of selected foods (Source: FLCCC)

Food Item	Glycemic Index
White rice	87
Watermelon	76
White bread	75
Orange juice	53
Banana	51
Pineapple	66
Papaya	60
Grape	46
Orange	42
Strawberry	40
Apple	34
Grapefruit	25
Fresh berries	25
Most vegetables	<20
Peanuts	7

Flattening the glucose curve

Apart from carbohydrate restriction/ketogenic diet and time-restricted eating, several simple interventions (or hacks) prevent the high glucose spikes that fuel cancer. The book "Glucose Revolution" by Jessie Inchauspe is highly recommended and provides more details on interventions to flatten the blood glucose curve, such as. (349)

Eat foods in the right order

Veggies (greens/fiber) should be eaten first, protein and fat second, and starch (sugars) last; this slows gastric emptying, as well as the breakdown and absorption of glucose. Eat fruit last; always preceded by fiber. Don't begin a meal with bread (starch).

- Begin all meals with a salad or green vegetables. Use olive oil and vinegar as salad dressing.
- Avoid starchy foods with no fiber.

- Avoid fruit juices and smoothies, which cause a large glucose spike.
- Skip breakfast. Breakfast is the worst time to eat sugar and starches; this results in a large glucose spike. Cereal for breakfast causes a rapid spike in glucose.
- Avoid snacking throughout the day.
- Drink a tablespoon of vinegar stirred into a tall glass of water before eating starch or something sweet. Apple cider vinegar is recommended. The acetic acid in vinegar decreases the enzymatic breakdown of starch, increases glycogen synthesis (and glucose uptake), and increases fatty acid oxidation. (354-357) Vinegar may be beneficial even if consumed up to 20 minutes after a starchy food. Apple cider vinegar is usually unpasteurized and should be avoided in pregnancy.
- If vinegar is not readily available, consume a few fiber tablets (esp. glucomannan tablets) before eating a starchy/sweet treat.
- Go for a 20-minute walk within an hour of eating/having starchy food. During exercise, muscles take up glucose for energy while increasing mitochondrial oxidative capacity. (358-360) Going to the gym or doing resistance exercise is an alternative. Climbing a few stairs is an option at work. If sedentary, do sitting calf raises (the soleal pump). The soleal pump is strongly recommended; it has been demonstrated to reduce postprandial glucose by about 50%, reduce hyperinsulinemia, and improved lipid metabolism. (361) If you exercise and you have not eaten, i.e., you are engaging in fasted exercise, your liver releases glucose into the bloodstream to fuel the mitochondria in your muscles; this causes a glucose spike. This is mediated by increased release of cortisol, epinephrine, and norepinephrine (with decreased glucagon); i.e., release of harmful stress hormones. If you exercise before eating, we would suggest a shake with 'superfoods,' including a plant protein, super green, Omega-3 fatty acids, vitamins and adaptogenic herbs, probiotics and fiber, super mushrooms, and berries (e.g., Ka'Chava ™ https://www.kachava.com/ or 310 Shakes™ https://310nutrition.com/collections/meal-replacement-shakes) instead of a regular protein shake.

Establishing/restoring a "normal" microbiome

The microbiome has a remarkable effect on blood sugar levels and insulin sensitivity. (362-368) Establishing a normal microbiome is important for regulating blood glucose levels and improving insulin sensitivity. Furthermore, alterations in the microbiome play an important role in both tumorigenesis and tumor propagation. Follow these suggestions to help establish a "normal microbiome":

- Eat a diverse range of foods.
- Eat lots of vegetables, legumes, and beans.
- Eat fermented foods like yogurt (unsweetened), kefir, apple cider vinegar, kombucha, pickles, sauerkraut, tempeh, and kimchi.
- Eat foods rich in polyphenols (dark fruits). Include resveratrol supplements.
- Eat prebiotic fiber. Glucomannan is a dietary fiber (soluble and insoluble) made from the root of the konjac plant.

- Eat chia seeds, high in insoluble and soluble fiber.
- Eat less sugar and sweeteners.
- Reduce stress.
- Avoid taking antibiotics unnecessarily.
- Stop snacking.
- Exercise regularly.
- Spend time outdoors in the natural world to expose yourself to millions of microbes, many of which can benefit microbiome diversity.
- Get enough sleep.

The consumption of fermented foods may be particularly important in restoring/maintaining a normal microbiome. Large cohort studies as well as limited interventional studies have linked the consumption of fermented foods with weight maintenance and decreased diabetes, cancer, and cardiovascular disease risks. (369)

The saturated fat-cholesterol hoax

The Cholesterol-Saturated fatty acid hoax (347, 370, 371) began to proliferate in the 1960s. Dr. Ancel Keys popularized the notion that saturated fats and high cholesterol were the primary causes of atherosclerotic heart disease — the so-called Diet-Heart Hypothesis. (372, 373) This concept has been vigorously studied, including in many randomized controlled trials, and has been convincingly proven to be false. (347, 374, 375) Indeed, replacing saturated fats with a diet high in vegetable oils (linoleic acid) was associated with higher rates of death, cardiovascular and coronary heart disease as well as a significantly increased risk of cancer. (376)

Healthy and unhealthy oils

Avoid seed oils high in linoleic acid. Linoleic acid is an Omega-6 fatty acid that our bodies require in small amounts. Unfortunately, many people eat up to 10 times the desired amount of linoleic acid, because of excess consumption of foods made with seed oils. Too much linoleic acid is associated with inflammation, obesity, heart disease, and other unfavorable conditions. Therefore, avoid:

- Soybean oil
- Corn oil
- Cottonseed oil
- Sunflower oil
- Sesame oil
- Grapeseed oil
- Safflower oil
- Rice bran oil
- Margarine

Instead, opt for healthy oils and fats such as the ones listed below. Use only high-quality products and check production and expiration dates.

- Olive oil (oleic acid, Omega-9 monounsaturated fatty acids); never heat olive oil to the point where it produces smoke.
- Avocado oil (oleic acid, Omega-9 monounsaturated fatty acids)
- Coconut oil (medium chain fatty acid)
- Flaxseed oil (alpha-linolenic acid, ALA Omega-3)
- Walnut and Pecan oils; should be refrigerated to avoid spoilage
- Butter (saturated fat)

2. Exercise (aerobic and resistance training)

Lifestyle modification — with an emphasis on exercise, a healthy diet, and stress reduction — plays a major role in reducing the risk of death from cancer and improving quality of life. (377, 378) As already discussed, obesity and metabolic syndrome increase the risk of death in patients with cancer. In a study involving early-stage breast cancer, patients with metabolic syndrome were at a significantly increased risk of distant metastasis (HR 2.45, 95% CI 1.24–4.82) compared with those without the syndrome. (379)

Regular exercise combining both aerobic activity and resistance training is recommended in patients undergoing treatment for cancer. Aerobic exercises such as walking, high-intensity interval training (HIIT), cycling, swimming, etc., improve overall cardiovascular fitness with improved indicators of quality of life, including better cognition and mood with less fatigue and reduced anxiety and depression. (380-385) Resistance training preserves lean body mass (muscle mass), which reduces insulin resistance and improves glucose control and may be an important factor in increasing overall survival as sarcopenia is a major negative prognostic factor in patients with cancer. (386)

The Combined Aerobic and Resistance Exercise (CARE) Trial compared different types and doses of exercise performed during breast cancer chemotherapy. (387) In this study a combined dose of 50-60 minutes of aerobic and resistance exercise performed three times weekly was significantly associated with better patient-reported outcomes and health-related compared to performing aerobic exercise alone. Meta-analyses that focused on specific types of cancer reported benefits in breast cancer treated with adjuvant chemotherapy and/or radiotherapy, colorectal cancer treated with chemotherapy, lung cancer treated with chemotherapy, prostate cancer treated with radiation therapy, and hematologic malignancies. (380) A meta-analysis of 22 prospective cohort studies found that breast cancer mortality was significantly reduced among women who reported participating in recreational physical activity after their breast cancer diagnosis (HR 0.59, 95% CI 0.45–0.78). (388)

Patients should be encouraged to engage in at least 30 minutes of moderate-intensity physical activity at least five days of the week, or 75 minutes of more vigorous exercise, along with two to three weekly strength training sessions, including exercises for major muscle groups. (377, 385) However, more hours of exercise (but not more vigorous activity) may have increased benefits. Two analyses showed a substantial inverse dose-response effect between hours per week engaged in physical activity and breast cancer mortality. (389, 390) Walking, particularly in the sunshine, has enormous physical, emotional, and psychological benefits. (391, 392)

3. Stress Reduction and Sleep

A substantial body of research has investigated the associations between stress-related psychosocial factors and cancer outcomes. (393) This data demonstrates that psychosocial stress is associated with a higher incidence of cancer and poorer survival in patients with diagnosed cancer. (393) It is critically important that patients engage in activities that reduce stress (meditation, yoga, mindfulness exercises, etc.) and get at least 8 hours of high-quality sleep (ensure adequate sleep hygiene). (246-251, 394) See section on propranolol and the use of propranolol to mitigate against catecholamine induced cancer proliferation and metastases (page 72).

Adaptogens are herbs that help in combating stress. These herbs normalize physiological processes and help the body adapt to stress. In Ayurvedic medicine (traditional medicine native to India), *Ashwagandha* has proven to be a safe and effective adaptogen. Randomized controlled trials have shown a significant benefit in terms of stress reduction, improved cognition and mood, and quality of sleep. (395-397) In a double-blind, placebo-controlled randomized controlled trial, participants who had chronic stress were randomized to ashwagandha extract (300 mg twice daily) or placebo for 60 days. (398) At the end of 60 days, participants in the active treatment group had a 44% ($p< 0.001$) reduction in stress scores and a 28% ($p< 0.001$) reduction in cortisol levels. In a similar study, Ashwagandha resulted in a marked improvement in the quality of sleep in patients with insomnia. (399) A meta-analysis of 12 RCTs demonstrated that Ashwagandha supplementation significantly reduced anxiety ($p = .005$) and stress levels ($p = .005$) compared to placebo. (400) In this study, the non-linear dose-response analysis indicated a favorable effect of Ashwagandha supplementation on anxiety up to 12,000 mg daily and on stress up to 300-600 mg daily.

As Ashwagandha is an immune system activator (inhibits NF-κB), it should not be used concomitantly with immunosuppressive drugs such as tacrolimus and cyclosporine. Furthermore, the safety of Ashwagandha has not been established during pregnancy and in breastfeeding women.

Healthy sleep is essential for neural development, learning, memory, cardiovascular, and metabolic regulation. Sufficient sleep is needed to provide recovery after preceding waking activities and to ensure optimal functioning during subsequent wakefulness. (401) As recommended by the National Sleep Foundation, in a healthy individual, the recommended sleep duration for younger adults is seven to nine hours, and for older adults is seven to eight hours. (402) Other than adequate duration, healthy sleep comprises good quality sleep.

The National Sleep Foundation endorses the following sleep quality indicators: 1) sleep latency of 15 minutes and less, 2) one or fewer awakening of more than five minutes per night, 3) wake time after sleep onset of 20 minutes and less, and 4) sleep efficiency of 85% and more. (403) Insomnia is defined by the complaints of difficulty initiating sleep, difficulty maintaining sleep, or early morning awakenings and is associated with one or more daytime symptoms such as fatigue, cognitive impairment, or mood disturbance (depression). (404) A systematic review demonstrated that short sleep duration, defined as less than six hours of sleep per 24 hours, is associated with a significant mortality increase. (405)

A meta-analysis of 5 RCTs demonstrated that Ashwagandha supplementation significantly improved sleep, particularly in a subgroup of adults diagnosed with insomnia; the treatment dosage was > 600 mg daily and the treatment duration was > 8 weeks. (404) Ashwagandha showed improvement in sleep compared to the placebo for the Sleep Quality Scale, sleep onset latency, total sleep time, wake time after sleep onset, and sleep efficiency. In addition, extensive studies have demonstrated that ashwagandha has potent in vivo and in vitro anti-cancer effects has been demonstrated to improve the quality of life in patients with breast cancer undergoing chemotherapy. (406) For this reason we strongly recommend supplementation with ashwagandha as adjuvant therapy in patients with cancer.

4. Comprehensive Lifestyle Changes

We recommend comprehensive lifestyle changes for both the prevention and treatment of cancer. A landmark prospective, randomized study evaluated the short- and long-term effects of a comprehensive lifestyle intervention on women with stage II or stage II breast cancer who had undergone surgery. (407-411) The intervention included techniques to reduce stress, improve the "quality of life," and promote healthy behaviors including guidance on diet, exercise, relaxation techniques, social support and healthy living. Patients in the intervention group attended regular sessions with follow-up appointments to ensure compliance with the lifestyle program. Eleven years later, women who participated in the intervention had a 45% lower risk of cancer recurrence than those in the control group and were 56% less likely to have died from breast cancer compared to women in the control group. Intervention patients were also 49% less likely than women in the control group to die from any cause. The study also demonstrated that women who took part in the intervention had significantly improved psychological, behavioral, and health outcomes, as well as improved immune function compared with patients in the control group.

5. Health Benefits of Sunshine

Sunlight has great therapeutic powers. Our forefathers roamed the earth and were exposed to sunlight on a daily basis, likely with profoundly important health benefits. (412) During the 1918 influenza pandemic, "open-air treatment of influenzae" appeared to be the most effective treatment for seriously ill patients. (413) A recent large prospective study demonstrated that avoiding sun exposure is a risk factor for all-cause mortality. (414) In this study, the mortality rate amongst avoiders of sun exposure was approximately twofold higher compared with the highest sun exposure group. A large epidemiological study found women with higher solar UVB exposure had only half the incidence of breast cancer as those with lower solar exposure and that men with higher residential solar exposure had only half the incidence of fatal prostate cancer.(415) The cancers for which solar UVB is significantly associated with reduced incidence are bladder, brain (males), breast, corpus uteri, esophageal, gastric, non-Hodgkin's lymphoma, pancreatic, and renal cancer. (416) Sunlight is critical for mental health; this is most well appreciated with depression but in reality the effects are far more broad reaching.

Apart from UV radiation stimulating vitamin D synthesis, near-infrared (NIR) radiation has a profound effect on human physiology. (417) Approximately 40% of the sun's radiation in the NIR spectrum (700- 1500 nm). NIR activates mitochondria to produce melatonin (locally). In addition, NIR enhances mitochondrial electron transport and the generation of ATP. We suggest that patients expose themselves to about 30 minutes of midday sunshine whenever possible (at least 3 times a week). A brisk midday walk has a doubly beneficial effect, the exposure to sunlight and the health benefits of walking. (391, 392)

6. Sunshine and skin cancer

Skin cancer is the most common cancer in the United States.(418) Current estimates are that one in five Americans will develop skin cancer in their lifetime. By far the most common type of skin cancer is basal cell carcinoma (comprising 80% of all skin cancers). (419, 420) The three primary risk factors for BCC are excessive sun exposure, fair skin (which makes you more susceptible to excessive sunlight penetrating your skin), and a family history of skin cancer. Because BCC almost never metastasizes it is generally a very benign cancer. Cutaneous Squamous Cell Carcinoma (SCC) is the second most common type of skin cancer, SCC is also caused by sunlight. (419) Unlike BCC, SCC can be dangerous, as it does metastasize. In turn, if it is removed prior to metastasizing, it has a 99% survival rate, but if removed after metastasis, this drops to 56%. Because the face is the most sun exposed area and the commonest site of BCC and SCC, we suggest wearing a hat when exposed to sunshine and avoiding sunscreens (see below). Melanoma comprises 1% of all skin cancer diagnoses, however, melanoma is responsible for most of the deaths from skin cancer. (421-423) Survival is greatly improved by early detection. The five-year survival rate for melanoma depends upon how far it has spread at the time of its diagnosis (ranging from 99% to 35% and averaging out to 94%)
Skin cancers are by far the most diagnosed cancers in the United States, so to prevent them, the public is constantly told to avoid the sun. However, while the relatively benign skin cancers

are caused by sun exposure (BCC & SCC), melanoma responsible for most skin cancer deaths are due to a lack of sunlight.(424, 425) This is unfortunate because sunlight is arguably the most important nutrient for the human body, as avoiding it doubles one's rate of dying and significantly increases their risk of cancer.

Paradoxically, while sun exposure (UVb) increases the risk of non-melanoma skin cancer, sun exposure reduces the risk of melanoma and the overall risk of dying from cancer. (424, 426) In 1937, Peller and Stephenson reported that soldiers of the U.S. Navy, intensively exposed to open air, sun rays, and salt water, had 8-fold higher frequency of skin cancer and lip cancer, but the death rate among these cases of cancer was 3-fold lower than expected. In addition, they reported a 44% lower incidence of other cancer-related deaths. (427) In patients with melanoma sun exposure is strongly negatively associated with death from melanoma. (428) An Italian study reported that sunbathing holidays after a diagnosis of melanoma were related to reduced rates of relapses (HR=0.3, 95% CI=0.1-0.9). (429) In the MISS study (Melanoma in Southern Sweden), there was a dose dependent increase in the risk of death with lower sun exposure, with a 40% higher risk of cancer-related death in the group with low sun exposure [sHR=1.4, 95% CI=1.04-1.6] as compared to those with greatest sun exposure. (426) It should be noted that Sunscreen users in Sweden have been reported to be at an 80% increased risk of skin cancer. (OR=1.8, 95%CI=1.1-2.9). (430) In addition, research suggests that using sunscreen either has no effect on the rates of malignant melanoma or increases the risk. A plausible explanation of this increased risk might be that the application of a sunscreen inhibits the redness of the skin but allows prolonged UV exposure.

It is critically important to understand that while melanoma is widely considered to be linked to sunlight exposure this conjecture is false:

- Most importantly, 87% of all SCC cases occur in regions of the body that have significant sunlight exposure, such as the face, while 82.5% of BCC occurs in those regions. Conversely, only 22% of melanomas occur in sun exposed regions. This indicates that SCC and BCC are linked to sun exposure, but melanoma is not.(424)
- Outdoor workers get 3–10 times the annual UV dose that indoor workers get, yet they have lower incidences of cutaneous malignant melanoma and an odds ratio (risk) that is half that of their indoor colleagues.(431)
- A study of 528 patients with melanoma found those who had solar elastosis (a common change in the skin that follows excessive sun exposure) were 60% less likely to die from melanoma. (428)
- A 1997 Meta-Analysis of the available literature found workers with significant occupational sunlight exposure were 14% less likely to get melanoma.(425)
- In many areas of the world there has been a significant increase in the incidence of melanoma, which argues against sunlight being the primary issue as sun-exposure has not significantly changed in the last few decades.(431, 432) As discussed elsewhere in this document this is likely due to insulin resistance, omega-6 vegetable oils, processed food and topical carcinogens

CHAPTER 6: REPURPOSED DRUGS

Remarkably, unlike conventional chemotherapeutic drugs that mostly act via a single cellular biological pathway, almost all the repurposed drugs/nutraceuticals used as adjunctive treatments for cancer have multiple modes of action. These mechanisms can generally be divided into two major groups, namely:

i. those that act directly on cancer cell pathways promoting cell death (apoptosis); and
ii. those that alter the tumor microenvironment (TME) restoring immune function and T cell cytotoxicity, limiting angiogenesis and metastatic spread, and inhibiting cancer stem cells.

Those nutraceuticals and repurposed drugs that have been demonstrated to reduce the risk of developing cancer are likely to be highly effective in treating cancer. Furthermore, it is likely that the metabolic pathways involved in cancer prevention play a major role in limiting cancer growth and spread. Consequently, an evaluation of a repurposed drug's efficacy in preventing cancer is important in considering the role of that drug in the treatment of cancer.

Most published studies demonstrating the benefit of nutraceuticals and repurposed drugs are *in vitro* mechanistic experiments and studies performed in animal models. Prospective clinical studies are generally small, focusing on mechanisms of action or surrogate markers of efficacy. Indeed, most of the published clinical data consists of epidemiological studies, retrospective observational studies, small case series, and case reports with few prospective clinical studies. This is not unexpected due to the "war on repurposed drugs" that is being waged by Big Pharma and its supporters; there is little funding to support well-designed clinical studies using cheap, potentially effective, and lifesaving drugs.

A 2014 ProPublica investigation found that "Big Pharma's focus on blockbuster cancer drugs squeezes out research into potential treatments that are more affordable." (433) A researcher at Harvard Medical School who has tried for many years to find funding for a study on the effects of aspirin on breast cancer told the reporter: "For some reason, a drug that could be patented would get a randomized trial, but aspirin, which has amazing properties, goes unexplored because it's 99 cents at CVS." (433)

Large, pharma-funded, randomized, double-blind controlled trials (RCTs) — considered by the medical establishment and those in the ivory towers to be the gold standard — have numerous limitations, however, and frequently don't reflect real-world clinical practice. Furthermore, there is now strong scientific data and a growing consensus that well-conducted observational studies produce results statistically similar to those of traditional RCTs. (434) It is, therefore, possible, and indeed desirable to design prospective observational studies to study the clinical efficacy of the metabolic approach to cancer and specifically the combined use of multiple repurposed drugs. As the metabolic approach to cancer necessitates a combination of interventions, including caloric reduction and a ketogenic diet, and multiple off-label anticancer drugs, it would be nearly impossible to design a double-blind randomized study; indeed, such an approach may be considered unethical.

The METRICS study (NCT02201381) is an example of an off-label drug protocol for the treatment of patients with glioblastoma. (257) METRICS is a novel, participant-funded, open-label, non-randomized, single-arm real-world study designed to gather high-quality evidence on the safety, tolerability, and effectiveness of the combination of four off-label metabolically targeted medicines (metformin, atorvastatin, mebendazole, and doxycycline) as an adjunctive cancer treatment for glioblastoma and other tumors. (257) The retrospective arm of the METRICS study has produced very encouraging results, with a significant increase in disease-free survival of patients compared to a control group.

The Repurposing Drugs in Oncology (ReDO) project has cataloged 268 approved drugs with anticancer effects. (5) See Appendix 2 for an abbreviated list of repurposed drugs, and nutraceuticals. In addition, over three thousand plant species have anti-cancer activity.(435) It would be impossible to review all the drugs in ReDo's database in this monograph; rather, we have focused on and evaluated the drugs that appear to have the greatest clinical utility. These repurposed drugs are listed in priority according to the strength of the supporting clinical and mechanistic evidence (see Appendix 1 which outlines the stratification methodology).

Patients with cancer should consider taking at least the first 8-10 listed interventions; this can be modified according to the patient's individual clinical response and preferences. Furthermore, it is important to recognize that many of these interventions act additively/synergistically with each other and with conventional chemotherapy. Metronomic chemotherapy dosing is preferred (see below). Patients should monitor the response to treatment with a PET scan (glucose uptake scan) every three months and then at least every 6 months once in remission/cancer stable. Patients should follow their tumor markers concomitantly. Circulating tumor DNA (in blood specimens) is an emerging technology that may prove useful for monitoring tumor progression. (436, 437) Patients and their healthcare providers should dynamically follow their tumor markers and adjust their treatment protocol accordingly. Patients who demonstrate a good clinical response should not stop their treatment protocol abruptly, as this may result in a relapse, (4) but rather reduce the number of interventions dynamically.

Antioxidant supplements (vitamins A, C, and E; coenzyme Q10, and N-acetyl cysteine) should be avoided in patients with cancer. In an experimental model, Wang et al demonstrated that vitamin C, vitamin E and n-acetylcysteine (NAC) increased tumor angiogenesis by BACH1 mechanism (redox-sensitive transcription factor BTB and CNC homology 1). (438)These antioxidants should specifically be avoided in patients undergoing chemotherapy and radiotherapy, as these interventions act largely by increasing oxidant injury, which is minimized by antioxidant supplements. (439, 440) Paradoxically, while oral vitamin C is a potent antioxidant, (441) high-dose intravenous vitamin C generates reactive oxygen species that potentiates the effects of chemotherapy and radiation therapy (see section on intravenous vitamin C).

SUMMARY OF REPURPOSED DRUGS TO CONTROL CANCER

Listed in order of priority, stratified based on the totality of evidence (see Appendix 1) and reviewed in detail below. The summary of the anticancer pathways of the repurposed drugs are listed in Table 5. A list of the ReDo drugs is provided in Appendix 2. (5)

TIER ONE REPURPOSED DRUGS: STRONG RECOMMENDATION

1. Vitamin D3: 20,000 to 50,000 IU daily – NOTE: dosage should be adjusted according to blood vitamin D levels, aiming for a 25-OH level of at least 55-90 ng/dl
2. Propranolol 40 – 180 mg daily
3. Melatonin: start at 1 mg and increase to 20-30 mg at night (extended/slow release)
4. Metformin: 1,000 mg twice daily
5. Curcumin (nanocurcumin): 600 mg daily or as per manufacturer's suggested dosing
6. Ivermectin 12-18 mg/ day
7. Mebendazole: 100-200 mg daily
8. Green tea catechins: 500-1,000 mg daily
9. Omega 3 fatty acids: 2-4 g daily
10. Berberine: A daily dose of 1,000-1,500 mg or 500-600 mg two or three times daily. (Depending on blood glucose levels, metformin and berberine can be used together or alternating months)
11. Atorvastatin: 40 mg twice daily. (Simvastatin 20 mg twice daily is an alternative.)
12. Disulfiram: 80 mg three times daily or 500 mg once daily
13. Cimetidine: 400-800 mg twice daily
14. Mistletoe: (given subcutaneously by an integrative oncologist)
15. Ashwagandha 600- 1200 mg daily
16. Sildenafil: 20 mg daily. (Tadalafil 5 mg daily is an alternative)
17. Itraconazole 100 -600mg/daily

TIER TWO REPURPOSED DRUGS: WEAK RECOMMENDATION

18. Low dose naltrexone: 1-4.5 mg daily
19. Doxycycline: 100 mg daily (for cycles of 2 weeks)
20. Spironolactone 50-100 mg /day
21. Resveratrol: 1,000 mg daily (bioavailable enhanced formulation)/Pterostilbene
22. Wheatgrass 3- 6 g/day
23. Captopril 25 mg twice/three times daily

TIER THREE REPURPOSED DRUGS: EQUIVOCAL EVIDENCE (NOT STRONGLY FOR OR AGAINST)

24. Cyclooxygenase inhibitors: aspirin 325 mg daily or Diclofenac 75-100 mg daily
25. Nigella sativa: 400-500 mg encapsulated oil twice daily
26. Ganoderma lucidum (Reishi) and other medicinal mushrooms
27. Dipyridamole: 100 mg twice daily
28. High-dose intravenous Vitamin C (50-75 g IV as per protocol)
29. Dichloroacetate 500 mg two or three times daily
30. Sulforaphane
31. Artemisinin
32. Cannabinoids
33. Fenofibrate
34. Niclosamide
35. Pao Pereira
36. Dandelion extract

TIER FOUR REPURPOSED DRUGS: NOT RECOMMENDED

37. B-complex vitamins
38 Colchicine
39. Shark cartilage
40. Laetrile (amygdalin)

PRE-OPERATIVE REPURPOSED DRUGS TO REDUCE METASTASES

Beta-adrenergic signalling is implicated in the post-surgical metastatic process and numerous in vivo studies have reported that peri-operative propranolol is associated with a reduced rate of metastases. (442) In a phase II randomized trial Hiller et al evaluated the use of preoperative β-Blockade with propranolol on metastatic tumor biomarkers in women undergoing surgery for breast cancer. (443) In this triple-blind placebo-controlled clinical trial, 60 patients were randomly assigned to receive an escalating dose of oral propranolol (n = 30; 80-160 mg daily) or placebo (n = 30) for 7 days prior to surgery. In this study, propranolol downregulated primary tumor expression of mesenchymal genes and altered intratumoral neutrophil, natural killer cell, and dendritic cell recruitment with elevated tumor infiltration of CD68(+) macrophages (M1 macrophage polarization) and CD8(+) T cells.

The combination of propranolol with a COX-2/PGE2 inhibitor, such as ketorolac or etodolac, and/or cimetidine has the potential to show synergism in a peri-operative setting. (444, 445)

Forget and colleagues reported on a retrospective analysis of breast cancer patients treated with conservative surgery, with and without intraoperative NSAIDs (DCF or ketorolac). (446) Patients treated pre-incisionally with ketorolac (20 mg -30 mg) or DCF (75 mg) showed improved disease-free survival (HR = 0.57, 95% CI: 0.37–0.89, $P = 0.01$) and an improved overall survival (HR = 0.35, CI: 0.17–0.70, $P = 0.03$), compared to patients not treated with NSAIDs. (447) The findings of this study were, however, not replicated in a prospective RCT (see section on NSAIDS). (448) Perioperative cimetidine reverses histamine-induced suppression of lymphocyte proliferation and increases the number of tumor-infiltrating lymphocytes (see section on cimetidine). (449, 450) It should be noted that cimetidine increases the plasma levels of propranolol, hence propranolol should be dosed carefully. (451)

NCT02596867 is a Phase II open-label 'window of opportunity' trial in newly diagnosed breast cancer.(452) Propranolol at a dose of 1.5 mg/kg BID, is administered for three weeks prior to surgical resection. The primary outcome is a reduction in the proliferative index (Ki-67), secondary outcomes relate to safety, toxicity and adherence. NCT00502684 and is a Phase III randomized, placebo-controlled trial of peri-operative propranolol and etodolac (a COX-2 inhibitor) in colorectal cancer patients undergoing resection.(452) Patients in the treatment arm receive etodolac 800 mg BID for the entire intervention period, propranolol 20 mg BID for 5 pre-operative days, 80 mg BID on the day of surgery, 40 mg BID for the first postoperative week, 20 mg PO BID for the second postoperative week. The primary clinical endpoint of this study is the rate of local and distant recurrence rate at three years.

Perioperative propranolol together with a COX-2 inhibitor and possibly low dose cimetidine (200 mg BID) given for 7-10 days prior to surgical resection of a tumor (including a biopsy) may reduce the risk of metastatic disease. A dose of propranolol of 40-80 mg BID to keep the resting pulse > 60-70 bpm is suggested. Careful dosage adjustment of propranolol is required in patients receiving cimetidine. The anesthesiologist should be aware the patient is taking a beta-blocker. The addition of vitamin D (20 000 IU/day) may have additional benefits. Postoperatively patients should continue a tapering dose of propranolol for 2 weeks (together with the COX-2 inhibitor) followed by a maintenance program of dietary management and repurposed drugs as based on the recommendations presented in this monograph. The clinician may elect to include propranolol, vitamin D and a COX-2 inhibitor in the maintenance regimen.

Table 5. Summary of the anti-cancer pathways of the repurposed drugs and nutraceuticals

	↑ Apoptosis	↑ autophagy	↓ cell proliferation	Cell cycle arrest	↑ Immune	↓ TME	Antiinflamm.	↓ Stem Cells	↓angiogenesis	↓ glucose	↓ glutamine
Vitamin D	+	+	+	+	+	+	+	+	+	-	-
Propranolol	+	+	+	+	+	+	+	+	+	+	-
Melatonin	+	+	+	+	+	+	+	+	+	+	-
Green Tea	+	+	+	-	+	+	+	+	+	+	+
Metformin	+	+	+	+	+	+	+	+	+	+	-
Curcumin	+	+	+	+	+	+	+	+	+	+	+
Ivermectin	+	+	+	+	+	+	+	+	+	+	-
Mebendazole	+	+	+	+	+	+	+	+	+	+	+
Omega-3 FA	+	+	+	+	+	+	+	+	+	+	-
Berberine	+	+	+	+	+	+	+	+	+	+	+
Atorvastatin	+	+	+	+	+	+	+	+	+	-	-
Disulfiram	+	+	+	+	+	+	+	+	+	+	-
Cimetidine	+	+	+	+	+	+	+	+	+	-	+
Mistletoe	+	+	+	+	+	+	+	+	+	+	-
Sildenafil	+	+	+	+	+	+	+	+	+	+	-
Itraconazole	+	+	+	+	+	+	+	+	+	+	-
LDN	+	+	+	+	+	+	+	+	+	-	-
Doxycycline	+	+	+	+	+	+	+	+	+	+	-
Spironolactone	+	+	+	+	+	+	+	+	+	-	-
wheatgrass	+	+	+	+	+	+	+	+	+	+	-
Resveratrol	+	+	+	+	+	+	+	+	+	+	+
COX inhibitor	+	+	+	+	+	+	+	+	+	+	-
Nigella sativa	+	+	+	+	+	+	+	+	+	+	+
Reishi	+	+	+	+	+	+	+	+	+	+	-

CHAPTER 7: TIER ONE REPURPOSED DRUGS – STRONG RECOMMENDATION

1. Vitamin D

Vitamin D is synthesized in human skin after the photoisomerization of 7-dehydrocholesterol to pre-vitamin D3 under the influence of UV B radiation (wavelength, 280-315 nm). (531) The major factors influencing this process are either environmental (latitude, season, time of day, ozone and clouds, reflectivity of the surface) or personal (skin type, age, clothing, use of sunscreen, genetics). (532) From the skin, parental vitamin D3 (*cholecalciferol*) finds its way into the general circulation, and it is then metabolized in the liver to 25-hydroxyvitamin D3 [25(OH)D3] (*calcifediol*). 25(OH)D3 is an immediate precursor metabolite to the active form of vitamin D3, 1,25-dihydroxyvitamin D3 [1,25(OH)2D3] (*calcitriol*), that is the product of the mitochondrial CYP27B1-hydroxylase confined primarily but not entirely to the proximal tubular epithelial cell of the kidney. (532, 533)

As vitamin D has a much shorter half-life than 25(OH)D3 (1-2 days versus 2-3 weeks), 25(OH)D3 is considered the best indicator of vitamin D status; hence 25(OH)D3 is the most widely used test indicating vitamin D status. (532, 533) A vitamin D level > 30 ng/ml is widely considered "normal" while a level between 20-30 ng/l is considered vitamin D insufficient and a level <20 ng/ml is considered vitamin D deficient. (532-534) However, more recent data suggests that a level > 50 ng/ml is desirable, and ideally targeting a level between 55- 90 ng/ml is preferable.(531, 535-537)

It may take many months or even years to achieve optimal levels in patients with low vitamin D levels (< 20 ng/ml) taking the standard recommended dose of 5,000 IU/day. It is therefore important that the optimal regimen for vitamin D supplementation be followed to achieve adequate circulating levels (see Table 6). (536, 537) Since the highest dose of commercially available vitamin D3 is 50,000 IU capsules, and due to its affordability (low cost) and better gastrointestinal absorption, we recommend using 50,000 IU D3 capsules for community setups.(531, 536, 537) Together, a number of these capsules can be taken as a bolus dose [i.e., single upfront doses such as 100,000 to 400,000 IU]. However, the liver has a limited 25-hydroxylase capacity to convert vitamin D to 25(OH)D: thus, taking 50,000 IU capsules over a few days provides better bioavailability. (531, 536, 537)

Vitamin D2 is manufactured through the ultraviolet irradiation of ergosterol from yeast, while vitamin D3 is synthesized trough the ultraviolet irradiation of 7-dehydrocholesterol from lanolin; both are used in over-the-counter vitamin D supplements. (532) Vitamin D2 has 30% of the biological activity of vitamin D3. It is best to include both Vitamin K2 (Menaquinone [MK7] 100 mcg/day, or 800 mcg/week) and magnesium (250-500 mg/day) when doses of vitamin D > 8 000 IU/day are taken. (538, 539) It should be noted that vitamin K2 itself has anticancer properties and an inverse relationship exists between vitamin K2 (and not K1) intake and cancer mortality. (540-543)

Table 6. Guidance on Upfront Loading Dose Regimens to Replenish Vitamin D Stores in the Body

When serum vitamin D levels are available, the doses provided in this table can be used for the longer-term maintenance of serum 25(OH)D concentration above 50 ng/mL (125 nmol/L). The table provides the initial bolus dose, weekly dose, frequency, and duration of administration of oral vitamin D in non-emergency situations, in a non-obese, 70 kg adult.

Serum Vitamin D (ng/mL) **	Vitamin D Dose: Using 50,000 IU Capsules: Initial and Weekly $		Duration (Number of Weeks)	Total Amount Needed to Correct Vit. D, Deficiency (IU, in Millions) #
	Initial Bolus Dose (IU)	Follow-Up: $$ The Number of 50,000 IU Caps/Week		
<10	300,000	×3	8 to 10	1.5 to 1.8
11–15	200,000	×2	8 to 10	1.0 to 1.2
16–20	200,000	×2	6 to 8	0.8 to 1.0
21–30	100,000	× 2	4 to 6	0.5 to 0.7
31–40	100,000	×2	2 to 4	0.3 to 0.5
41–50	100,000	×1	2 to 4	0.2 to 0.3

(Source Nutrients – Special Issue: "Vitamin D – Calciferol and COVID" (536) Reproduced with permission from the author.

More than half of human tissues express the gene for the vitamin D receptor, with vitamin D having pleiotropic functions in pathways of energy metabolism, immunity, and cellular growth and differentiation that clearly extend the control of calcium homeostasis. (544) The biologically active form of vitamin D, 1,25(OH)D3, regulates over 1200 genes within the human genome. (531) The most important extra-skeletal function of vitamin D is its role in the modulation of the immune system. Vitamin D receptors are present on immune cells, with this vitamin playing a critical role in both innate and adaptive host immunity. (545, 546)

Vitamin D has anticancer effects both directly *via* controlling the differentiation, proliferation, and apoptosis of neoplastic cells as well as indirectly through regulating immune cells that affect the microenvironment of malignant tumors. Evidence from observational and randomized controlled studies indicates that low vitamin D status is associated with higher mortality from life-threatening conditions such as cancer and cardiovascular disease. (547, 548) In a real-world analysis of 445,601 participants, aged 40–73 years, from the UK Biobank cohort, both vitamin D deficiency and insufficiency were strongly associated with all-cause mortality.(549) A Cochrane analysis demonstrated that supplementation with vitamin D3 (cholecalciferol) decreased all-cause mortality (RR 0.94, 95% CI 0.91 to 0.98, p = 0.002); however, supplementation with vitamin D2, calcifediol, and calcitriol did not affect mortality. (550)

Vitamin D deficiency has been demonstrated to increase the risk of breast cancer while supplemental vitamin D intake had an inverse relationship with this outcome. (551) Both prospective and retrospective epidemiologic studies indicate that levels of 25-hydroxyvitamin D below 20 ng per milliliter are associated with a 30 to 50% increased risk of incident colon, prostate, and breast cancer, along with higher mortality from these cancers. (532) People living at higher latitudes are at increased risk for vitamin D deficiency and are reported to have an increased risk of Hodgkin's lymphoma as well as colon, pancreatic, prostate, ovarian, breast, and other cancers and are more likely to die from these cancers, as compared with people living at lower latitudes. (335, 532) Vitamin D supplementation likely plays an important role in the prevention of cancer, as highlighted in the prospective study by Bischoff-Ferrari et al (see section on Primary Cancer Prevention). (231, 232) Furthermore, in a meta-analysis of 50 trials with a total of 74,655 participants, Zhang et al reported that Vitamin D supplementation significantly reduced the risk of cancer death (0.85,0.74 to 0.97, 0%). (552) In subgroup analyses, all-cause mortality was significantly lower in trials with vitamin D3 supplementation than in trials with vitamin D2 supplementation. An analysis of 25(OH)D-cancer incidence rates suggests that achieving a vitamin D level of 80 ng/mL vs. 10 ng/mL would reduce cancer incidence rates by 70 ± 10%. (335)

The VITamin D and OmegA-3 TriaL (VITAL) was a nationwide, randomized, placebo-controlled, 2X2 factorial trial of vitamin D3 (cholecalciferol, 2000 IU/day) and marine omega-3 fatty acids (1 g/day) for the prevention of cancer and cardiovascular disease. (553) The primary endpoints of this study were total invasive cancer and major cardiovascular events. While the hazard ratios for cancer deaths comparing vitamin D to placebo were HR 0.83 (0.67–1.02) none of the primary or secondary endpoints reached statistical significance. It should be recognized that in this study both the dose of vitamin D and omega 3 fatty acids were absurdly low; and it is likely that this study was designed to fail. Nevertheless, the results of the VITAL study differ significantly from the DO-HEALTH trial which used similarly low doses of vitamin D and omega-3 fatty acids. (231, 232) In this study the HR for the prevention of cancer with vitamin D3 and omega 3 fatty acids compared to placebo was 0.53 (0.28-1.0).

Anticancer pathways and mechanisms

Experimental evidence indicates that vitamin D has diverse antineoplastic activity (see Figure 8). Binding of vitamin D to its target, the vitamin D receptor, leads to transcriptional activation and repression of target genes and results in induction of differentiation and apoptosis, inhibition of cancer stem cells, and decreased proliferation, angiogenesis, and metastatic potential. (554) Vitamin D induces apoptosis of cancer cells, (555) counteracts aberrant WNT-β catenin signaling, (556) and has broad anti-inflammatory effects via downregulation of nuclear factor-Kβ and inhibition of cyclooxygenase expression. (557) In colon, prostate, and breast carcinoma cells, 1,25-(OH)2D3 upregulates several pro-apoptotic proteins (BAX, BAK, BAG, BAD, G0S2) and suppresses survival and anti-apoptotic proteins (thymidylate synthase, survivin, BCL-2, BCL-XL). (558) In this way, it favors the release of cytochrome C from mitochondria and the activation of caspases 3 and 9 that lead to apoptosis. 1,25-(OH)2D3 and metformin have additive/synergistic antiproliferative and proapoptotic effects in colon carcinoma and other types of cells. (559)

In many cancer cell types, 1,25-(OH)2 D3 directly arrests the cell cycle in the G0/G1 phase by downregulating cyclin-dependent kinases and repressing genes that encode cyclins D1 and C. (560) 1,25-(OH)2D3 decreases the expression of epidermal growth factor receptor (EGFR) and interferes with the insulin-like growth factor (IGF)-I/II pathway. (335) Vitamin D has activity against human breast cancer cell lines by targeting Ras/MEK/ERK pathway. (558) In addition, 1,25-(OH)2D3 diminishes the proliferation of breast cancer cells by inhibiting estrogen synthesis and signaling through estrogen receptor (ER)α. (561) In colon carcinoma cells, 1,25-(OH)2 D3 upregulates an array of intercellular adhesion molecules that are constituents of adherens junctions and tight junctions, including E-cadherin, occludin, claudin-2 and -12, and ZO-1 and -2. (562) The Wnt/β-catenin pathway plays an important role in cancer. Antagonism of the Wnt/β-catenin pathway by 1,25-(OH)2 D3 was reported in colon carcinoma cells by a double mechanism: (a) liganded VDR binds nuclear β-catenin, which hampers the formation of transcriptionally active β-catenin/TCF complexes, and (b) induction E-cadherin expression that attracts newly synthesized β-catenin protein to the plasma membrane adherens junctions. In that way, it decreases β-catenin nuclear accumulation. (563)

1,25-(OH)2 D3 is an important modulator of the immune system, as reflected by the expression of vitamin D receptors by almost all types of immune cells. 1,25-(OH)2D 3 is an enhancer of innate immune reactions against tumor cells by activating macrophages, natural killer (NK) cells, and neutrophils. (335) An important mechanism of 1,25-(OH)2D3 is the inhibition of the NF-KB pathway. In turn, this causes the downregulation of multiple cytokines and their effects. 1,25(OH)2 D3 reduces the protumorigenic effect of PG E2 in prostate cancer cells by inhibiting COX-2 and so decreasing the levels of PG E2 and two PG receptors (EP2 and FP). (564)

Autophagy is a process of elimination of cytoplasmic waste materials and dysfunctional organelles that serves as a cytoprotective mechanism but that, when excessive, leads to cell death. (335) In cancer, VDR ligands trigger autophagic death by inducing crucial genes in several cancer cell types. Thus, 1,25-(OH)2 D3 de-represses the key autophagic MAP1LC3B (LC3B) gene and activates 50-AMP-activated protein kinase (AMPK). In Kaposi's sarcoma cells and myeloid leukemia cells, vitamin D compounds inhibit PI3K/AKT/mTOR signaling and activate Beclin-1-dependent autophagy. 1,25-(OH)2D3 has a pro-differentiation effect on several types of carcinoma cells either by direct upregulation of epithelial genes and/or the repression of key epithelial mesenchymal transcription factors (EMT-TFs). (565)

In diverse types of carcinoma cells (colon, prostate, and breast), the antiangiogenic action of 1,25-(OH)2 D3 relies to a great extent on its ability to inhibit two major angiogenesis promoters: it suppresses the expression and activity of hypoxia-inducible factor (HIF)-1α, a key transcription factor in hypoxia-induced angiogenesis, and of vascular endothelial growth factor (VEGF). (335) 1,25-(OH)2D3 also has inhibitory effects on tumor-derived endothelial cells. It reduces their proliferation and sprouting in vitro and diminishes the blood vessel density in cancer models. (566)

Clinical studies
Data suggest that the majority of patients with cancer are vitamin D deficient (level < 20 ng/ml).(548, 554, 567, 568) Several prospective observational studies have shown that higher levels of plasma 25-hydroxyvitamin D were associated with improved survival among patients with colorectal cancer. (567, 569-571) Similarly, elevated 25-OH D levels were associated with better overall survival in patients with breast and gastric cancer and lymphoma. (572) In a population-based study of patients with cancer of the breast, colon, lung, and lymphoma a 25-OHD level below 18 ng/ml at diagnosis experienced shorter survival. (573) In a meta-analysis of 19 studies Robsahm et al reported an inverse relationship between 25-Hydroxyvitamin D and cancer survival. (574)

Chen performed a meta-analysis of observational cohort studies and randomized trials which assessed the role of post-diagnosis vitamin D supplement intake on survival among cancer patients. (575) The meta-analysis included 11 publications consisting of 5 RCTs and 6 observational cohort studies. The summary relative risk (SRR) for overall survival of vitamin D supplement use vs. non-use, pooling cohort studies and randomized trials, was 0.87 (95% CI, 0.78–0.98; p = 0.02). Vaughan-Shaw et al performed a meta-analysis of 7 studies evaluating the use of supplemental vitamin D in patients with colorectal cancer. (576) The study reported a 30% reduction in adverse outcomes and a beneficial effect on progression-free survival (HR = 0.65; 95% CI: 0.36–0.94). In a meta-analysis by Kuznia et al, subgroup analysis revealed that vitamin D3 administered daily, in contrast to bolus supplementation, reduced cancer mortality by 12 %. (577) It should be recognized that a daily dose of between 800 IU and 4000 IU was administered in the studies included in this meta-analysis and that vitamin D levels were not monitored. A more dramatic reduction in mortality would likely be realized if patients were dosed more appropriately.

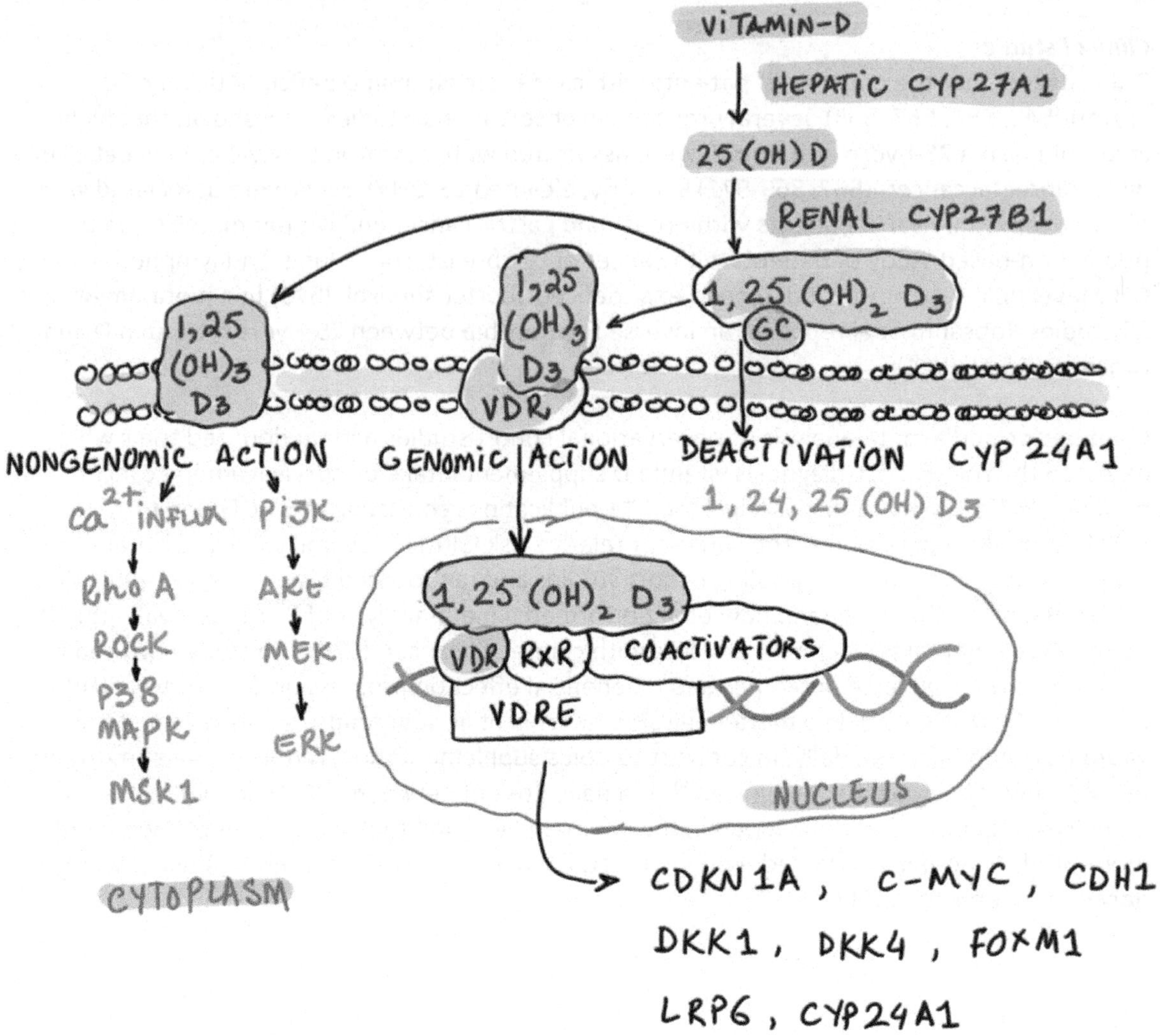

Figure 8. Overview of metabolic pathways of Vitamin D. (Source: Dr. Mobeen Syed}

Footnote for Figure 9: CYP27A1: Cytochrome P450 family 27 subfamily A member 1, CYP27B1: Cytochrome P450 family 27 subfamily B member 1, 25(OH)D: 25-hydroxyvitamin D, 1,25(OH)2 D3: 1,25-dihydroxyvitamin D3, GC: Vitamin D-binding protein (Gc protein), VDR: Vitamin D receptor, RXR: Retinoid X receptor, VDRE: Vitamin D response element, CDKN1A: Cyclin-dependent kinase inhibitor 1A, C-MYC: Cellular Myelocytomatosis oncogene, CDH1: Cadherin-1, DKK1: Dickkopf-1, DKK4: Dickkopf-4, FOXM1: Forkhead box protein M1, LRP6: Low-density lipoprotein receptor-related protein 6, PI3K: Phosphatidylinositol 3-kinase, Akt: Protein kinase B, MEK: Mitogen-activated protein kinase kinase, ERK: Extracellular signal-regulated kinase, Rho A: Ras homolog gene family member A, ROCK: Rho-associated protein kinase, P38: p38 mitogen-activated protein kinase, MAPK: Mitogen-activated protein kinase, MSK1: Mitogen- and stress-activated protein kinase 1

SUNSHINE was a double-blind, multicenter, randomized clinical trial designed to evaluate the efficacy of "high dose" vitamin D3 compared with standard-dose vitamin D3 given in combination with standard chemotherapy in patients with metastatic colorectal cancer. (554) The high-dose group received a loading dose of 8,000 IU per day of vitamin D3 (two 4,000 IU capsules) for cycle 1 followed by 4,000 IU/d for subsequent cycles. The standard dose group received 400 IU/d of vitamin D3 during all cycles. In this underpowered (n=139) RCT, multivariable HR for progression-free survival or death was 0.64 (95% CI, 0-0.90; p = .02) in favor of the high dose group. Comparison of progression-free survival between the high-dose and standard-dose vitamin D3 groups using a log-rank test stratified by ECOG performance status was statistically significant (p = .03). At baseline, median plasma 25-hydroxyvitamin D levels were deficient in both the high-dose vitamin D3 group (16.1 ng/mL [IQR, 10.1 to 23.0 ng/mL]) and in the standard-dose vitamin D3 group (18.7 ng/mL [IQR, 13.5 to 22.7 ng/mL]). Only 9% of the total study population had sufficient levels (≥30 ng/mL) of 25-hydroxyvitamin D at baseline. At treatment discontinuation, patients in the high-dose vitamin D3 group had a median 25-hydroxyvitamin D level of 34.8 ng/mL (IQR, 24.9-44.7 ng/mL), whereas those in the standard-dose vitamin D3 group were still deficient in vitamin D and had a median 25-hydroxyvitamin D level of 18.7 ng/mL(IQR, 13.9-23.0ng/mL) (difference, 16.2 ng/mL [95% CI, 9.9-22.4 ng/mL]; *P* < .001). It is important to note that based on these levels the "high dose" group was profoundly underdosed. As indicated above, vitamin D dosing should be based on a serum level aiming for a level of > 50 ng/ml (target 55-90 ng/ml). Based on the data from this study we would suggest a daily dose of vitamin D3 of 20,000 to 50,000 IU/day until a vitamin D level is obtained. It is possible that patients with cancer may require an even higher level, approximating 150 ug/dl.

Wang et al demonstrated that postoperative vitamin D supplementation in esophageal cancer patients undergoing esophagectomy was associated with improved quality of life and with improved disease-free survival. (578) Similarly, vitamin D use post-diagnosis was found to be associated with a reduction in breast cancer-specific mortality. (579) Two recent clinical trials in prostate cancer patients suggest that vitamin D supplementation may prevent prostate cancer progression. (580, 581) Vitamin D has additive or synergistic effects when combined with conventional chemotherapy. (559) Zeichner et al demonstrated that use of vitamin D during neoadjuvant chemotherapy in HER2-positive nonmetastatic breast cancer was associated with improved disease-free survival (HR, 0.36; 95% CI, 0.15-0.88; p=0.026). (582)

Types of cancers that Vitamin D may be beneficial for

Vitamin D supplementation is likely beneficial in most cancers, but particularly in patients with breast, colorectal, gastric, esophagus, lung, and prostate cancer as well as those with lymphomas and melanoma.

Dosing and cautions

As almost all patients with cancer are severely vitamin D deficient. A high loading dose of Vitamin D is suggested followed by dose titration according to vitamin D blood levels, aiming for a level of > 50 ng/ml (target 55-90 ng/ml). However current data suggest that levels up to 150 ng/mL are necessary for certain types of cancer to stop growth and metastasis. Vitamin D intoxication is observed when serum levels of 25-hydroxyvitamin D are greater than 150 ng per milliliter (374 nmol per liter). (532) Hypercalcemia will usually not occur until levels exceed over 250 ng/ml. We, therefore, suggest a daily dose of 20,000 to 50,000 IU/day until a vitamin D level is obtained. With the suggested doses, serum 25(OH)D concentrations rise above 100 ng/mL within a week or two, but unless a suitable higher maintenance dose is used (~ 10,000 IU/day), the level will start to drop to baseline after three weeks or so, and the benefit of vitamin D will be lost. If measuring vitamin D levels is not feasible/possible, we would suggest a loading dose of 100,000 IU followed by 10,000 IU/day. Doses of 10,000 IU of vitamin D3 per day for up to 5 months were reported to be safe and without toxicity. (532, 535) It should be noted that dosages of vitamin D up to 80,000 IU/day have been reported to be safe. (583, 584) We recommended vitamin D3 over D2 as vitamin D2 is approximately 30% as effective as vitamin D3 in maintaining serum 25-hydroxyvitamin D levels. (532) Furthermore, vitamin D3 should be dosed daily rather than large intermittent bolus dosing. It is best to include both Vitamin K2 (Menaquinone [MK4/MK7] 100 mcg/day, or 800 mcg/week) and magnesium (250-500 mg/day) when doses of vitamin D > 8 000 IU/day are taken. (538, 539) Patients taking coumadin need to be closely monitored and the need to consult with their PCP before taking vitamin K2. Further, we suggest measuring PTH (parathyroid) levels and calcium levels and titrating the dose of Vitamin D according to the PTH levels as follows (Coimbra Protocol): (585, 586) i) if the PTH level is below the lower end of the reference range, reduce the dose of Vitamin D ii) if the PTH level is at (or close too) the lower end of the reference range, maintain dose, iii) if PTH is within the reference range but not near to the low end of the reference range increase the dose of Vitamin D.

2. Propranolol

This chapter is based in part on the chapter on propranolol from the book by Jeffrey Dach, MD entitled *Cracking Cancer Toolkit*.(146) Chronic stress activates the sympathetic nervous system, which secretes catecholamines which feed cancer growth.(587, 588) Accumulating data indicate that the psychological stress caused by chronic stressors is a major risk factor for cancer occurrence, growth and metastasis.(587, 588) "*Experimental analyses with in vivo animal models have now shown that behavioral stress can accelerate the progression of breast, prostate, and ovarian carcinomas, neuroblastomas, malignant melanomas, pancreatic carcinoma and some hemopoietic cancers such as leukemia. In many of these experimental models, the biological effects of stress could be efficiently blocked by beta-adrenergic antagonists and mimicked by pharmacologic beta agonists.*"(589) In a mouse ovarian cancer model chronic stress promoted cancer progression.(590) Similarly chronic stress enhanced metastatic spread in a mouse model of Lewis lung cancer. (591) Partecke et al demonstrated that chronic stress increases experimental pancreatic cancer growth, reduces survival and could be antagonized by beta-adrenergic receptor blockade.(592)

Anticancer pathways and mechanisms

Propranolol is a commonly used non-selective, beta-adrenergic receptor antagonist used in the treatment of hypertension, angina, anxiety, cardiac arrhythmia, hyperthyroidism, essential tremor and as a prophylaxis against migraine, variceal bleeding and myocardial infarction. First developed in the 1960s, the drug is now available globally in generic form and is on the WHO List of Essential Medicines.(593)

Propranolol is a well-known and widely used beta-blocker with a range of actions which are of interest in an oncological context. Propranolol displays effects on cellular proliferation and invasion, on the immune system, on the angiogenic cascade, and on tumour cell sensitivity to existing treatments. Both pre-clinical and clinical evidence of these effects exist, in multiple cancer types. (593)

Propranolol blocks activation of the sympathetic nervous system. In a murine model of acute lymphoblastic leukemia (ALL) Lamkin et al found that chronic stress enhanced tumour growth and dissemination and that the effect could be inhibited by propranolol.(594) In a mouse model, Sloan et al reported that stress induced beta-adrenergic signaling increased macrophage infiltration into the tumor (M2 polarization), induced pro-metastatic gene expression and induced a 30-fold increase in distant metastatic lesions. (595) In this study, pharmacologic activation of β-adrenergic signaling induced similar effects, and treatment of stressed animals with the β-antagonist propranolol reversed the stress-induced macrophage infiltration and inhibited tumor spread to distant tissues.

Beta-adrenergic receptors are overexpressed in many cancers, playing a key role in invasion and metastatic behavior.(596) In addition, beta-adrenergic signaling plays a role in the tumor micro-environment, inducing immunosuppression, and enhancing tumor evasion by impairing host anti-tumor immunity. (597) Infiltration by nerve fibers is a feature of the tumor microenvironment that is associated with aggressiveness and involves nerve growth factor (NGF) production by cancer cells.(598) Catecholamines expressed in the tumor microenvironment greatly potentiate the pro-inflammatory milieu. Adrenergic signalling impairs anti-tumor CD8+ T cell responses which is reversed by propranolol.(597) Propranolol down-regulates hexokinase 2 and inhibits glucose metabolism.(599, 600) In a late stage breast cancer patient treated with neoadjuvant propranolol, propranolol decreased the expression of the pro-proliferative and pro-survival markers, while increasing pro-apoptotic p53 expression.(600) In addition, propranolol has pro-apoptotic activity in cancer cells lines independent of p53 status.(601)

Neuroblastoma is a pediatric tumor of the sympathetic nervous system, which is often associated with elevated catecholamines. Wolter et al demonstrated that propranolol inhibited growth of a panel of fifteen neuroblastoma cell lines and treatment induced apoptosis and decreased proliferation. Activity was dependent on inhibition of the β2, and not β1, adrenergic receptor, and treatment resulted in activation of p53 and p73 signaling in vitro.(601) Furthermore, β-blockers increase the response to chemotherapy via direct antitumor and anti-angiogenic mechanisms in neuroblastoma. (602)

The most important function of propranolol acting via multiple mechanisms is to reduce metastatic spread. (603) Propranolol has been shown to inhibit the expression of the tissue remodelling factor matrix metalloproteinase-2 (MMP-2), MMP-9 and the pro-angiogenic vascular endothelial growth factor (VEGF) (604-606) The anti-angiogenic effect of propranolol, via down-regulation of

VEGF has also been shown in a range of cancer cell lines including nasopharyngeal carcinoma, melanoma, pancreatic cancer, leukemia, head and neck squamous cell carcinoma and infantile hemangiomas. (593) Guo et al observed that norepinephrine promoted the invasiveness of a pancreatic cell line in a concentration dependent manner and that norepinephrine increased the expression of MMP-2, MMP-9, and VEGF.(606) In this model these effects were inhibited by propranolol. Xia et al demonstrated that catecholamines contribute to the neovascularization of lung cancer via tumor-associated macrophages.(607) Park *et al* showed that hypoxia-inducible factor 1α (HIF-1α) expression is upregulated by norepinephrine and abrogated by propranolol. (608, 609)

Propranolol reduces migratory activity of breast cancer cells. In a breast cancer model the combination of metformin and propranolol reduced cancer progression, metastases, and reduced migratory and invasive behavior of cancer cells.(610) In this study the metabolic pathway of the cancer cell was skewed away from mitochondrial oxidative phosphorylation and towards glycolysis. In an experimental model, Brohee et al demonstrated that propranolol sensitizes prostate cancer cells to glucose metabolism inhibition and prevents cancer progression.(611)

In a number of cancer cell lines propranolol exerts synergistic anti-tumor activity when combined with conventional chemotherapy. (593, 602) Pasquier et al demonstrated that propranolol potentiates the anti-angiogenic effects and anti-tumor efficacy of chemotherapy agents.(612)

Clinical studies

Chang et al reviewed the use of propranolol in a database of 24,238 patients over a 12-year follow-up period. (613) These authors reported that propranolol treatment significantly lowered the risk of cancers of the head and neck (HRL 0.58), esophagus (HR:0.35), stomach (HR: 0.54) colon (HR 0.68) and prostate cancer (HR:0.52).

In an observational study of 800 women who underwent removal of a triple-negative breast cancer, the hazard ratio for women on beta-blockers was 0.32 for metastases and 0.42 for death from breast cancer, compared to controls not on beta-blockers.(614) Melhem-Bertrandt reported relapse-free survival in a cohort of women using beta-blockers (HR=0.32). (615) In a meta-analysis of 4 studies the risk of death from breast cancer was reduced by half with the use of beta-blockers (HR 0.5; 95% CI 0.32-0.8). (616) In a meta-analysis of 13 studies evaluating the use of beta-blockers in early stage breast cancer, the use of beta-blockers was associated with a significant improvement in the recurrence free survival (RFS) in the overall population (HR 0.73; 95% CI, 0.56-0.96; P = 0.025) and in patients with triple-negative disease (HR 0.53; 95% CI, 0.35-0.81; P = 0.003).(617)

Data from a National Cancer Registry demonstrated that the cumulative probability of breast cancer-specific mortality was significantly lower for propranolol users compared with matched nonusers (hazard ratio, 0.19; 95% CI, 0.06 to 0.60). (452) A long term epidemiological study of breast cancer patients demonstrated that those patients receiving propranolol had a 57% reduction in distant metastases and a 71% reduced risk of dying from breast cancer compared to control patients.(618) In a 10 year follow up study of patients with breast cancer, patients treated with beta-blockers showed a significant reduction in metastasis development (p=0.026), tumour recurrence (p=0.001), and longer disease free interval (p=0.01).(618)

In patients with ovarian cancer users of non-selective beta blockers had more than double the overall survival time when compared to non-users (90 months vs. 38.2 months, p<0,001).(619) In a retrospective evaluation of 1971 patients with multiple myeloma, the intake of beta-blockers was associated with a reduced risk of disease-specific death (0.53, 95% CI 0.42-0.67 in comparison to non-BB).(620) Multivariable analysis showed the same pattern for overall survival. In a non-randomized prospective study in patients with melanoma, the use of propranolol (80 mg daily) at the time of diagnosis was significantly inversely associated with recurrence of melanoma (80% risk reduction; hazard ratio, 0.18; 95% CI, 0.04-0.89; P = .03).(621)

Types of cancers propranolol may be beneficial for
It is likely that propranolol is effective against a broad range of cancers but may have particular activity against the following tumors: neuroblastoma, breast, melanoma, angiosarcoma, lung cancer, multiple myeloma, cervical cancer, hepatocellular carcinoma, ovarian cancer, prostate cancer, pancreatic cancer and brain sarcoma.(146, 593) In light of the positive clinical experience of propranolol in the treatment of infantile hemangioma, most recently confirmed in a large multi-center randomized controlled trial, (622) and evidence of beta-adrenergic receptor expression in a range of vascular tumors including angiosarcomas propranolol is indicated in the management of these tumors.(623)

Dosing and cautions
The anti-hypertensive dose of propranolol is in the range 160 – 240 mg/day, starting at 80 mg and increasing as required to a maintenance dose that is generally 160 mg – 240 mg.(593) In patients with cancer we suggest a starting dose of 40 mg twice a day increased to 80 mg twice daily as tolerated. Propranolol should be avoided in patients with severe asthma, uncontrolled heart failure, and those with symptomatic bradycardia. Sudden termination of treatment is not advised,

3. Melatonin

Melatonin, N-acetyl-5-methoxytryptamine, is a small lipophilic molecule that is secreted by the pineal gland and its synthesis shows a circadian pattern. Melatonin is mainly produced by the pineal gland in response to darkness. (624) At night, melatonin levels increase, then start to decrease in the early morning and throughout the day. Elevated levels of melatonin at night stimulate target organs to enter into suitable homeostatic metabolic rhythms, which help protect the body from developing different diseases. (245)

Exposing the body to light at night may result in disruption of melatonin production and the circadian rhythm. Peak melatonin levels in the blood vary between individuals and depend on age, with levels decreasing rapidly after age 40. (625)

Melatonin has specific receptors to regulate many physiological functions namely MT1 and MT2; both are members of the seven transmembrane G-protein coupled receptor family. (626) Melatonin receptors are found throughout the body, which explains its multiple biological functions. (624) In addition, mitochondria of all cells produce melatonin in an autocrine fashion under the influence of near-infrared irradiation. (627, 628) Melatonin has numerous biological properties acting both directly and indirectly as a potent antioxidant. (624) Melatonin plays a critical role in normal mitochondrial function, being a strong inducer of oxidative phosphorylation.

Anticancer pathways and mechanisms

Low melatonin levels have been implicated in the etiology of cancer. Several studies have shown reduced levels of melatonin in patients with certain types of cancers, compared with normal, healthy people of the same age. (625) Disruption of nocturnal melatonin secretion in night shift workers has been associated with a modestly increased risk for breast and other cancer types. A meta-analysis of 26 observational studies found significantly increased breast cancer incidence among female airline cabin crew. (629) The International Agency for Research on Cancer reclassified "shiftwork that involves circadian disruption" from a possible to a probable human carcinogen, in recognition of this relationship. (630)

In experimental models, melatonin has demonstrated a broad spectrum of anticancer activity with multiple underlying mechanisms being proposed (see Figure 9). (222, 245) Melatonin exerts cytotoxic, anti-mitotic, and pro-apoptotic actions in breast cancer cells. The antiproliferative activity of melatonin has been demonstrated in both ER-positive and ER-negative human breast cancer cell lines. In most of these reports, melatonin acted via the MT1 membrane receptor. In addition, melatonin activates cancer cell apoptosis; this may be mediated by PUMA up-regulation. Melatonin increases the expression of pro-apoptotic mediators such as BAX/BAK, Apaf-1, caspases, and p53. (631) Melatonin has been demonstrated to inhibit the proliferation of cancer stem cells and to reduce the expression of Ki67 and matrix metalloproteinase 9. (632) Melatonin can cause cancer cells to switch from anaerobic glycolysis to conventional oxidative phosphorylation via the Krebs cycle. This slows down the proliferative activity of cancer cells, reduces their metastatic potential, and directs the cells to undergo apoptosis. Melatonin stimulates the synthesis of acetyl-CoA from pyruvate by inhibiting the mitochondrial enzyme pyruvate dehydrogenase kinase. (633) A study demonstrated that melatonin altered Ewing sarcoma metabolic profile by inhibiting the Warburg effect. (634) In prostate cancer cells, melatonin was able to reduce glucose metabolism via the downregulation of glycolysis and the pentose phosphate pathway. (635) The antiestrogenic action of melatonin could also enhance the ability of this hormone to limit the proliferation of hormone-sensitive breast cancer. (222)

Anti-angiogenesis is one of the major mechanisms by which melatonin exerts its anticancer effects. Melatonin inhibits hypoxia-induced factor 1-α thereby preventing vascular endothelial growth factor (VEGF) expression. Melatonin also inhibits endothelial cell migration, endothelial cell invasion, and endothelial cell tube formation. It also prevents cancer cell migration via alteration of PI3K and MAPK signaling pathways in both receptor-dependent and independent manner. (632) Melatonin has been demonstrated to stimulate T cell and natural killer (NK) production and reduce regulatory T cells (Tregs). (636, 637)

Melatonin may benefit cancer patients who are also receiving chemotherapy, radiotherapy, supportive therapy, or palliative therapy by improving survival and ameliorating the side effects of chemotherapy.

Clinical studies

In addition to case studies, (638, 639) the clinical benefit of melatonin in patients with cancer is supported by the highest level of evidence, namely meta-analyses of RCTs. (640, 641) Seely et al systematically reviewed the effects of melatonin in conjunction with chemotherapy, radiotherapy, supportive care, and palliative care on 1-year survival, complete response, partial response, stable disease, and chemotherapy-associated toxicities. (641) This analysis included 21 randomized studies all of which studied solid tumors. The pooled relative risk (RR) for 1-year mortality was 0.63 (95% CI = 0.53-0.74; $P < 0.001$). Improved effects were found for complete response, partial response, and stable disease. In trials combining melatonin with chemotherapy, adjuvant melatonin decreased 1-year mortality (RR = 0.60; 95% CI = 0.54-0.67).

Types of cancers that melatonin may be beneficial for

Melatonin may be active in several cancers including cancers of the breast, ovary, pancreas, liver, kidney, mouth, stomach, colon/rectum, brain, lung, prostate, head and neck, and various leukemias and sarcomas. (222, 245)

Dosing and cautions

Providers should advise patients to begin with 1 mg at night; a slow-release/extended-release preparation is suggested to minimize REM sleep-induced nightmares (best taken an hour before retiring). The dose should be increased up to 20-30 mg, as tolerated. Melatonin is probably the safest medical compound available, with a LD50 of infinity (it is impossible to kill an animal with industrial doses of melatonin). The only side effects reported are early morning drowsiness and "bad dreams" (when the dose is increased too rapidly). (624)

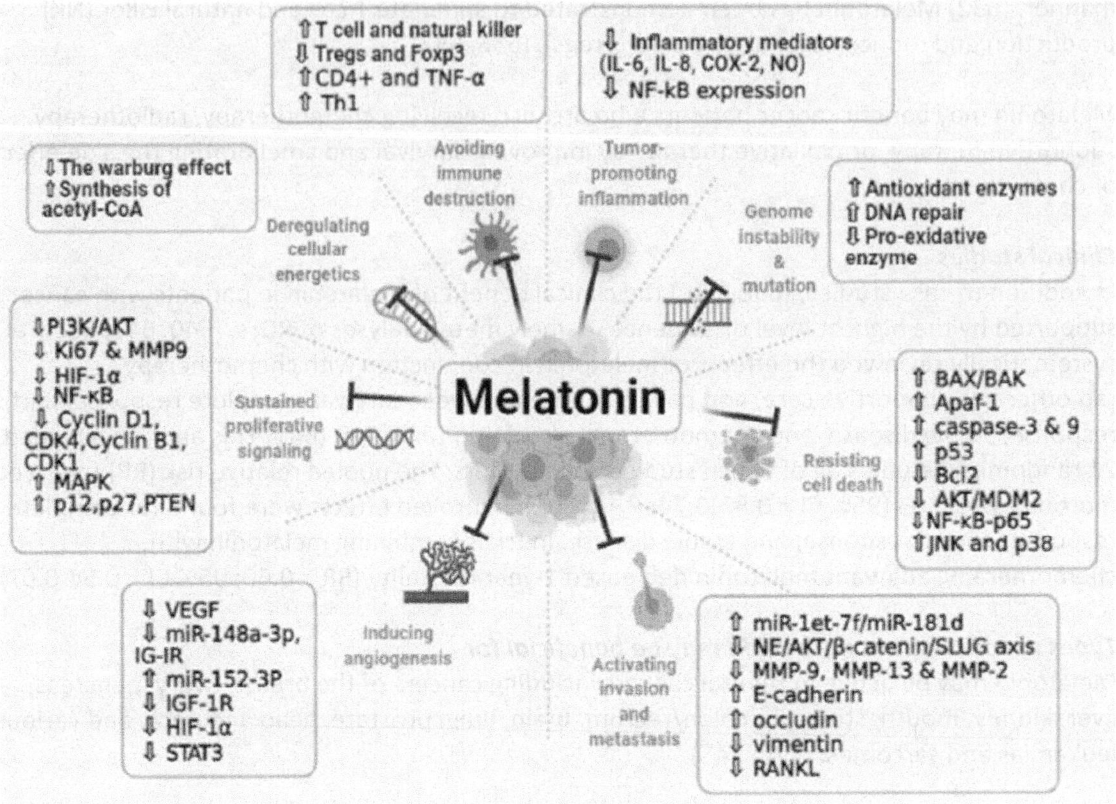

Figure 9. Multiple anticancer pathways affected by melatonin (Source: Reproduced from Talib et al under Creative Commons 4.0 license). (245)

4. Metformin

Numerous trials have shown that metformin, routinely used to treat diabetes, also inhibits the development of cancer cells, and reduces cancer cell proliferation.

Anticancer pathways and mechanisms

Metformin has been shown to have anticancer activity both in vivo and in vitro. (642) It has been proposed that the anticancer properties of metformin result from both direct effects on cancer cells, particularly through inhibition of the AMPK/mTOR pathway, (643) and indirect effects on the host, by its blood glucose-lowering properties and anti-inflammatory effects. Metformin inhibits complex I of the electron transport chain in mitochondria, putting cancer cells under bioenergetic stress and forcing them to rely on glycolysis for ATP synthesis. (644) Metformin's inhibition of GPD2 activity alters the cytosolic redox balance, which prevents redox-dependent substrates from entering the gluconeogenic pathway. (645) Metformin suppresses protein synthesis and cell development by activating ATM (ataxia telangiectasia mutated), LKB1 (liver kinase B1), and adenosine monophosphate-activated kinase (AMPK). This reduces mTOR action. (646) By turning on AMPK, metformin can activate p53, which ultimately stops the cell cycle. (646) Peroxisome proliferator-activated receptor-gamma coactivator 1-alpha (PGC-1), a distinct molecular pathway, is upregulated due to AMPK activation following metformin exposure. Low levels of PGC-1 have been linked to poorer outcomes, and it is a transcriptional coactivator involved in mitochondrial biogenesis. Metformin boosts PGC-1 and suppresses gluconeogenesis activation. (645) Metformin interacts with the S1RT1 pathway: The sirtuin 1 (SIRT1) route, which is activated by the NAD (+)-dependent protein sirtuin 1 (SIRT1) with deacetylase activity, is another significant mechanism that connects metabolism with cell proliferation. (645) Unlike most standard chemotherapy, metformin suppresses cancer stem cells, the root of cancer. (647)

Metformin regulates the EGFR and IGFR pathways, which are involved in cell growth, proliferation, and the coordination of several metabolic processes. A similar circuit performs profound functions in apoptosis and cell proliferation and is a critical axis for metabolism and cell growth. Additional research has revealed that a poor prognosis, metastasis, and disease progression are linked to elevated IGF-1 and IGF-2 expression and IGFBP-3 abnormalities. Evidence suggests that metformin treatment may prevent some of these alterations and exert an antitumor effect. Both the EGFR and IGFR pathways can boost metabolic cell modifications in a coordinated manner, acting as neoplasm promoters and forming a feedback system. (645)

Clinical studies

Meta-analyses have examined the role of metformin in the primary prevention of cancer, where it was found to significantly reduce overall cancer incidence. (238, 239) Lega et al performed a meta-analysis of 21 observational studies, evaluating the outcomes of diabetic patients with cancer who were receiving metformin. (648) In this study, metformin was associated with a reduction in all-cause mortality [HR, 0.73; 95% confidence intervals (CI), 0.64-0.83] and cancer-specific mortality (HR, 0.74; 95% CI, 0.62-0.88); patients with colorectal cancer demonstrated the greatest benefit. In a similar analysis performed by Yin et al, metformin improved overall survival in patients with lung, breast, and prostate cancer. (649) In diabetic patients with colorectal cancer Mei et al demonstrated that metformin reduced the risk of all causes of death by 44% and the specific risk of colorectal cancer death by 34%. (650) Coyle et al performed a meta-analysis of 27 observational studies which investigated the use of metformin as an adjunctive treatment for cancer. (651) The findings of this study suggested that metformin was associated with significant benefit in the early treatment of patients with colorectal and prostate cancer, particularly in those receiving radical radiotherapy.

Types of cancers that metformin may be beneficial for

Various malignancies can be prevented with the use of metformin. In general, metformin can: i) lower cancer incidence, ii) lower cancer mortality, iii) improve cancer cell response to radiotherapy and chemotherapy, iv) optimize tumor migration and lower malignancy, v) lower relapse risk, and vi) lessen the harmful effects of androgen derivatives. (645, 646) Collective findings show that metformin has a broad spectrum of anticancer activity against breast, pancreatic, gastric, colorectal, endometrial, pancreatic prostate, non-small cell lung cancer (NSCLC), and bladder cancers. (645, 650-656) However, the greatest benefit may be in patients with colorectal and prostate cancer, (650, 656), particularly when used as an adjunctive therapy.

Dosing and cautions
A dose of metformin of 1,000 mg twice daily is suggested. Metformin is a remarkably safe drug with very few side effects. The most common adverse effects include abdominal or stomach discomfort, cough, hoarseness, decreased appetite, and diarrhea. Prolonged use is associated with vitamin B12 deficiency; supplementation with a B complex vitamin is therefore suggested. Metformin may cause very low blood glucose when combined with berberine; hence the blood glucose should be very closely monitored in patients taking this combination; if low glucose does occur, we would suggest alternating metformin and berberine (monthly).

5. Curcumin

Curcumin, popularly called "curry powder" or turmeric, is a polyphenol extracted from Curcuma longa. Curcumin has antioxidant, anti-inflammatory, antimicrobial, antiviral, and anticancer properties. (657)

Anticancer pathways and mechanisms
Curcumin has been shown to interfere with multiple cell signaling pathways in cancer cells, including (see figure 10): (658-675)

i. Cell cycle (cyclin D1 and cyclin E)
ii. Apoptosis (activation of caspases and down-regulation of antiapoptotic gene products), proliferation (HER-2, EGFR, and AP-1)
iii. Survival (PI3K/AKT pathway)
iv. Invasion (MMP-9 and adhesion molecules)
v. Angiogenesis (VEGF)
vi. Metastasis (CXCR-4)
vii. Inflammation (NF-kappa B, TNF, IL-6, IL-1, COX-2, and 5-LOX)

Aberrant activation of NF-κB is characteristic of cancer, with NF-κB playing a major role in cancer angiogenesis, proliferation, metastasis, inflammation, and through the induction of cell survival pathways and inhibition of apoptosis. Phosphorylated NF-KB binds DNA and starts the transcription of oncogenes that block apoptosis and initiates cellular proliferation and angiogenesis. (657) Curcumin suppresses NF-KB activity by inhibiting the phosphorylation by I kappa B kinase and impeding nuclear translocation of the NF-KB p65 subunit. STAT3, is a common target for several signaling pathways regulating oncogenes, as well as modulating the transduction of pro-inflammatory cytokines and growth factors. (657) STAT3 contributes to the growth and survival of the cancer cell, increasing the expression of anti-apoptotic proteins such as Bcl-2 and Bcl-xL, thereby blocking apoptosis. Several factors, such as IL-6, as well as EGFR and PDGF, are reported to be STAT3 activators. (676) STAT3 is reported to be a molecular target of curcumin in several tumors, both directly and indirectly by inhibition of IL-6. (677) The accumulation and activation of immune suppressive cells like Treg, Th17, and MDSCs, the differentiation of macrophages toward the M2 phenotype, and the absence of functional DCs are all caused by STAT3 activation. Curcumin significantly decreases STAT3 phosphorylation. (666) Curcumin inhibits breast cancer cell lines through inhibiting HER2-tyrosine kinase. (678) Curcumin inhibits the phosphorylation of Akt, mTOR, and their downstream proteins, resulting in cell cycle arrest in various breast cancer cell lines. (679)

Curcumin downregulates hexokinase-2 and dissociates HK-2 from the mitochondria inducing apoptosis. (680) Curcumin is also able to interfere with the cell signaling pathway of EGFR, a family of receptor tyrosine kinases, that is reported to be associated with the proliferation, adhesion, migration, and differentiation of cancer cells. (681, 682) Curcumin inhibited the growth and proliferation of breast cancer cells by reducing EGFR signaling and decreasing EGFR and Akt levels. (681) Curcumin has been demonstrated to induce apoptosis of triple-negative breast cancer cells by inhibition of EGFR expression. (682) In pancreatic cancer cells, curcumin potentiates the anticancer activity of gemcitabine via inhibition of NF-κB, proliferation, angiogenesis, and expression of Cdc20, which is associated with enhanced cell proliferation and invasion. (683)

Curcumin has an impact on the tumor microenvironment by inhibiting angiogenesis even under the hypoxic status within the tumor microenvironment. (663) Furthermore, curcumin has activity against cancer stem cells in addition to promoting apoptosis. (663, 667, 674, 684) Curcumin induces apoptosis in tumor cells, (658) through ROS-mediated endoplasmic reticulum (ER) stress and mitochondrion-dependent pathways. (663) In addition, curcumin acts through the Wnt/-catenin pathway. (665, 675)

Clinical studies

Despite the broad anticancer activities of curcumin in experimental models, its clinical use has been limited by its poor bioavailability. Its oral bioavailability is low due to its poor absorption, extensive phase I and II biotransformation, and rapid elimination through the gall bladder. (685) Due to its low solubility in water and poor absorption, it is traditionally taken with full-fat milk and black pepper, which enhance its absorption. To improve the bioavailability, various curcumin analogs and novel drug delivery systems (e.g., phospholipids, lecithinized curcumin, nanoparticles, and liposomes) are under investigation.

While a few case series describing the use of curcumin in cancer have been published, (659, 672, 686-690) the clinical efficacy of curcumin has been evaluated in a limited number of studies. In a pilot randomized clinical trial in patients with multiple myeloma, the addition of curcumin (4 g twice daily for 28 days) to treatment with melphalan and prednisone increased the rates of remission ([75% vs. 33.3%, p=0.009]. (661) In this study NF-KB, VEGF, and TNF levels were significantly lower in the curcumin group with TNF levels being strongly correlated with remission [OR=1.35; 95% CI=1.03-1.76, p=0.03]. In a phase IIa, open-labeled trial patients with metastatic colorectal cancer were randomized to fluorouracil/oxaliplatin chemotherapy (FOLFOX) compared with FOLFOX + 2 g oral curcumin/d (CUFOX). (691) In the intention-to-treat population, the HR for overall survival was 0.34 (95% CI: 0.14, 0.82; P = 0.02) (median of 200 and 502 days for FOLFOX and CUFOX, respectively). In a prospective, single-arm phase II study, Pastorelli et al evaluated the use of a phytosome complex of curcumin (2 g/day) as adjunctive therapy with gemcitabine in patients with advanced pancreatic cancer. (692) The median overall survival of patients treated with gemcitabine as a single agent is 5.7 months. (693) These investigators reported a 27.3% of response rate with 34.1% of cases having stable disease, with a total disease control rate of 61.4%. The median progression-free survival and overall survival were 8.4 and 10.2 months, respectively. Saghatelyan et al randomized 150 women with advanced metastatic breast cancer to receive either paclitaxel plus placebo or paclitaxel plus curcumin once per week for 12 weeks with 3 months of follow-up. (694) In this study, the curcumin was given intravenously. The intention-to-treat analysis revealed that the objective response rate of curcumin was significantly higher than that of the placebo (51% vs. 33%, p<0.01) at 4 weeks of follow-up. The difference between the groups was even greater when only patients who had completed the treatment (61% vs. 38%, odds ratio =2.64, p<0.01) were included.

In dose escalation studies, up to 10 g of curcumin taken daily has been shown to be well tolerated. Patients with breast cancer taking 6 g/day of curcumin for 7 weeks, and patients with prostate cancer who took 3 g/day of curcumin for 9 weeks exhibited no adverse effects. [301,353,389]

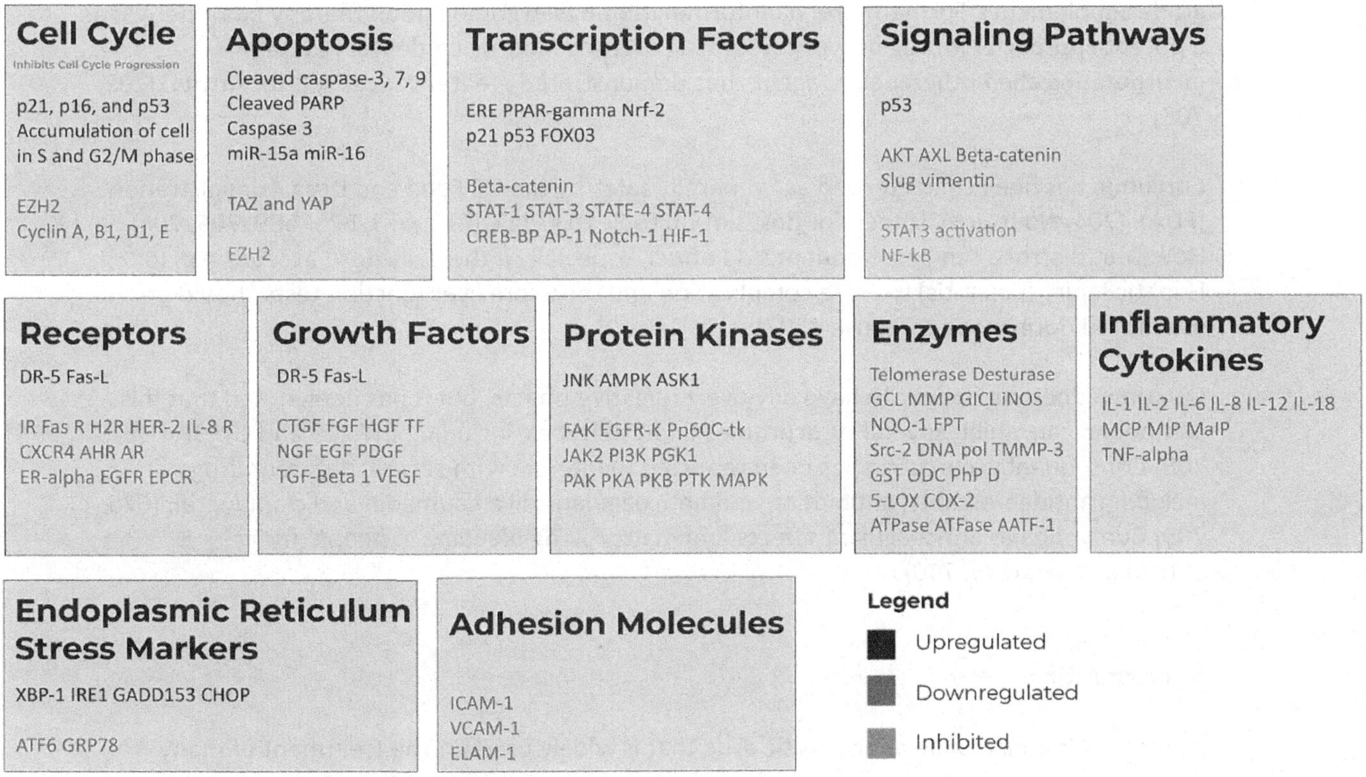

Figure 10. Curcumin - a multifaceted anticancer agent [Source: Dr. Mobeen Syed]
Footnote for Figure 10. See Appendix 3.

***Types of cancers that curcumin (turmeric) may be beneficial** for*
Colorectal, lung, pancreatic, breast, prostate, chronic myeloid leukemia, liver, gastric, brain tumors, ovarian, skin, head and neck, lymphoma, esophageal cancer, and myeloma. (657, 675)

Drug formulations and cautions
The use of curcumin has been limited by its poor solubility, absorption, and bioavailability. The manipulation and encapsulation of curcumin into a nanocarrier formulation can overcome these major drawbacks and potentially may lead to a far superior therapeutic efficacy. In a murine Hodgkin's Lymphoma model, formulating curcumin in solid lipid nanoparticles exhibited greater anticancer activity compared to curcumin alone. (695) Nano-curcumin preparations or formulations designed to enhance absorption are therefore recommended. (696-699)

In the U.S., a large share (55%) of the turmeric dietary supplement market is comprised of products formulated to enhance curcumin bioavailability, including proprietary products where curcuminoid extracts are often combined with some type of lipophilic carrier to increase absorption, or products combining curcumin with piperine to decrease metabolism. (700)

However, as the quality of these products may vary, we would recommend the use of USP-grade supplements. Furthermore, nanoformulation-based combination therapy has emerged as a potent approach for drug delivery systems. (701) A nanodrug co-delivery system incorporating chemotherapeutic agents has demonstrated greater cancer cell sensitivity. (702, 703)

Curcumin has been characterized as "generally safe" by the US Food and Drug Administration (FDA). (704) No toxicity is seen for doses of up to 8–10 g/day. (672, 673, 675, 689, 705, 706) However, diarrhea can be a frequent side effect, especially if the daily dose exceeds 4 g. (672) Hepatic injury (hepatitis) is a rare complication and therefore liver function tests should be monitored during long-term use. (707)

Curcumin does not appear to have any overt negative effects, but it has been noted that this compound can inhibit several cytochromes P450 subtypes, including CYP2C9 and CYP3A4. (675, 708) Consequently, curcumin has been reported to interact with several different drugs, including antidepressants, antibiotics, and anticoagulants like coumadin and clopidogrel. (675, 709) Curcumin has anticoagulant effects and may prolong bleeding in people using anticoagulants. (675, 710)

6. Ivermectin

Ivermectin is a macrolide antiparasitic drug that is widely used for the treatment of many parasitic diseases, such as river blindness, elephantiasis, and scabies. Satoshi Omura and William C. Campbell won the 2015 Nobel Prize in Physiology or Medicine for the discovery of the efficacy of ivermectin against parasitic diseases. Ivermectin was approved by the FDA for use in humans in 1978. Recently, scientists have discovered that ivermectin has strong anticancer effects. Ivermectin has been reported to inhibit the proliferation of several tumor cells by regulating multiple signaling pathways. (711-713)

Anticancer pathways and mechanisms

In 1996, Didier et al. found that ivermectin may effectively reverse tumor multidrug resistance, this is the first reported antitumorigenic activity of ivermectin.(714) Since then, many studies revealed that ivermectin exerted antitumor effects through multiple targets including chloride channel, PAK1 protein, Akt/mTOR signaling, P2X4/P2X7 receptors, WNTTCF pathway, SIN3 domain, NS3 DDX23 helicase and Nanog/Sox2/Oct4 genes. (715)

Experimental data demonstrated that ivermectin inhibited the proliferation of multiple breast cancer cell lines. (716) The mechanism involved the inhibition by ivermectin of the Akt/mTOR pathway to induce autophagy. Ivermectin has been demonstrated to inhibit the proliferation of canine breast tumor cell lines by blocking the cell cycle related to the inhibition of the Wnt pathway. (717) In a study that screened Wnt pathway inhibitors, ivermectin inhibited the proliferation of multiple cancers, including the colorectal cancer cell, and promoted apoptosis by blocking the Wnt pathway. (718) Other cancers that show an active WNT pathway and are inhibited by ivermectin include carcinomas of the lung, stomach, cervix, endometrium, and lung, as well as melanomas and gliomas. (718)

Triple-negative breast cancer (TNBC) refers to cancer that is negative for estrogen receptor, progesterone receptor, and human epidermal growth factor receptor 2 (HER2) and is the most aggressive subtype of breast cancer with the worst prognosis. (719) In addition, there is also no clinically applicable therapeutic drug currently available. A drug screening study of TNBC showed that ivermectin resulted in impairment of clonogenic self-renewal in vitro and inhibition of tumor growth and metastasis in vivo by blocking the SIN3-interaction domain.(720) Ivermectin exerts an antitumor effect through the autophagy pathway. Using the autophagy inhibitors chloroquine and wortmannin or knocking down Bclin1 and Atg5 by siRNA to inhibit autophagy, the anticancer activity of ivermectin reduced significantly. (716)

Ivermectin induces cancer cell apoptosis mainly through the mitochondrial pathway. (711) Chen et al demonstrated that ivermectin inhibited the viability and induced apoptosis of esophageal squamous cancer cells through a mitochondrial-dependent pathway. (721) Heat shock protein-27 (HSP27) is highly expressed in and supports oncogene expression of many cancers. Ivermectin inhibits MAPKAP2-mediated HSP27 phosphorylation and depolymerization, thereby blocking HSP27-regulated survival signaling and client-oncoprotein interactions. (722) Chen et al demonstrated that ivermectin inhibited the viability and induced apoptosis of esophageal squamous carcoma cells through a mitochondrial-dependent manner. In addition, Sharmeen et al demonstrated that ivermectin induced chloride-dependent membrane hyperpolarization and cell death in leukemia cells. (723) Li et al demonstrated that Ivermectin induces nonprotective autophagy by downregulating PAK1 and apoptosis in lung adenocarcinoma cells. (715) Hu et al demonstrated that ivermectin augmented the efficacy of chemotherapy in an osteosarcoma cell line. (724)

Ivermectin has anticancer activity by influencing the tumor microenvironment. Ivermectin decreases MDSC and Tregs and targets cancer stem cells. (225, 725) Furthermore, ivermectin acts to suppress the action of TAMs, which otherwise produce aberrant cytokine signals that act to suppress tumor apoptosis via a number of pathways, particularly TGF-β, and also upregulates the expression of the p53 tumor suppressor gene.

Although a number of antiparasitic drugs including ivermectin, mebendazole and niclosamide have proven anti-cancer effects it is important to recognize that cancer is NOT a parasitic disease as has been suggested in the "popular press" and by misguided clinicians. There is no evidence that cancer is caused by or related to any parasitic disease. These drugs act via specific biochemical pathways specific to the cancer cell which are distinct from their anti-parasitic mechanisms of action.

Clinical studies

While many in vitro studies have demonstrated the effectiveness of ivermectin against multiple cancers, the reported clinical effectiveness is limited to small case series. (726, 727) However, it appears that ivermectin is widely prescribed across the world for cancer. Further, I am aware of multiple "anecdotal" reports of solid tumors that have shown a dramatic response to repurposed drug regimens that included ivermectin.

Types of cancers ivermectin may be beneficial for
Ivermectin has shown in vitro activity against breast cancer (including TNBC), as well as lung, stomach, cervix, esophageal, endometrium, liver, prostate, kidney and ovarian cancer as well as cholangiocarcinoma, melanomas, leukemia, lymphoma and gliomas. (711)

Dosing and cautions
The optimal dosing strategy with ivermectin is unclear. De Castro et al reported the use of 1mg/kg/day for up to 6 months in three pediatric patients with refractory AML without untoward side effects. (726) Ishiguro et al reported the use of ivermectin 12 mg twice weekly.(727) Anecdotal evidence suggest that a daily dose of 12-18 mg may be effective (prescribed indefinitely). As ivermectin has a remarkable safety record long term treatment at this dose appears safe. As mentioned previously, ivermectin may be synergistic with mebendazole. As ivermectin does not cross the blood-brain barrier this drug is likely ineffective for brain tumors. Furthermore, caution is advised in patients with disruption of the blood-brain barrier.

7. Mebendazole/ Fenbendazole/Albendazole

Anticancer pathways and mechanisms
A compound originally developed as a treatment for parasitic worms, mebendazole (MBZ) works by fatally disrupting the cellular microtubule formation in abnormal cancer cells that occurs as the cell is attempting to divide. Like the other benzimidazoles, Mebendazole binds to the tubulin colchicine-binding domain and appears to act by both p53-dependent and independent mechanisms. (728) MBZ inhibits many factors involved in tumor progressions such as tubulin polymerization, angiogenesis, pro-survival pathways, matrix metalloproteinases, and multi-drug resistance protein transporters. (729) MBZ inhibits cancer stem cells; this mechanism of action is critical in preventing metastasis. (223, 729) In addition, in a juvenile glioblastoma mouse model MBZ reduced tumor cell growth and invasion when evaluated under *in-vitro* and *in-vivo* conditions through inhibition of both the glutaminolysis and the glycolysis pathways. (304) In this study the effect of ketosis and MBZ were synergistic in inhibiting tumor growth.

MBZ decreases the activity of the Hedgehog pathway, which is common in gliomas, melanomas, lung cancers, ovarian cancers, and colorectal cancer. (155) MBZ inactivates Bcl-2 and activates caspases to promote apoptosis in cancer cells and the release of cytochrome c which has also been shown to trigger apoptosis in malignant cells. Benzimidazole modulates the typically overactivated MAPK pathway, switching it to activate the apoptotic pathway, rather than the anti-apoptotic pathway; it also destabilizes microtubules, structural proteins required to maintain a cell's integrity during the process of mitosis, among other functions; it *also* interferes with cancer cells' glycolysis-dependent metabolism, upon which *most* cancers are heavily preferentially dependent, as well as functioning as an inhibitor of mitochondrial oxidative phosphorylation, or OXPHOS, which reduces the residual energy available via the ordinary metabolic ATP production pathway.

MBZ can cross the blood-brain barrier and has been demonstrated to slow the growth of gliomas by targeting signaling pathways involved in cell proliferation, apoptosis, invasion, and migration, as well as by making glioma cells more susceptible to conventional chemotherapy and radiotherapy. (730)

MBZ can also sensitize cancer cells to conventional therapy, such as chemotherapeutics and radiation, enhancing their combined antitumor potential, confirming that MBZ may be useful as an adjuvant therapeutic combined with traditional chemotherapy. (730) When combined with low-dose chemotherapy there is also evidence these drugs help to destroy the tumor-associated macrophage cells that may help maintain a favorable environment for the cancer to flourish.

Clinical studies

The use of benzimidazoles in cancer is limited to a few case reports (731, 732) and a small case series. (733) Mebendazole is a component of the multidrug cocktail used in the METRICS study.(257) The use of benzimidazoles, and in particular fenbendazole, has achieved much attention as a repurposed drug for cancer due to the reported experience of Joe Tippens. (146) In 2016, Tippens was diagnosed with non-small-cell lung cancer with extensive metastatic disease. At the advice of a veterinarian friend, he took Fenbendazole together with nanocurcumin, and three months after starting these drugs his PET scan was completely clear. He remains alive and disease-free up until the present; however, some questions surround his apparent cure.

Types of cancers that mebendazole may be beneficial for

A wide variety of cancers, including non-small cell lung cancer, adrenocortical, colorectal, chemo-resistant melanoma, glioblastoma multiforme, colon, leukemia, osteosarcoma/soft tissue sarcoma, acute myeloid sarcoma, breast (ER+ invasive ductal), kidney, and ovarian carcinoma, have been shown to be responsive to benzimidazoles, including MBZ. (252, 728-730, 734-743)

Dosing and cautions

We suggest Mebendazole 100-200 mg/day. The cost of mebendazole in the U.S. skyrocketed once this drug was discovered to have activity against cancer ($555 for a single 100 mg tablet?). However, mebendazole is available from international (India) and local compounding pharmacies for between 25c to $2 for a 100 mg tablet. Ivermectin can be considered an alternative if mebendazole is unavailable. However, it I likely that both drugs combined may have additive or synergistic anticancer activity.

8. Green Tea

Anticancer pathways and mechanisms

Green tea is a significant source of a type of flavonoid called catechin, which includes epigallocatechin gallate (EGCG), epigallocatechin (EGC), epicatechin gallate (ECG), and epicatechin (EC). The most abundant individual catechin in fresh tea leaves is EGCG, which is more than 40% of the total content of catechins. (234) Green tea catechins (GTCs) have been proven to be effective in inhibiting cancer growth in several experimental models. (744-746) In addition, GTCs may have synergistic anticancer activity when combined with other phytochemicals, particularly resveratrol. (747, 748) GTCs, particularly EGCG, may have a role in both the prevention and treatment of cancers, (749) specifically those dependent on the glutamate pathway as a source of energy. Mitochondrial glutamate dehydrogenase (GDH) catalyzes the oxidative deamination of L-glutamate. Activation of GDH is tightly correlated with increased glutaminolysis. Furthermore, glutamate serves as a mitochondrial intracellular messenger when glucose is being oxidized and the GDH participates in this process by synthesizing glutamate. (750) Li and colleagues demonstrated *in vitro* that EGCG allosterically inhibits GDH in nanomolar concentrations. (301, 302)

GTCs have an important anticarcinogenic role by promoting and/or inhibiting signal transmission through the targeted regulation of multiple links in the signal pathways that are activated or inhibited in cancer cells. (234) EGCG regulates signaling pathways by interacting with membrane receptors. EGCG significantly inhibited the expression of VEGF and reduced VEGF receptors. Inactivation of the VEGF signaling pathway suppresses angiogenesis, a common strategy for inhibiting carcinogenesis. EGCG activates PKA, which dephosphorylates related proteins such as the tumor suppressor Merlin and inhibits the proliferation of cancer cells. (751) EGCG inhibits STAT3 phosphorylation by blocking JAK2 phosphorylation. STAT3 suppresses anti-tumor immune responses and promotes the proliferation and migration of cancer cells. EGCG inhibits the MAPK signaling by competing for the phosphorylation sites of downstream proteins. EGCG inhibits the Wnt pathway by phosphorylating β-catenin and promoting its degradation. EGCG inhibits transcription factors involved in activating the Sonic hedgehog pathway. EGCG inhibited the activities of MMP2 and MMP9 and promoted the expression of tissue inhibitor of MMPs (TIMp1/2) to suppress the invasion and metastasis of tumor cells. (751) Green tea extract has been demonstrated to suppress cancer stem cells. (752, 753)

GTCs have anticancer effects via additional pathways. (234) GTCs exert potent and selective *in vitro* and *in vivo* pro-apoptotic activity in cancer cells via several pathways. (744, 745, 754) GTC inhibits A549 cells by regulating its cell cycle arrest, increasing the expressions of p21 and p27, and inhibiting the expressions of p-AKT and cyclin E1 in a dose-dependent manner in the cancer cells. (755) EGCG inhibited the proliferation of human lung cancer cells by targeting the epidermal growth factor receptor (EGFR) signaling pathway.

GTCs have been demonstrated to alter the tumor microenvironment (TME) thereby attenuating immunosuppression and the risk of metastases. (748) Flavonoids including GTCs (and resveratrol) are potent modulators of pro-inflammatory gene expression being, therefore, of great interest as agents selectively suppressing molecular targets within pro-inflammatory TME. GTCs have been demonstrated to increase the ratio of active cytotoxic T lymphocytes to Tregs in tumors, indicating a switch of "cold" tumors to "hot" with significantly improved anti-tumor immune therapeutics. (756) GTCs have anticancer effects by enhancing anticancer immunity via PD-1 axis and TLR4 pathways. (757, 758) In addition, GTCs repolarize tumor-associated macrophages (M2 to M1 macrophages), triggering an immune response and limiting metastases. (759) GTCs have been demonstrated to attenuate MDSC-mediated immunosuppression and increased the proportions of CD4+ and CD8+ T cells. (760)

Studies have shown that 20% of cancer-related deaths were directly due to TLR-induced cancer cachexia, in which cancer cells released heat shock proteins that acted as TLR-4 agonists in macrophages, skeletal muscle, and fat cells, causing downstream signal transduction. EGCG effectively downregulates the TLR-4 signal pathway. (758)

GTCs inhibit the accumulation of MDSCs, leading to restoration of the IFN-γ, enhancing the activity of CD8+ T-cells, and improvement of the ratio of CD4(+) to CD8(+) T-cells, which is beneficial to the improvement of the immune system's attack on tumor cells. (234) In addition, a phytochemical mixture including GTCs exerted anti-tumor activity by repolarization of M2-polarized macrophages and induced the production of IL-12, which recruit cytotoxic T lymphocytes and natural killer cells (NK) with the tumor microenvironment. (759)

In addition to all these beneficial effects, GTCs potentiate the effects of conventional chemotherapeutic agents. Due to their effects on the important signaling pathways in vivo, catechins are often used as sensitizing agents in combination with chemotherapeutic drugs. The combination of anticancer drugs with catechins, whether before or after drug administration, reduced the toxicity of these drugs and enhanced the clinical efficacy by accelerating apoptosis of cancer cells. (234) Importantly, the combination of a number of chemotherapeutic drugs with GTCs will improve the chemotherapeutic sensitivity of cells to the drug, allowing a reduction in the dose of the chemotherapeutic drug. (234)

Clinical studies

Numerous experimental models have explored the mechanistic anticancer effects of GTCs; this data is supported by epidemiologic data, a case series of patients with B cell malignancies,(761) several case reports,(762, 763) and a RCT. A meta-analysis including 18 prospective cohorts and 25 case-control studies showed a significant inverse association between intake of tea catechins and risk of various cancers, with a relative risk (RR) being 0.935 (95% CI = 0.891-0.981). (234) Similarly an umbrella review and meta-analysis by Kim et al, which included 64 observational studies (case-control or cohort) demonstrated that GTC significantly reduced the risk of gastrointestinal cancer (oral, gastric, colorectal, biliary tract, and liver), breast cancer, and gynecological cancer (endometrial and ovarian cancer) as well as leukemia, lung cancer, and thyroid cancer. (243) In a phase I dose finding study in patients with Chronic Lymphocytic Leukemia EGCG was well tolerated and a decline in the absolute lymphocyte count and/or lymphadenopathy was observed in the majority of patients. (764) Lemanne et al reported on a patient who demonstrated a complete and durable remission of chronic lymphocytic leukemia (CLL) following high dose EGCG. (763) In a randomized, double-blind, placebo-controlled study, treatment with 600 mg/day of green tea catechins reduced the risk of prostate cancer from 30% to 3% in men with high-grade prostate intraepithelial neoplasia. (303)

Types of cancers that green tea may be beneficial for
Green tea catechins may be effective against a range of tumors including cancers of the prostate, breast, uterus, ovary, colorectal, glioma, liver and gallbladder, melanoma, and lung cancers. (234) GTCs appear to be particularly beneficial for prostate cancer as well as breast cancer. (299, 303, 744-747, 760, 765)

Dosing and cautions
Green tea catechins should be taken in a dose of 500-1000 mg/day. Green tea extract should be taken during/after a meal rather than on an empty stomach. (244) Green tea extract has rarely been associated with liver toxicity. (766) The safety of green tea extract was evaluated by the US Pharmacopeia (USP) Dietary Supplement Information Expert Committee (DSIEC). (244) The DSIEC concluded that *"when dietary supplement products containing green tea extracts are used and formulated appropriately the Committee is unaware of significant safety issues that would prohibit monograph development."* (244) Based on this data we suggest that green tea exacts be taken in the dosages recommended by the manufacturer. Regular liver function tests are suggested in patients taking green tea extract and green tea exact should be avoided/used cautiously in those with underlying liver disease.

9. Omega-3 Fatty Acids

The term omega-3 polyunsaturated fatty acids (omega-3 FAs) refers to a group of polyunsaturated fatty acids (PUFA) which contain a double carbon bond at the third carbon atom (n-3 position) from the methyl end of the carbon chain. Alpha-linolenic acid (ALA, 18-carbon PUFA obtained from plant sources), eicosapentaenoic acid (EPA, 20-carbon PUFA form fish) and docosahexaenoic acid (DHA, 22-carbon PUFA obtained from marine source) are the most common omega-3 FAs. (767)

Over the past decades, extensive studies have addressed the therapeutic effects of omega-3 polyunsaturated fatty acids (omega-3 FAs) against different human diseases such as cardiovascular and neurodegenerative diseases and cancer. (767) These studies have demonstrated the clinical utility and safety of these natural occurring substances. Furthermore, more recently, omega-3 FAs have been demonstrated to improve the outcome against certain types of cancer, improve the efficacy and tolerability of chemotherapy and improve quality of life indicators. (767) In addition, omega 3 FA improve cancer cachexia.

Anticancer pathways and mechanisms
The four main antineoplastic activities omega-3 FA that have been proposed are (i) modulation of cyclooxygenase (COX) activity; (ii) alteration of membrane dynamics and cell surface receptor

function, (iii) increased cellular oxidative stress, and iv) the production of novel anti-inflammatory lipid mediators including resolvins, protectins and maresins. (768, 769)

Omega-3 FAs compete with linoleic acids (LA) as a key nutrient in cancer. The ratio of the two classes of FAs is important since omega-3 and omega-6 share the same biochemical pathways and can compete between them to generate imbalances. The precursor of the omega-6 FA, LA, is associated with pro-inflammatory response. Cancer progression seems to be influenced by the ratio omega-3/omega-6 FA in the diet, rather than by their singular intake. (767) While LA promotes the survival of tumor cells preventing their death, omega-3 FAs promote the self-destruction of the tumor cells, thus limiting the expansion of cancer. Omega-3 FAs, especially EPA and DHA, affect cancer cell replication, cell cycle, and cell death. In this context, in vitro and in vivo studies have shown that omega-3 FAs sensitize tumor cells to anticancer drugs. Omega-3 FAs also modulate several pathways including modulating gene expression involved in multiple signaling pathways including NF-κB, Notch, Hedgehog, Wnt, and mitogen-activated protein kinases (MAPKs). (770) Omega-3 FAs suppress the formation of arachidonic acid derived prostanoids (prostaglandin E2), which are responsible for inflammatory response, cell growth, apoptosis, angiogenesis, and metastasis. (771) EPA and DHA induce apoptosis in breast cancer cell lines by activation of Bcl2 expression and pro-caspase 8, together with reduction of EGFR activation. (771) Omega-3 FAs can block the activity of self-renewing colon cancer stem cells (CSC). (772, 773)

Clinical studies

In a prospective RCT, the intake of omega-3 FAs and vitamin D was associated with a dramatic reduction in the risk of developing cancer. (232) In the VITAL cohort study conducted in postmenopausal women, the current use of fish oil was associated with reduced risk of breast cancer (HR 0.68, 95% CI: 0.50-0.92). (774) A meta-analysis of 16 prospective cohort studies examining marine omega-3 FAs intake suggests a reduction in breast cancer risk when individuals with highest intakes are compared with those with lowest intakes of marine PUFA. (775) Two large observational studies have demonstrated significant inverse relationships between omega-3 FAs intake and the risk of colorectal neoplasia. (776, 777)

A recent meta-analysis of six prospective case–control studies and five cohort studies evaluated the omega-3:omega-6 intake ratio and/or omega-3:omega-6 ratio in serum phospholipids in relation to the risk of developing breast cancer. (778) The authors concluded that each 1/10 increment in the dietary n-3:n-6 ratio was associated with a 6% reduction in breast cancer risk, and each 1/10 increment in the serum n-3:n-6 phospholipid ratio was associated with a 27% reduction in breast cancer risk.

Patients with familial adenomatous polyposis who had previously undergone colectomy and ileorectal anastomosis were randomized to 2g EPA/day or placebo. In this RCT there was a 22.4% reduction in polyp number in the EPA group (p=0.01). (779) A phase II study evaluated addition of 1.8 g DHA daily to an anthracycline based chemotherapy regimen for metastatic breast cancer. The DHA group had a significantly longer time to disease progression and overall survival (median 34 months vs 18 months). (780) In a small RCT, supplementation with fish oil increased first line chemotherapy efficacy in patients with advanced non-small cell lung cancer.(781)

Higher intakes of EPA and DHA from dietary sources were reported to be associated with a 25% reduction in breast cancer recurrence and improved overall mortality in a large cohort of over 3,000 women with early-stage breast cancer followed for a median of 7 years. (782) Cohort studies assessing the risk of prostate cancer mortality and fish omega-3 FAs intake suggest an association between higher intake of fish and decreased risk of prostate cancer–related death.(783) In a small RCT, patients with leukemia or lymphoma concurrently receiving chemotherapy were randomized to receive 2g /day of fish oil or placebo for 9 weeks. (784) Overall long-term survival was greater in the fish oil group ($p < 0.05$). In a meta-analysis which included 12 RCT and 1184 patients with cancer cachexia, the use of omega-3 FAs was associated with a significant improvement in quality of life and duration of survival (median survival ratio, 1.10; 95% CI, 1.02-1.19; P = .014). (785)

Types of cancers that omega-3 fatty acids may be beneficial for
Omega-3 FAs may be beneficial for breast cancer, colorectal cancer, leukemia, gastric cancer, pancreatic cancer, esophageal cancer, prostate cancer, lung cancer, and head and neck cancer.(767)

Dosing and cautions
We suggest a dose of 2-4 g omega-3 FAs daily. Omega-3 fatty acids may increase the risk of bleeding and should be used cautiously in patients on anticoagulants.

10. Berberine

Depending on the patient's blood glucose levels, providers can consider using metformin and berberine together or alternating (switching back and forth for one month at a time).

Anticancer pathways and mechanisms
Berberine's anticancer mechanisms include reducing the growth of cancer cells, preventing metastasis, inducing apoptosis, activating autophagy, controlling the microbiota in the gut, and enhancing the effects of other cancer treatments by focusing on antibacterial action, which includes controlling the microbiota in the gut and preventing intratumoral microbes. (786-790)

Berberine may prevent the growth of cancer cells through the upregulation of miR-214-3p, the downregulation of SCT protein levels, the regulation of catenin, the inhibition of telomerase activity, and the deactivation of MAPK signaling pathways. (791-793) By increasing p21, p27, and p38 and lowering CDK1, CDK4, cyclin A, and cyclin D1, berberine may inhibit the growth of cancer cells. (786, 794) Through the AMPK-p53, PI3K/AKT/mTOR, miR19a/TF/MAPK signaling pathways, and modulation of the CASC2/ AUF1/B-cell/Bcl-2 axis, berberine promotes cancer cells apoptosis. (788, 795-797) Berberine downregulates many TME-related genes, including

PDGFRB, COL1A2, and BMP7, and upregulating E-cadherin, thereby inhibiting metastatic spread. (798-800)

Berberine has anticancer effects by influencing the gut microbiota. For example, berberine increases the Firmicutes/Bacteroidetes ratio and the relative abundance of Clostridiales, Lactobacillaceae, Bacteroides, and Akkermansia muciniphila. (789, 790)

Berberine increases radiation sensitivity and enhances the effects of anticancer medications such as cisplatin, 5-fluorouracil, doxorubicin, niraparib, and icotinib. (801-804)

Clinical studies

While there is limited clinical data on the benefits of berberine, a randomized, double-blind study demonstrated that berberine in a dose of 300 mg twice daily significantly reduced the risk of recurrent colorectal adenomas following polypectomy. (805)

Types of cancers that berberine may be beneficial for

Berberine shows anticancer effects on various cancers, such as breast, lung, gastric, liver, colorectal, ovarian, cervical, and prostate. (786-788, 791-797, 799-804, 806)

Dosing and cautions

A total daily dose of 1000-1500 mg (take 500 mg two or three times daily or 600 mg twice daily) is suggested. As insulin release is glucose-dependent hypoglycemia has not been reported with this herb; however, blood glucose should be monitored and the additive/synergistic effect of metformin on the blood glucose profile should be determined. Berberine should not be taken in patients taking cyclosporine as this combination will increase cyclosporine levels (absolute contraindication). Berberine may alter the metabolism of the following drugs, which should be used with caution (monitor effects): anticoagulants, dextromethorphan, tacrolimus (Prograf), phenobarbitone, losartan (inhibits effect) and sedative drugs (see https://www.webmd.com/vitamins/ai/ingredientmono-1126/berberine). If you are scheduled for surgery, please notify your anesthesia team if you are taking Berberine. You may need to stop taking Berberine one week prior to surgery.

11. Atorvastatin or simvastatin.

The lipophilic statins appear to be highly effective in the management of several cancers.

Anticancer pathways and mechanisms

Statins may affect tumor cells directly in four main ways: i) growth suppression, ii) apoptosis induction, iii) anti-invasive and anti-metastatic effects, and iv) anti-angiogenic effects. A primary effect is that statins block activity of the cholesterol-producing enzyme HMG CoA, which means less cholesterol is available to produce new cell walls in rapidly proliferating tumors. Rapidly multiplying cancer cells require more cholesterol to allow the creation of cell membranes. (807, 808) A reduction in the availability of cholesterol may limit the cellular proliferation required for cancer growth and metastasis. In addition, statins alter the expression of genes regulating the balance between life-promoting and death-promoting proteins in cancer and may have a number of benefits in killing cancer cells. Studies have shown statins also reactivate caspases and upregulate the production of PPARγ, another protein that programs cell death. Statins also reduce the number of cell surface GLUT-1 glucose receptors, thus reducing cancer cell activity by limiting the amount of energy available. Additionally, statins' direct inhibition of HMGCR depletes the body's stores of isoprenoids, which play a crucial role in controlling the growth and spread of cancer cells. (809)

Clinical studies

Lipophilic statins have been demonstrated to reduce the incidence and all-cause mortality from a number of cancers. A 10-year retrospective cohort study by Farwell et al compared statin usage in a veteran population taking antihypertensive medications and found that, on average, statin users had a 31% lower risk of prostate cancer incidence. (810) NSAIDs have been found to significantly reduce prostate cancer risk and may act synergistically with statins to prevent prostate cancer. (811)

Nielsen et al assessed mortality among patients from the entire Danish population who had received a diagnosis of cancer between 1995 and 2007. (812) In this study multivariable-adjusted hazard ratios for statin users, as compared with patients who had never used statins, was 0.85 (95% CI, 0.82 to 0.87) for death from cancer. The reduced cancer-related mortality among statin users as compared with patients who had never used statins was observed for 13 cancer types. Zhong et al demonstrated that patients who used statins after a diagnosis of cancer had an HR of 0.81 (95% CI: 0.72–0.91) for all-cause mortality compared to non-users; the benefit was most marked for colorectal, prostate, and breast cancer. (813)

In a population-based retrospective cohort study that looked at the usage of statins after a prostate cancer diagnosis, (814) the post-diagnostic use of statins was associated with a decreased risk of prostate cancer mortality (HR, 0.76; 95% CI, 0.66 to 0.88) and all-cause mortality (HR, 0.86; 95% CI, 0.78 to 0.95); longer and higher dosages led to a lower incidence in mortality, as well as distant site metastasis.

In a meta-analysis of 10 studies, statin use was associated with improved recurrence-free survival (RFS; HR 0.64; 95% CI 0.53–0.79) in women with breast cancer. (815) Furthermore, this survival benefit appeared to be confined to use of lipophilic statins. Similarly, Ahern et al performed a population study of women with stages I–III breast cancer; they reported a 10% reduction in breast cancer recurrence among women who were prescribed a lipophilic statin (most commonly simvastatin). (816) Similarly, in colorectal and hepatocellular cancer, statin usage reduces cancer-specific mortality, in particular when used either prior to diagnosis or prior to recurrence. (817-819) In lung cancer, retrospective studies have shown that statins reduce cancer-specific mortality. (820)

Types of cancers that statins may be beneficial for

Breast, prostate, colorectal, hepatocellular, lung, testicular, pancreatic, gastric, ovarian, leukemia, brain, and kidney. (653, 809, 812, 821)

12. Disulfiram

As an inhibitor of aldehyde dehydrogenase (ALDH), disulfiram (DSF) inhibits all the currently identified cytosolic and mitochondrial ALDH isoforms, resulting in the specific accumulation of acetaldehyde, which causes unpleasant effects when alcohol is consumed, and thus it functions as an anti-alcoholism drug. Recently, DSF has been repurposed because of its potent effect as a cancer treatment in preclinical studies.

Its anti-tumor effect has been reported in many preclinical studies and recently on seven types of cancer in humans: non-small cell lung cancer (NSCLC), liver cancer, breast cancer, prostate cancer, pancreatic cancer, glioblastoma (GBM) and melanoma and has a successful breakthrough in the treatment of NSCLC and GBM. (822)

Anticancer pathways and mechanisms

DSF inhibits NF-kB signaling, proteasome activity, and aldehyde dehydrogenase (ALDH) activity. It induces endoplasmic reticulum (ER) stress and autophagy and has been used as an adjuvant therapy with irradiation or chemotherapy drugs. DSF not only kills the normal cancer cells but also targets cancer stem cells. (823) Disulfiram binds to nuclear protein localization protein 4 (NPL4), induce its immobilization and dysfunction, ultimately leading to cell death.

The cytotoxicity of DSF depends on copper (Cu). (824) DSF penetrates cancer cells and chelates Cu intracellularly. Compared with normal tissues, many cancers exhibit higher levels of intracellular Cu (2–3 fold). (825) Copper plays a crucial role in redox reactions and triggers the generation of reactive oxygen species (ROS). DSF/Cu is a strong inducer of ROS production and an effective proteasome inhibitor, resulting in the inhibition of NF-κB. NF-κB is an ROS-induced transcription factor with strong anti-apoptotic activity, which in turn reduces the pro-apoptotic effect of ROS. (824, 826) DSF/Cu simultaneously activate the ROS-JNK pro-apoptotic pathway and downregulate anti-apoptotic pathways such as NF-kB signaling. (827) The activation of executioner caspases, such as an increased ratio of Bax and Bcl2 proteins, indicated that the intrinsic apoptotic pathway may be involved in DSF/Cu-induced apoptosis. (828) As a bivalent metal ion chelator, DSF has been considered to form a complex with Cu (DSF/Cu), which is more readily taken up by cells and exerts cytotoxic effects on a variety of cancer cells while sparing normal cells. When chelated with copper, DSF down-regulates the expression of several genes involved in DNA repair pathways.

Recently, an increasing number of clinical trials have verified the hypothesis that the binding of disulfiram or its metabolites to copper produces antitumor effects. In a study of head and neck squamous cell carcinoma, a DSF/Cu injection markedly inhibited tumor growth at a concentration of 50 mg/kg, while DSF alone showed limited efficacy compared to DSF in combination with copper. (829) DSF ultimately exerted inhibitory effects on head and neck carcinoma cell lines mainly by inducing autophagic cell death and inhibited tumor progression in xenograft model.

DSF shows cytotoxicity towards several model cancer cell lines in vitro, including breast, lung, pancreatic, prostate, liver, and ovarian cancer, as well as acute myeloid leukemia, glioblastoma and melanoma, effectively inducing apoptosis in cancer cells. For example, DSF inhibits the growth of temozolomide-resistant glioblastoma (GBM) cells, (IC90 = 100 nM), but does not affect normal human astrocytes. These classically temozolomide-resistant cells were sensitive to 500 nM DSF, a sufficient concentration to suppress tumor cell growth over 72 h, and the self-renewal ability of these cells was also completely inhibited. (830, 831) Tumor-associated macrophages (TAM) affect tumor progression and resistance to chemotherapeutic agents. FROUNT is highly expressed in macrophages, and its myeloid-specific deletion impairs tumor growth. Further, DSF acts as a potent inhibitor of FROUNT and decreases macrophage tumor-promoting activity. (832)

In preclinical studies, when administered in combination with other conventional therapies, DSF exerts a synergetic therapeutic effect on cancer. According to in vivo studies, the activities of chemotherapeutic drugs such as cisplatin, temozolomide cyclophosphamide, 5-fluorouracil, sunitinib and auranofin are all potentiated by DSF. (822)

Clinical studies

In a double blind trial, 64 women with breast cancer were treated with sodium ditiocarb (diethyldithiocarbamate) or a placebo. (833) After 6 years, a significantly higher overall survival rate was observed in the ditiocarb group than in the placebo group (81 vs 55%, respectively). The disease-free survival rates were 76 and 55% in the ditiocarb and placebo groups, respectively. Ditiocarb is the main DSF metabolite in the human body that contributes to its mechanism of action.

In a phase IIb clinical trial the addition of DSF to a combination regimen of cisplatin and vinorelbine was well tolerated and appeared to prolong survival in patients with newly diagnosed non-small cell lung cancer. (834) The addition of DSF plus copper to temozolomide appears to prolong the disease-free survival in patients with glioblastoma. (835-837)

Types of cancers disulphiram may be beneficial for

DSF may be beneficial in the following cancers: breast, lung, pancreatic, prostate, liver, and ovarian cancer, as well as acute myeloid leukemia, glioblastoma, and melanoma. DSF and copper may have a particular role in patients with glioblastoma. (822, 824)

Dosing and cautions

DSF is inexpensive, and its tolerability and safety have been demonstrated over years of clinical experience with many patients. DSF is generally administered at a dose of 80 mg three times a day or 250 mg once daily, which appears to be the maximal tolerable dose. (835, 837) Copper at a dose of 2 mg three times a day should be added. (836)

13. Cimetidine

Anticancer pathways and mechanisms

Cimetidine, commonly used to treat ulcers and gastroesophageal reflux disease, has been demonstrated to have four different anti-tumor effects, namely: Anti-proliferative, immunomodulatory, anti-cell adhesion, and anti-angiogenic effects on cancer cells. (838)

Anti-proliferative: Histamine, the principal mast cell mediator, and its receptors (HR1-HR4) were increased in several malignancies and associated with cancer survival, metastasis, and recruitment of suppressive cells to the TME. Mast cells and their mediators have previously been linked with tumor progression and metastasis. (839)

L-histidine decarboxylase (HDC), an enzyme that produces histamine, is expressed by a variety of tumor types both in vitro and in vivo. Tumors are also capable of secreting large amounts of histamine in a paracrine and/or autocrine manner. Histamine has a wide range of actions, including inflammatory and immunological effects. Four histamine receptors, of which H2 and H4 are involved in cancer cell proliferation, invasion, and angiogenesis, mediate these physiological effects. By blocking H2 receptors, cimetidine reduces cancer cell proliferation.(838, 840-842) In addition, cimetidine upregulates Caspase 3 level to induce apoptosis of cancer cells and has synergistic activity when combined with vitamin C. (840)

Immunomodulation: Cimetidine has been demonstrated to kill myeloid-derived stem cells (MDSCs), decrease Tregs, and increase natural killer cells (NKs). Histamine has been linked to an immunosuppressive tumor microenvironment in cancer, which includes increased CD4+CD25+ regulatory T cell (Treg) activity, decreased dendritic cell (DC) antigen-presenting activity, decreased NK cell activity, and increased myeloid-derived suppressor cell (MDSC) activity. (838, 843, 844). MDSCs express H_1–H_3 receptors, and there is in vitro and in vivo evidence that blockade of H_1 (using the H_1RA cetirizine) or H_2 (using cimetidine), can reverse the immunosuppressive action of these cells. (838, 844) Cimetidine causes an increase in NK activity compared to non-cimetidine-treated controls in patients undergoing cardiopulmonary bypass surgery. (838, 845)

Additionally, it has been demonstrated that in patients with colorectal and gastric cancer, perioperative cimetidine reverses the histamine-induced suppression of lymphocyte proliferation and increases the number of tumor-infiltrating lymphocytes (TIL). (449, 450) Increased tumor-infiltrating lymphocytes were linked to improved prognosis in these studies and are also thought to be significant in several other cancer types, such as breast, ovarian, brain, and head and neck cancers. (838)

The heterodimeric cytokine interleukin-12, which is mostly produced by monocytes and macrophages, is a crucial inducer of cell-mediated immunity because it promotes the growth, proliferation, and activity of Th1 cells. (838) IL-12 overproduction may have a role in the etiology of autoimmune disease. Histamine binding to the H2 receptor, which is connected to the suppression of IL-12 and enhancement of IL-10 production, is associated with a shift in the Th1/Th2 balance toward Th2-dominance of the immune response. Studies showed that cimetidine prevented this effect in human peripheral blood mononuclear cells. (838, 846-848)

Anti-cell adhesion: It has been demonstrated that cimetidine inhibits cancer cells' ability to adhere to endothelial cells without affecting their H2RA activity. (838)

Anti-angiogenesis: Angiogenesis accelerates the development and progression of tumors. (840) Evidence from mouse and rat bladder cancer models suggested that the anti-angiogenic impact of cimetidine may be connected to a decreased expression of platelet-derived endothelial growth factor (PDECGF) and vascular endothelial growth factor (VEGF) via the H2R/cAMP/PKA pathway. (449, 838, 840, 849, 850) TNF-α plays a variety of roles within the TME and promotes tumor growth through several methods. Cimetidine has anti-angiogenic effects by downregulating TNF-α. (840)

Clinical studies

There is limited data on the clinical benefits of cimetidine in patients with cancer. Most of the studies have been performed in the post-operative period in patients undergoing colorectal surgery. (838) In a Cochrane meta-analysis of five studies (n=421) that prescribed cimetidine as an adjunct to curative surgical resection of colorectal cancers, a statistically significant improvement in overall survival (HR 0.53; 95% CI 0.32 to 0.87) was demonstrated. (851) In two small series of patients with melanoma, the combination of cimetidine and interferon was associated with a clinical response ranging from complete regression to partial regression and prolonged disease stabilization. (852, 853) A report from Denmark assessed overall survival of gastric cancer patients treated with oral cimetidine 400 mg twice daily for 2 years. In this double-blinded study, 181 patients were randomized to cimetidine or placebo immediately after surgery. Median survival in the cimetidine group was 450 days and 316 days in the placebo group (p = 0.02). (854) Relative survival rates (Cimetidine/placebo) were 45%/28% at 1 year.

Types of cancers cimetidine may be beneficial for

While cimetidine appears to be beneficial in patients with colorectal cancer (449, 838, 848, 855-857), melanoma (838, 858), and gastric cancer (449, 450, 838, 841, 856), this drug may have some benefit in patients with pancreatic cancer (838, 859), ovarian carcinoma (838, 860), prostate cancer (838), Kaposi's Sarcoma (838), salivary gland tumors (838, 861), renal cell carcinoma (838, 858, 862, 863), breast cancer (838, 840, 864), glioblastoma (838, 865) and bladder cancer (838, 850). Cimetidine may have a role as part of a pre-operative protocol to reduce metastases (see section under propranolol).

Dosing and cautions

Most studies used a standard dose of 400 mg twice daily. Cimetidine has few side effects, with the most frequent being gynecomastia. However, Cimetidine has a number of potentially serious drug-drug interactions by interfering with the CYP450 metabolizing enzymes; drug-drug interactions should therefore be evaluated before prescribing cimetidine. Cimetidine should not be combined with itraconazole and metformin. In addition, cimetidine should be used with caution in patients with renal and hepatic impairment.

14. Mistletoe

The European white-berry mistletoe (Viscum album L.), an evergreen plant that grows as a semi parasite on trees, has a long tradition in the treatment of cancer patients, particularly in continental Europe. A large percentage of patients with cancer use adjunctive mistletoe extracts to reduce disease- and treatment-related symptoms and to improve quality of life. (866) Mistletoe extracts are aqueous, total plant extracts from European mistletoe, manufactured and marketed as injectable drugs with indications in oncology. Mistletoe extracts are administered subcutaneously, normally two to three times per week. They may also be administered intravenously by integrative oncologists.

Anticancer pathways and mechanisms

Mistletoe extracts mediate numerous antitumor, antiapoptotic, anti-proliferative and immunomodulatory effects in models of cancer. Mistletoe contains biologically active molecules including lectins, flavonoids, viscotoxins, oligo- and polysaccharides, alkaloids, membrane lipids and other substances. (867) Although the exact pharmacological mode of action of mistletoe is not completely elucidated, there is a growing number of biological studies with a clear focus on lectins. Lectins mediate many immunological activities including increasing the natural killer cytotoxicity and the number of activated lymphocytes; they increase the antioxidant system and mistletoe stimulated the production of granulocyte-macrophage colony-stimulating factor (GMCSF), Interleukin 5 and Interferon gamma. (868, 869) Cytotoxic effects of the mistletoe extract are reported to be a result of protein synthesis interference, cell-cycle inhibition, and induced apoptosis. (870, 871) Ben-Arye et al demonstrated that mistletoe exhibited significant anti-cancer activity in cisplatin- sensitive and resistant ovarian cells and increased chemosensitivity in both cancer cell lines. (872) It has also been suggested that mistletoe has antiangiogenic properties.

Clinical studies

Over 50 prospective studies, including over 30 RCTs, have evaluated the role of mistletoe in patients with cancer. A Cochrane review published in 2008 which included 21 studies demonstrated a benefit in terms of QoL, performance index, symptom scales and reduction of adverse effects of chemotherapy. (873) In 2010 Kienle and Kiene reported the results of a systematic review assessing the effect of mistle extract on the QoL in patients with cancer. (874) This study included 26 RCTs' and 10 non-RCTS. Half of the studies investigated mistletoe concomitant with chemotherapy, radiotherapy, or surgery. Almost all the studies included in this review reported that mistletoe improved QoL. In an update meta-analysis published in 2020 Loef and Walach reported that the pooled standardized mean difference for global QoL after treatment with mistletoe extracts vs. control was SMD = 0.61 (95% CI 0.41–0.81, $p < 0{,}00001$). (867) The authors performed an additional meta-analysis evaluating the effect of mistletoe on survival in patients with cancer. (875) For RCTs, the pooled effect estimate of mistletoe on survival was HR = 0.81 (95% CI 0.69-0.95, $P = .01$). A meta-analysis which included 12 RCT demonstrated that mistletoe reduced cancer related fatigue (SMD -0.48; 95% CI -0.82 to -0.14; *p* = 0.006). (876) A phase I trial of intravenous mistletoe extract in patients with advanced cancer demonstrated a disease control rate (percentage of complete/partial response and stable disease) of 23.8% with improved indicators of QoL. (877) In summary, mistletoe is used by integrative oncologists to improve the QoL, increase the tolerability of chemotherapy, and exert a possible benefit on tumor control and survival.

Types of cancers mistletoe may be beneficial for

Mistletoe improves the QoL in patients with most cancers. Mistletoe has been used in breast cancer, bladder cancer, gynecological cancers (cervical cancer, corpus uteri cancer, and ovarian cancer), colorectal cancer, gastric cancer and pancreatic cancer, glioma, head and neck cancer, lung cancer, melanoma, and osteosarcoma.

Dosing and cautions

The limitation of mistletoe is that it is administered parenterally (subcutaneously or intravenously) and is therefore administered under the supervision of an integrative oncologist used as a component in a personalized treatment protocol. (878)

15. Ashwagandha

Anticancer pathways and mechanisms

Ashwagandha (*Withania somnifera*, WS) has been used in the Mediterranean region and Ayurvedic medicine for millennia as a functional food and a medicinal plant with anticancer activity. (879) The plant is an erect, grayish, evergreen shrub with long tuberous roots, short stems, ovate and petiolate leaves, and greenish axillary and bisexual flowers The leaves, roots, stems, and flowers bear medicinal values with 29 common metabolites derived from the leaves and root extracts. (879) Its active substances that play a crucial role in pharmacological action are withanolides and alkaloids. (880)

Preclinical studies have demonstrated the ability of this plant to regulate mitochondrial function and apoptosis and reduce inflammation by inhibiting inflammatory markers such as cytokines (including IL-6 and TNF-a), nitric oxide, and reactive oxygen species. Ashwagandha plays a major role in the induction of cancer cell apoptosis, it inhibits cell proliferation and inhibits cell migration. (880-882) In glioblastoma cells ashwagandha triggers cell cycle arrest and apoptosis. (883) In a human head and neck cell line ashwagandha showed dose-dependent growth-inhibitory activity attributed to caspase-dependent apoptosis. (884) Loss of mitochondrial membrane potential, release of cytochrome c, and activation of caspase 9 suggested that ashwagandha leads to activation of mitochondria-mediated apoptosis.

Widodo et al demonstrated cancer killing activity of ashwagandha mediated by p53, apoptosis and insulin/IGF signaling pathways linked to the ROS signaling and that the selective killing of cancer cells was mediated by induction of oxidative stress. (885) The anti-cancer effects of ashwagandha on the proliferation and migration of colorectal cell lines has been shown to be due to reduced transcriptional activity of STAT3. (886) In addition, Notch 1 and

Notch/AKT/mTOR signaling is inhibited by ashwagandha in a colon cell line. (152) In an experimental adenomatous polyposis coli model ashwagandha was associated with a 59% reduction of tumor and polyp initiation and progression. (253)

Ashwagandha has potent anti-inflammatory activity that likely has a major effect on the tumor microenvironment inhibiting angiogenesis and metastasis. In a study using the HaCaT human keratinocyte cell line, an aqueous solution from Ashwagandha root was found to inhibit the NF-KB and MAPK (mitogen-activated protein kinase) pathways by decreasing the expression of proinflammatory cytokines, including interleukin (IL)-8, IL-6, tumor necrosis factor (TNF-α), IL-1β, and IL-12, and increasing the expression of anti-inflammatory cytokines. (887)
In an vivo and in vitro model, Jawarneh et al. demonstrated that a combination of Ashwagandha extract and intermittent fasting has potential as an effective breast cancer treatment that may be used in conjunction with cisplatin. (882) The combination was found to decrease cancer cell proliferation through apoptosis induction, while also reducing cisplatin-induced toxicity in the liver and kidney.

Clinical studies
In the setting of cancer, Ashwagandha has been studied almost exclusively in experimental models, with limited clinical data regarding its clinical efficacy. Biswell et al performed an open-label prospective non-randomized comparative trial on 100 patients with breast cancer to receive either a combination of chemotherapy with Ashwagandha or chemotherapy alone.(406) *Withania somnifera* root extract was administered to patients in the study group at a dose of 2 g every 8 hours, throughout the course of chemotherapy. Patients in the treatment group had significantly less fatigue and higher quality of life scores. The 24-month overall survival for all stages in study and control group patients were 72% versus 56%, respectively; however, the result was not significant.

As discussed under the section of stress reduction and sleep *Ashwagandha* has proven to be a safe and effective adaptogen. Randomized controlled trials have shown a significant benefit in terms of stress reduction, improved cognition and mood, and quality of sleep. (395-397) A meta-analysis of 12 RCTs demonstrated that Ashwagandha supplementation significantly reduced anxiety (p = .005) and stress levels (p = .005) compared to placebo. (400) While ashwagandha has not been proven to improve the outcome of patients with cancer, because of its effects on stress reduction, sleep, and quality of life we have included this herb as a recommend therapy in patients with cancer.

Types of cancers that ashwagandha may be beneficial for
Ashwagandha may be effective against cancers such as breast, colon, lung, prostate, glioblastoma multiforme, melanoma and blood cancers. (879, 880) Ashwagandha can be used to treat cancer alone or in combination with other chemotherapeutic agents.

16. Phosphodiesterase 5 inhibitors: sildenafil, tadalafil, and vardenafil

Selective phosphodiesterase 5 inhibitors, including sildenafil, tadalafil, and vardenafil, are widely used in the treatment of erectile dysfunction and pulmonary arterial hypertension. These drugs may also be effective cancer treatments.

Anticancer pathways and mechanisms

Sildenafil treatment affects HSP90 expression, a chaperone protein that promotes degradation of PKD2, a serine threonine kinase with an important role in cancer cell proliferation and viability. (888) Sildenafil and tadalafil were shown to inhibit the development and progression of aflatoxin B1 induced hepatocellular carcinoma. (889) PDE5 inhibitors can reduce the incidence of intestinal cancer by altering epithelial homeostasis via cGMP. In a rodent model, sildenafil-treated mice showed less polyp formation with greater differentiation, less proliferation, and less inflammation. (890)

Booth et al demonstrated that PDE5 inhibitors interacted in a greater than additive fashion with numerous cytotoxic agents to cause cell death. (891) The most potent PDE5 inhibitor was sildenafil. In this study, treatment with PDE5 inhibitors and chemotherapy drugs promoted autophagy with knock out of Beclin1 reducing the drug combination lethality by about 50%. Furthermore, these authors demonstrated that celecoxib (an NSAID) and PDE5 inhibitors interacted in a greater than additive fashion to kill multiple tumor cell types including human glioma cells. (892) The effects of celecoxib were COX2 independent. The drug combination inactivated mTOR and increased the levels of autophagy and activated the JNK pathway. The combined use of platinum-based chemotherapeutic agents and PDE inhibitors have a higher antiproliferative effect on lung cancer cells than platinum monotherapy. (893) Sildenafil combined with curcumin increases the efficacy of 5-Fluorouracil in controlling colorectal tumors. (894)

Sildenafil could inhibit colonic tumorigenesis via blocking the recruitment of MDSCs. (895) Treatment with sildenafil reduced MDSC numbers infiltrating primary tumors and metastatic lesions and increased CD8+ T cells. (896) PDE5 inhibitors reduce Tregs and cancer stem cells and impair MDSC function. (896, 897) Klutzny et al demonstrated that PDE5 inhibition eliminates cancer stem cells via induction of PKA signaling. (898)

Clinical studies

In a study of 192,661 patients, the use of PDE5 inhibitors was shown to be associated with a decreased risk of developing colon cancer. (899) The use of PDE5 inhibitors is associated with a lower risk of colorectal cancer in men with benign colorectal neoplasms. (254) Two recent clinical trials, conducted among patients with head and neck squamous cell carcinoma, reported that tadalafil can enhance systematic immune responsiveness as well as tumor-specific immunity by reducing MDSCs, regulatory T cells, and improving T-cell function. (900, 901) Huang et al demonstrated that in patients with colorectal cancer, the post-diagnostic use of PDE5 inhibitors was associated with a decreased risk of cancer-specific mortality (adjusted HR = 0.82, 95% CI 0.67-0.99) as well as a decreased risk of metastasis (adjusted HR = 0.85, 95%

CI 0.74-0.98). (902) In a retrospective cohort analysis of 3100 patients with prostate cancer treated with radical prostatectomy between 2003 and 2015, patients were divided into those receiving a PDE-5 inhibitor or non-recipients (controls). In this study, multivariate analysis documented that PDE-5 inhibitor administration was associated with a lower risk of biochemical recurrence and death. (903)

Types of cancers that phosphodiesterase 5 inhibitors may be beneficial for
Prostate, breast, hepatocellular, colorectal, lung, head and neck, glioblastoma, and leukemias. (896)

Dosing and cautions
Sildenafil 20 mg daily or tadalafil 5mg daily. PDE5 inhibitors are contraindicated in patients receiving nitrates or with a previous history of non-arteritic anterior ischemic optic neuropathy. Despite its wide therapeutic window, sildenafil may show serious cardiovascular side effects in patients.

17. Itraconazole

Itraconazole is a common anti-fungal agent that was developed in the 1980s, which decreases ergosterol synthesis by inhibiting lanosterol 14α-demethylase, resulting in the destruction of the fungal membrane. (904) The anti-fungal effect of itraconazole is unlikely to be associated with its anticancer activity; which appears to be mediated by reversing chemoresistance mediated by P-glycoprotein, modulating the signal transduction pathways of Hedgehog, mechanistic target of rapamycin (mTOR) and Wnt/β-catenin in cancer cells, inhibiting angiogenesis and lymphangiogenesis, and possibly interfering with cancer-stromal cell interactions. (904)

Anticancer pathways and mechanisms
Itraconazole's anticancer mechanisms likely entail blocking the resistant protein P-glycoprotein, interfering with the tumor microenvironment, and mediating other signaling pathways linked to tumor formation. (904-906) Itraconazole prevents the growth and spread of tumor cells by blocking the abnormally active Hedgehog and Wnt/-catenin signaling pathways. (904, 905, 907-909) Itraconazole also inhibits angiogenesis, reduces the proliferation of endothelial cells, and triggers cell cycle arrest and autophagocytosis. (905, 906, 909-914) Itraconazole slows down the progression of cancer by preventing the phosphorylation of proteins in the PI3K/AKT/mTOR/S6K signaling pathway, which in turn prevents the growth and proliferation of cancer cells. (905, 909, 915) Furthermore, by inhibiting the PDGF/PI3K/Akt/mTOR pathway, itraconazole dramatically reduced angiogenesis. (905, 916)

Itraconazole binds to the sterol-sensing domain of NPC1, a lysosomal protein closely associated with cholesterol trafficking, resulting in a thorough inhibition of cell proliferation and angiogenesis. Itraconazole also directly targets the mitochondrial protein voltage-dependent anion channel 1 (VDAC1) to regulate AMP-activated protein kinase pathway and mTOR activity. (904, 905, 915, 917)

The receptor tyrosine kinase known as human epidermal growth factor receptor 2 (HER2) is a member of the HER family. (918) The HER signaling pathways involved in cell survival, proliferation, adhesion, migration, differentiation, and death are phosphoinositide-3-kinase (PI3K)/Akt signaling, protein kinase C (PKC), and mitogen-activated protein kinase (MAPK) pathway activation. (918) Itraconazole inhibits the growth of cancer cells by blocking the HER2/Akt signaling pathway. In esophageal cancer cells, it reduces the phosphorylation of downstream ribosomal protein S6, transcriptional expression of the upstream receptor tyrosine kinase HER2, and phosphorylation of upstream PI3K. (918)

Itraconazole activates the ROS pathway, which in turn activates downstream caspase and PAPR proteins, causing apoptosis. (909) This is accomplished by controlling the ratio of pro- and anti-apoptotic proteins. (909) Itraconazole also stimulates the pathway of the death receptor. It enhances the activation of the promoter caspase-8, which in turn promotes the activation of caspase-3, ultimately resulting in apoptosis, by up-regulating the production of FAS protein. (909)

Tumor growth is dependent on angiogenesis, which is driven by the secretion of growth factors from the tumor itself. Itraconazole prevents vascular endothelial growth factor/basic fibroblast growth factor-dependent angiogenesis in vivo and inhibits endothelial cell cycle progression at the G1 phase in vitro. (912, 915) Itraconazole dramatically reduces the ability of vascular endothelial growth factor (VEGF) to bind to VEGF receptor 2 (VEGFR2), preventing the activation of both VEGFR2 and phospholipase C1, a direct downstream substrate of VEGFR2. (912, 915)

Clinical studies

Itraconazole preclinical or clinical data suggested potential anticancer efficacy in single-agent or combination therapy. (905-908, 910, 911, 913, 914, 916, 919-925) Itraconazole with conventional chemotherapy (pemetrexed) significantly increased both progression-free and overall survival for lung cancer patients, according to a phase II clinical study, indicating that the drug's antiangiogenic qualities are responsible for the positive results. (905)

Retrospective studies supported the survival advantage of itraconazole treatment in refractory malignancies including ovarian clear cell, triple-negative breast, pancreatic and biliary tract cancer, as compared with the previous reports. (924-927)

In pancreatic cancer, itraconazole treatment combined with chemotherapy was conducted in progressive disease during chemotherapy. (924) A total of 38 patients received docetaxel (35 mg/m2), gemcitabine (1,000 mg/m2) and carboplatin (4 mg/min/ml) in combination with itraconazole (400 mg), following which a median OS of 11.4 months was observed. One complete response and 13 partial responses were observed, for a response rate of 37%.

In a randomized phase II clinical trial of metastatic castration-resistant prostate cancer, 46 chemotherapy-naïve patients were enrolled, of whom 29 received high-dose (600 mg/day) and 17 received low-dose (200 mg/day) itraconazole treatment. (910) Prostate-specific antigen progression free survival (PFS) rates at 24 weeks were 48.0 and 11.8% with median PFS of 11.9 and 35.9 weeks in the high-and low-dose arm, respectively.

Itraconazole exhibits concentration-dependent early anti-vascular, anti-metabolic, and anticancer effects in patients with non-small cell lung cancer (NSCLC), according to a cohort study. (919)

Types of cancers that Itraconazole may be beneficial for

Itraconazole may be helpful as an adjuvant drug in the treatment of prostate cancer, pancreatic, lung cancer, hemangioma, breast cancer, acute myeloid leukemia, basal cell carcinoma, medulloblastoma, biliary tract cancer Hepatocellular carcinoma, esophageal cancer, gastric cancer. (904, 905, 907-909, 911, 914, 918, 921, 922, 924)

Dosing and cautions

Itraconazole in a dose of 100 mg /day is recommended. The dose may be escalated to 400 mg/day however with this dosage liver function tests must be closely monitored due to hepatotoxicity. Itraconazole is a conventional antifungal drug that has received FDA approval and has an excellent safety record. (905) However, several studies have suggested that itraconazole has some contraindications, particularly when it comes to interactions with other cancer medications including rituximab, cimetidine and statins. (928, 929)

CHAPTER 8: TIER TWO REPURPOSED DRUGS – WEAK RECOMMENDATION

18. Low Dose Naltrexone (LDN)

Naltrexone is an opiate receptor antagonist preventing opiate stimulation; it has been used for decades as a treatment for addiction to opiates as it prevented the euphoria induced by recreational use of morphine and heroin. It was noted that in certain patients being treated with naltrexone for an opioid addiction many reported significant secondary benefit when being weaned off naltrexone. This group of patients had chronic inflammatory and autoimmune conditions and reported improvements whilst using the lower dosages of naltrexone. There have also been recent anecdotal reports of cancer resolution following the use of low doses of naltrexone (LDN). (930) Of note, a number of these anecdotal reports of response to LDN have been reported both administered as single agents or more usually in combination with another agent.

Anticancer pathways and mechanisms

In vivo studies performed in 1980s, highlighted the importance of dose in determining the overall effect of naltrexone as mice that were treated with clinically conventional doses of 10mg/kg induced a continuous occupancy of the opioid receptors, which was associated with increased tumor growth. (931) However, if doses were reduced to 1 or 0.1 mg/ kg, the receptor blockade was incomplete. Binding sites were thus available to exogenous opiates and endogenous endorphins, resulting in activation of their anti-tumor actions. In addition to dose, the schedule of naltrexone administration was also crucial, with intermittent administration of low-dose naltrexone achieving the greatest anti-tumor response.

LDN can influence cancer progression via three mechanisms; namely, (a) antagonism of receptors to which LDN binds, which include toll-like receptors 7-9 that lead to IL-6 suppression b) modulation of immune function in patients; and c) direct inhibition of signaling pathways involved in cancer cell control, including the priming of pro-apoptotic pathways. (930)

LDN has potent anti-inflammatory qualities, it appears to modulate and modify different elements of the immune system. *In vitro* investigations using models of individual components of immunity have described naltrexone altering the intracellular signaling in and subsequent cytokine output of immune cells. (930) In patients administered LDN, the systemic levels of cytokines that drive both humeral and cell mediated inflammation, such as G-CSF, IL-4, IL-6, IL-10, IFN-α and TNF-β, were significantly reduced after eight weeks. (932) Naltrexone can disrupt immune responses by inhibiting cytokine production by peripheral blood mononuclear cells by antagonizing TLRs. (933) More specifically, Liu et al screened a panel of available inflammation receptors and confirmed that naltrexone could completely block TLR-9 on immune cells, with some activity in TLR-7 and TLR-8. (930) Additionally, LDN is also thought to improve adaptive immune responses by enhancing the maturation of professional antigen presenting cells, as studies have shown increased expression of maturation markers on dendritic cells (DCs) following culture with LDN. (934)

Naltrexone in low doses can reduce tumor growth by interfering with cell signaling. The μ-opioid receptor (MOR) is up-regulated in several types of cancer including non-small cell lung cancer. MOR is an important regulator of cancer progression. In an in vitro model MOR overexpression increased Akt and mTOR activation, cell proliferation, tumor growth and metastases. (935) Liu et al demonstrated that the anticancer action of LDN is associated in part with changes to pERK and PI3-K signaling. (936) Tripold et al demonstrated that opioid-exposed breast cancer cells showed enhanced migration and strong STAT3 activation, which was efficiently blocked by an opiate receptor antagonist. (937) Furthermore, opioid treatment resulted in down-regulation of E-Cadherin and increased expression of epithelial-mesenchymal transition markers.

LDN is alters the balance of pro and antiapoptotic proteins that regulate cell killing. Specifically, *in vitro* and *in vivo* models show how the pro-apoptotic proteins BAX and BAD can be enhanced by a short-term exposure to LDN. (930, 938) LDN acts as an Opioid Growth Factor receptor (OGFr) antagonist and the OGF-OGFr axis is an inhibitory biological pathway present in human cancer cells and tissues, being a target for the treatment with naltrexone low-dose (LDN). (939) In an in vitro model, Ma et al demonstrated that LDN reduces tumor size by increasing levels of M1-like macrophages and activating the Bax/Bcl-2/caspase-3/PARP signaling pathway to induce apoptosis. (938)

Clinical studies

The benefit of LDN in patients with cancer is limited to several case reports and a small case series. Case reports have described the benefit of LDN in patients with lung adenocarcinoma, adenoid cystic tongue carcinoma (in combination with vitamin D3), renal cell cancer (together with Alpha Lipoic Acid (ALA)), B cell lymphoma (with ALA) and pancreatic cancer (with ALA).(940-945) Lissoni et al. report four partial responses and one stable disease in nine patients with renal cell cancer treated with IL-2 and LDN. (946) Significantly, however, these patients had disease progression when using IL-2 alone.

Types of cancers LDN may be beneficial for

LDN shows promising results for people with primary cancer of the bladder, breast, liver, lung, lymph nodes, colon, and rectum. (939)

Dosing and cautions

A dose of between 2 mg and 4.5 mg daily is suggested. Begin with 2 mg/day and increase to 4.5 mg/day. The dose should not be increased beyond 4.5mg as this paradoxically reduces the anti-inflammatory effects of LDN. Furthermore, the use of traditional doses of opiates for pain control in patients with cancer may activate oncogenic pathways. (937)

19. Doxycycline

Anticancer pathways and mechanisms

Doxycycline and minocycline were introduced into medicine as more potent, active, and stable semisynthetic tetracycline antibiotics. In general, the incidence of adverse effects caused by minocycline and doxycycline is very low. In addition, they show many non-antibiotic properties, including anti-inflammatory, antioxidant, neuroprotective, immunomodulatory, and anticancer effects. (947, 948) Recently published studies and analyses considered the repurposing of minocycline and doxycycline as anti-melanoma agents. (949, 950)

Mechanisms of the anticancer activity of doxycycline and minocycline involve reduction of STAT3 phosphorylation, prevention of NF-KB activation, repression of tumor necrosis factor (TNF) - α expression and inhibition of matrix metalloproteinases. (948, 951) Minocycline and doxycycline have been demonstrated to exert anti-melanoma effects. (949, 950) These drugs inhibited cell proliferation, decreased cell viability, and induced apoptosis. Rok et al demonstrated similar findings in amelanotic melanoma cells. (947) In this study, the treatment caused changes in the cell cycle profile and decreased the intracellular level of reduced thiols and mitochondrial membrane potential. In addition, exposure of melanoma cells to minocycline and doxycycline triggered the release of cytochrome c and activated initiator and effector caspases. In this study, doxycycline was a more potent drug than minocycline in mediating these anticancer effects.

Doxycycline blocks the activity of metalloproteinases, which would otherwise be involved in the breakdown of the extracellular matrix that allows individual cancer cells to break free and seed new metastatic cancer growth around the body. Considering the potent inhibitory effects of tetracyclines against metalloproteinases, their anticancer potential has been studied in a variety of cancers, including melanoma, lung, breast, and prostate cancers. (952) When combined with celecoxib, minocycline inhibited the osseous metastasis of breast cancer in nude (hairless) mice, by increasing tumor cell death and decreasing tumor expression of MMP-9 and VEGF. (953) Minocycline has been shown to inhibit *in vitro* invasion and experimental pulmonary metastasis in mouse renal adenocarcinoma. In addition, these drugs have been demonstrated to inhibit angiogenesis in vitro by a non-metalloproteinase-dependent mechanism. (954)

Weiler et al demonstrated that minocycline inhibited the TNF-α-induced fusion of cancer cells with breast epithelial cells; (951) this may have an important role in limited metastatic cancer spread. Minocycline has been demonstrated to act synergistically with cisplatin in the treatment of hepatocellular carcinoma. (955) Anti-proliferative and anti-metastatic properties of minocycline have also been demonstrated in various other types of cancer, including renal adenocarcinoma, (956) breast cancer, (953) and malignant gliomas. (957)

Clinical studies

Despite the numerous experimental models, there are no published reports that have investigated the clinical benefits of these drugs in patients with cancer.

Types of cancers doxycycline may be beneficial for

Despite the absence of clinical data, doxycycline may have clinical efficacy in the following cancers: melanoma, renal adenocarcinoma, breast cancer, prostate, and malignant gliomas.

Dosing and cautions

The standard dose of doxycycline is 100 to 150 mg daily. The duration of therapy in patients with cancer has not been studied; therefore, a course lasting no longer than 2 weeks is suggested. Serious adverse effects are uncommon, with the most common adverse effects being headache and nausea. Because of the effects of antibiotics on the microbiome a prolonged course of doxycycline should be avoided.

20. Spironolactone

Anticancer pathways and mechanisms

Spironolactone's primary mechanism of action in the therapy of cancer seems to be the regulation of DNA damage response. Spironolactone affects the hallmarks of immune protection, invasion, and metastasis activation, and cell death resistance. (958) Through the prevention of DNA damage repair, spironolactone also affects the genomic instability that is a contributing factor in the development of cancer. (958) Cancer cells can be made more susceptible to platinum-base substances by spironolactone. (905)

The worst kind of DNA damage is called a double-strand break (DSB). DSBs are repaired using homology-directed repair (HDR) or non-homologous end-joining (NHEJ) pathways. (959) Many malignancies have mutant or aberrantly expressed HDR pathways, and spironolactone decreases HDR activity, which limits the ability of cancer cells to survive. Additionally, spironolactone reduces the development of Rad51 foci and makes cancer cells more susceptible to substances that damage DNA, such as PARP inhibitors and cross-linking agents. (959)

Spironolactone has recently been discovered to be a DNA nucleotide excision repair (NER) inhibitor. (960) The multi-subunit complex known as transcription factor II-H (TFIIH), which is crucial for both the start of transcription and NER, contains the enzyme xeroderma pigmentosum group B (XPB). Spironolactone can prevent cancer cells from repairing DNA damage by inducing the proteolytic degradation of the TFIIH complex's (XPB) protein. (905, 960-963)

Given the crucial roles that XPB and TFIIH play in the DNA repair process, mutagenesis could result from the loss of XPB caused by spironolactone. (963) However, the negative effects of spironolactone's ability to reduce the incidence of cancer may be partially offset by its capacity to increase the death of cancer stem cells and facilitate immune identification. (961, 963)

Additionally, spironolactone can interfere with cisplatin-induced DNA crosslinks in lung cancer by inhibiting SIRT2-mediated transcription-coupled nucleotide excision repair. (905)

In patients with colon cancer, tumor metastasis and absence of NKG2D ligand (NKG2DL) expression are linked to a poor prognosis. (964) By activating the ATM-Chk2-mediated checkpoint pathway, spironolactone can increase the expression of NKG2DL in a variety of colon cancer cell lines, enhancing the removal of tumors by natural killer cells. (964) It can also up-regulate the expression of metastasis-suppressor genes TIMP2 and TIMP3, thereby reducing tumor cell invasiveness. (964)

Hepcidin is a regulating hormone produced by the liver that modifies iron fluxes to match body iron needs. Since cancer cells have abnormally high requirements for iron, starving them with iron-sequestering medications prevents the growth of tumors. (965) Hepcidin expression is primarily and most effectively stimulated by bone morphogenetic proteins (BMPs). (965) A component of cancer cells' metastatic invasion strategy seems to involve the overexpression of hepcidin by some BMPs. (965) When BMP signaling is blocked, the ability of cancer cells to spread through lymphatic and blood arteries is reduced. (965)Spironolactone inhibits the expression of hepcidin, hence preventing metastasis. (966)

Spironolactone reduces oxidative stress, cellular death, and inflammation. When spironolactone is given to PCOS mice, inflammation biomarkers such NF-kB, TNF-, and IL-6 in adipose tissues drastically decrease. (967)

Spironolactone chemosensitizers cancer cells and cancer stem cells to anticancer drugs like gemcitabine and osimertinib while suppressing the expression of survivin, an anti-apoptotic protein, at a dose that was safe for non-cancer cells. (968)

Clinical studies

Given that spironolactone is a progesterone derivative, and it has a secondary affinity for both androgen receptor and progesterone receptor, it was thought that spironolactone might have some clinical value in the treatment of prostate cancer. (958) Spironolactone dramatically decreased the incidence of prostate cancer in clinical investigations. (969-971) At first, spironolactone was said to further lower testosterone levels in men with prostate cancer who had undergone orchidectomy in the 1970s, indicating that the medication would be helpful as an adjuvant in these individuals. (958) More recently, a French case report describing the normalization of prostate-specific antigen in a patient with prior prostate cancer following spironolactone therapy was published. (958)

Researchers discovered that spironolactone exposure significantly decreased the occurrences of prostate cancer among 18,562 males with newly diagnosed heart failure (95% confidence interval 0.31-0.98, P =.043). (969) Additionally, Spironolactone is proven to be connected with a low rate of prostate cancer in a meta-analysis by Bommareddy et al.(971) Spironolactone was linked to a significantly decreased incidence of prostate cancer in a score-matched cohort analysis of 74,272 participants in the UK (hazard ratio 0.69; 95% confidence interval 0.60-0.80, P 0.001). (970)

Spironolactone can pass the blood-brain barrier because it is a lipophilic medication. (961, 972) Data shown that spironolactone has a cytotoxic effect on U87-MG glioblastoma cancer cells through a mechanism reliant on the activation of apoptosis. (961)

Types of cancer Spironolactone may be beneficial in treating.
In addition to treating prostate cancer, spironolactone may also be helpful for treating lung cancer, (905), colon cancer, (964) invasive bladder cancer, (973) glioblastoma, (961) and breast cancer. (974)

Dosing and cautions
While the optimal dose of spironolactone for the treatment of cancer is unknown, a dose of 50-100 mg/day is suggested. Potassium levels should be monitored particularly when using a higher dose and the concomitant use of other drugs that interfere with potassium elimination. There was concern that spironolactone use might raise the incidence of bladder, breast, and ovarian cancer. To date, however, the results of meta-analyses indicated that spironolactone use was not significantly linked to an increased risk of cancer and was instead linked to a lower risk of prostate cancer. (971)

21. Resveratrol

Resveratrol (3,40,5-trihydroxy-trans-stilbene) is a non-flavonoid polyphenol that occurs naturally in many species of plants, including peanuts, grapes, and berries. (528) Pterostilbene is a naturally occurring analog of resveratrol.

A significant amount of research, including preclinical, clinical, and epidemiological studies, has indicated that dietary consumption of polyphenols, found at high levels in vegetables and fruits, may prevent the evolution of an array of diseases, including cancer. (528) Resveratrol and other flavonoids (quercetin, turmeric) have numerous anticancer activities.

Anticancer pathways and mechanisms
Resveratrol has also been reported to possess a significant anticancer property in various preclinical animal models. (528) Resveratrol affects a variety of cancer stages, from initiation and promotion to progression, by affecting the diverse signal-transduction pathways that control cell growth and division, inflammation, apoptosis, metastasis, and angiogenesis. It has been shown that resveratrol has in vitro cytotoxic effects against a large range of human tumor cells, including myeloid and lymphoid cancer cells, and breast, skin, cervix, ovary, stomach, prostate, colon, liver, pancreas, and thyroid carcinoma cells. (528, 975-977)

Studies conducted in vitro have discovered that resveratrol exerts an anti-proliferative activity by inducing apoptosis. Resveratrol modifies the balance of cyclins as well as cyclin-dependent kinases (CDKs), resulting in cell cycle inhibition at G0/G1 phase. (978) Resveratrol causes activation of the p53-dependent pathway. (979) The inhibition of anti-apoptotic proteins of the

Bcl-2 family, and activation of pro-apoptotic proteins such as Bad, Bak or Bax, by resveratrol has also been shown to be a mechanism for caspase activation and cytochrome c release. (980) It has also been shown that resveratrol induces apoptosis via inhibiting the PI3K/Akt/mTOR pathway, modulating the mitogen-activated protein kinase pathway (MAPK) and inhibiting NF-KB activation. (528) Resveratrol also causes inhibition of signal transducers and activators of transcription 3 (STAT3), which adds to its pro-apoptotic and anti-proliferative potential. (981) In addition, resveratrol may inhibit cancer stem cells. (982)

Flavonoids, as antioxidants, inhibit regulatory enzymes and transcription factors important for controlling inflammatory mediators. Moreover, they modulate cellular oxidative stress by interacting with DNA and enhancing genomic stability. (748) Resveratrol also augments the activity and expression of antioxidant and phase-II detoxifying enzymes through the activation of nuclear factor E2–related factor 2 (Nrf2).

Preclinical research has demonstrated the effectiveness of flavonoids against inflammation-associated cancer progression. (748) Due to the association between inflammation and angiogenesis in tumor cells, experimental models demonstrate that flavonoids decrease angiogenesis and tumor metastasis. Resveratrol has been suggested to inhibit metastatic spread by inhibiting the expression of MMP (mainly MMP-9) and angiogenesis markers such as VEGF, EGFR, or FGF-2. (528, 983). Luteolin showed a potent capacity to target HIF-1α/VEGF signaling and angiogenesis. (529)

It has been reported that resveratrol can reverse multidrug resistance in cancer cells, and, when used in combination with clinically used drugs, it can sensitize cancer cells to standard chemotherapeutic agents. (528) In addition, it is likely that resveratrol has synergic activity against cancers when combined with GTCs.

Pterostilbene appears to be the most promising of the resveratrol analogs and significantly inhibited tumor growth, progression, local invasion and spontaneous metastasis in a mouse model of prostate cancer.(984) Studies have confirmed that pterostilbene exerts anti-proliferative and pro-apoptotic effects in various cancer cell types including lung, gastric, prostate, colon, breast cancers and CML and CLL.(985-987)

Clinical studies

Although resveratrol has shown excellent anticancer properties, most of the studies were performed in cell culture and pre-clinical models. Furthermore, resveratrol's poor bioavailability is a significant issue regarding extrapolating its effects on humans. (528) Pterostilbene may be the preferred formulation.

Types of cancers that resveratrol may be beneficial for

Resveratrol likely has anticancer effects in patients with breast, prostate, colorectal, hepatocellular, pancreatic, lung, and ovarian cancer. (528)

Dosing and cautions

Various approaches have been created to enhance the bioavailability of resveratrol, including consuming it with various foods, using it in combination with an additional phytochemical — piperine — and using a prodrug approach, micronized powders, or nanotechnological formulations. (528) A resveratrol dose of 500 mg twice daily is suggested. A bio-enhanced formulation containing trans-resveratrol from Japanese Knotweed Root appears to have improved bioavailability.

22. Wheatgrass

A wide range of health benefits have been attributed to wheatgrass, the young grass of the common wheat plant Triticum aestivum. Its components include chlorophyll, flavonoids, and vitamins C and E. Wheatgrass is also known as "green blood" because of its high chlorophyll content, i.e., 70% of its chemical composition. (988) Moreover, it has structural similarity with hemoglobin. Wheatgrass also contains the antioxidant enzymes superoxide dismutase and cytochrome oxidase that have the potential to convert reactive oxygen species to hydrogen peroxide and oxygen molecule. Forms of wheatgrass include fresh juice, frozen juice, tablets, and powders, with compositions varying according to their production processes, as well as to the growing conditions of the wheatgrass. Laboratory in vitro studies, mostly using the fermented wheat germ extract, have demonstrated anti-cancer potential and have identified apoptosis as a possible mechanism. (989) There is limited clinical data on the role of wheatgrass in patients with cancer.

In a study with colon cancer patients, after six-month supplementation of wheat germ extract to anticancer treatments, lower recurrences of metastatic disease and mortality were reported in the intervention group. (990) This open-label cohort trial compared anticancer treatments plus wheatgrass vs anticancer treatments alone. Sixty-six patients received wheatgrass supplement for more than 6 months and 104 patients served as controls. End-point analysis revealed that progression-related events were significantly less frequent in the wheatgrass group; new recurrences: 3.0 vs 17.3%, P= 0.01; new metastases: 7.6 vs 23.1%, P=0.01; deaths: 12.1 vs 31.7%, P=0.01). Survival analysis showed significant improvements in the wheatgrass group regarding progression-free (P=0.0184) and overall survivals (P=0.0278). In a controlled prospective trial of 100 patients with stage II–III colorectal cancer Avisar et al examined the effect of daily wheatgrass juice intake in addition to chemotherapy on immune parameters including IL-6, IL-8, IL-10, and IL-12 and white cell count (WBC). (991) In this study the anti-inflammatory cytokine IL-10 concentrations were significantly higher and the decline in WBC counts between was significantly lower in the wheatgrass group. The higher levels of IL-10 and the attenuating of WBC decline during chemotherapy may constitute preliminary evidence of the beneficial effects of wheatgrass on immune parameters, when given as a supplement to standard care. In a study of patients with breast cancer receiving adjuvant chemotherapy wheatgrass was associated with a reduction in neutropenic fever events and in neutropenic infections. (992)

23. Captopril

The angiotensin converting enzyme (ACE) inhibitors are used widely as antihypertensive agents, and it has been suggested that they have anti-cancer. (993) Angiotensin II, the product of ACE, has oncogenic and pro-proliferative qualities, which suggests that ACE inhibitors may have anti-cancer activity. (994) Captopril is unique among ACE inhibitors as it appears to reduce the risk of prostate cancer and possibly other cancers. (995) Liu *et al.* demonstrated that lisinopril extends the median survival time of patients with non-metastatic pancreatic ductal adenocarcinoma from 19.3 to 36.3 months. (996)

The efficacy of ACE inhibitors in reducing angiogenesis and tumor growth has been largely attributed to the overexpression of angiotensin II type I receptor (AGTR1). In fact, it has been widely studied that the overexpression of AGTR1 has been found in liver, breast, renal, pancreatic, bladder, prostate, ovarian, cervical, laryngeal, head and neck, and skin squamous cell cancer. (994) In cancer, angiotensin II up-regulates *AGTR1*, which in turn activates the extracellular signal-related kinase/protein kinase B pathways, resulting in increased VEGF production. As a result, inhibition of AGTR1 through ACE inhibitors is theorized to reduce not only VEGF but also angiogenesis and tumor growth. (994) Captopril has been demonstrated to be an inhibitor of angiogenesis and block neovascularization and may therefore play a role in decreasing metastases. (741)

In a mouse model injected with highly tumorigenic LNM35 human lung cells as xenografts captopril resulted in a significant reduction of tumor growth (58%, $P < 0.01$) and lymph node metastasis (50%, $P = 0.088$). (993) In this study captopril inhibited the viability of LNM35 cells by inducing apoptosis. The Wnt/β-catenin pathway plays an important role in tumorigenesis. Wnt signaling modulates multiple genes of the renin-angiotensin system (RAS), and Wnt inhibition can improve cancer outcomes via diverse mechanisms. Captopril induces significant down-regulation of Wnt target genes, c-myc and cyclin D1. (997) In addition, captopril's known anti-cancer effects include inhibition of matrix metalloproteinase-2 (MMP-2), an endopeptidase which selectively breaks down the extracellular matrix to promote cell migration. (998) in a rat intracranial gliosarcoma model captopril decreased gliosarcoma cell migration, mediated by reduction in MMP-2 protein expression. (998) The effect of captopril on MMP-2 may be potentiated by the addition of disulfiram as well as other repurposed drugs. (999) In a rat cirrhosis model captopril prevented fibrotic liver disease and progression toward hepatocellular carcinoma. (1000) In this model captopril suppressed the expression of pathways mediating fibrogenesis, inflammation, and carcinogenesis, including epidermal growth factor receptor (EGFR) signaling. While a number of *in vivo* and *in vitro* studies support the anticancer activity of captopril and other ACE inhibitors there are limited clinical studies to support the use of these drugs. (995, 996)

CHAPTER 9: TIER THREE REPURPOSED DRUGS - EQUIVOCAL EVIDENCE

24. Cyclooxygenase inhibitors – Aspirin (ASA) and NSAIDs (Diclofenac)

There are more than 20 different nonsteroidal anti-inflammatory drugs (NSAIDs), from six major classes determined by their chemical structures; they differ in their dose, drug interactions, and side effects. The primary effect of NSAIDs is to inhibit cyclooxygenase (COX), thereby impairing the transformation of arachidonic acid to prostaglandins, prostacyclin, and thromboxanes. COX inhibition is central to the mechanism of action of both aspirin and the non-salicylate NSAIDs.

Two related isoforms of the COX enzyme have been described, namely COX-1 and COX-2. COX-1 is expressed in most tissues but variably and is described as a "housekeeping" enzyme, regulating normal cellular processes. COX-2 is a highly regulated enzyme that is constitutively expressed in the brain, kidney, and bone. Its expression is increased during states of inflammation. The extent of enzyme inhibition varies among the different NSAIDs. The degree to which a particular NSAID inhibits an isoform of cyclooxygenase affects both its activity and toxicity.

NSAIDs have additional modes of action beyond that of COX inhibition, including Inhibition of neutrophil activation, Inhibition of the expression of inducible nitric oxide synthase (iNOS), Inhibition of the activation of nuclear factor (NF)-kappa β, and inhibition of Erk kinase activation. While there has long been an interest in the use of aspirin (ASA) and NSAIDs in chemoprevention, there is now emerging evidence that such drugs may have activity in a treatment setting.

Aspirin

Aspirin, also known as acetylsalicylic acid (ASA), is an NSAID that exhibits a broad range of pharmacologic activities, including analgesic, antipyretic, and antiplatelet properties. Low doses (typically 75 to 81 mg/day) irreversibly acetylate cyclooxygenase (COX)-1. This effect inhibits platelet generation of thromboxane A2, resulting in an antithrombotic effect. Intermediate doses (650 mg to 4 g/day) inhibit COX-1 and COX-2, blocking prostaglandin production, and have anti-inflammatory, analgesic, and antipyretic effects. High doses (between 4 and 8 g/day) are effective as anti-inflammatory agents in rheumatic disorders; however, the usefulness of aspirin at these high doses is limited by toxicity, including tinnitus, hearing loss, and gastric intolerance. ASA 325 mg daily appears to be at least as effective as 75 mg daily in terms of cardiovascular and cerebrovascular protection. Furthermore, there does not appear to be a difference in safety across the low dose range of 75-325 mg. (1001) Leukocytes, endothelial cells, mucosal cells, and vascular smooth muscle cells express COX-2. Selective targeting of COX-2 suppresses the prostaglandins, particularly prostacyclin, at sites of vascular inflammation. In cancer, the possible mechanisms by which aspirin may provide benefit range from a direct inhibitory effect on cancer cells themselves to antiplatelet effects, including reducing platelet–tumor cell interactions or reducing platelet secretion of proangiogenic and growth factors, cytokines, and chemokines. (1002) Malignant tumors within the proinflammatory and antiapoptotic tumor microenvironment have been shown to aberrantly express COX-1 and COX-2. (1003, 1004) Therefore, aspirin may exert an antitumor effect by way of a COX-related inhibition of inflammation and apoptosis. (1005) The extent of this effect would likely vary by tumor subtype; for instance, the relative expression of COX-1 and COX-2 in ovarian cancer was shown to vary by the histological grade and subtype of the cancer. (1004) In addition, COX-independent mechanisms have been suggested, including the suppression of signaling by IκB kinase β and extracellular signal regulated kinase, leading to reduced inflammation and proliferation. (1006, 1007)

Clinical studies

The Cancer Prevention Study II, published in 1991, showed a 40% reduction in colon cancer mortality associated with the regular use of aspirin in a cohort of 662,424 patients. (1008) Subsequently, two trials published in the *New England Journal of Medicine* in 2003 demonstrated clear benefits of low-dose aspirin (81 -325 mg/day) in secondary prevention of colorectal cancer. (1009, 1010) The issue becomes more complex as these trials were followed by negative studies, (1011, 1012) and in 2007 the U.S. Preventive Services Taskforce (USPSTF) recommended against the routine use of aspirin for any cancer prevention. (1013)

Shortly after the USPSTF recommendation, large meta-analyses of prospective trials of aspirin for cardiovascular disease were published, which found a clear benefit of aspirin in reducing both cancer incidence and mortality. (209, 1014) In 2016, the USPSTP reversed its position, stating that adults between the ages of 50 and 69 years would in fact derive cancer benefits from the preventive use of low-dose aspirin, defined as ≤325 mg per day. (1015) However, the benefit in patients without a history of cancer was small and outweighed by the risk of major bleeding. (1016)

This was followed by the ARRIVE trial, which was published in 2018. The ARRIVE trial enrolled nearly 13,000 patients with a mean age of 64 years. Patients in ARRIVE were randomly assigned to 100 mg of enteric-coated aspirin or placebo and followed up for an average of 5 years. Differences in cancer incidence were not significant but favored placebo. (526) Published one month later, the ASPREE trial was larger than ARRIVE and enrolled an older population, presumably at higher risk for cancer; 19,114 patients were randomly assigned to 100 mg of enteric-coated aspirin vs placebo. (1017, 1018) Surprisingly, aspirin was associated with an increase in all-cause mortality (HR, 1.14; 95% CI, 1.01-1.29), which was driven largely by an increase in deaths resulting from cancer (HR, 1.31; 95% CI, 1.10-1.56).

In the most recent USPSTF guideline, the use of aspirin was not associated with reductions in cardiovascular disease mortality or all-cause mortality. (1019) While the studies for colorectal cancer were highly heterogenous, for events occurring within the RCT periods only, low-dose aspirin had no statistically significant association with colorectal cancer incidence at 5 to 10 years of follow-up. In summary, the role of aspirin for the prevention of colorectal cancer is uncertain.

Clinical evidence supporting the role of aspirin in cancer prevention is greatest in those at high risk of colorectal cancer, as was demonstrated in the CAPP2 trial for patients with Lynch syndrome. (527) However, there is suggestive evidence in several other cancer types as well. Hepatocellular carcinoma rates were lower among patients with chronic viral hepatitis with low-dose aspirin use. (1020) The use of aspirin may be associated with a lower risk of pancreatic cancer. (1021, 1022) Until additional studies are available, the use of aspirin for cancer prevention is limited to specific high-risk patients.

The role of ASA in the treatment of cancer is equally as contradictory as for the prevention of cancer. Observational studies tend to demonstrate a survival advantage with the use of ASA; however, this benefit has not been replicated in prospective studies. In an observational study that included 70 studies with 18 different cancers, Elwood reported aspirin to be associated with a 20% reduction in cancer deaths (HR of 0.79; 95% confidence intervals: 0.73- 0.84). (1023) Wang et al evaluated 13 published cohort studies with 65,768 patients in order to estimate the overall risk of cancer-specific mortality associated with post-diagnosis low-dose aspirin use.(1024) The authors reported a significant decreased cancer-specific mortality with an odds ratio (OR) of 0.84 (95% CI 0.75-0.93). However, these findings have not been replicated in prospective clinical trials. (1025, 1026) The ABC trial was a randomized, phase III, double-blind placebo-controlled trial of aspirin as adjuvant therapy for high-risk, HER2-2 negative breast cancer. In this study, 3,021 patients were randomized to 300 mg aspirin or placebo daily for 5 years. (1026) The HR for invasive disease-free survival comparing aspirin to placebo was 1.27, which exceeded the prespecified HR of futility.

A011502 was a RCT conducted in the United States and Canada with 3020 participants who had high-risk nonmetastatic breast cancer. (1027) Participants were randomized to receive 300 mg of aspirin (n = 1510) or placebo once daily (n = 1510) for 5 years. The study was closed after the first interim analysis due to futility. All invasive disease–free survival events, including death, invasive progression, and new primary events, were numerically higher in the aspirin group, although the differences were not statistically significant. There was no difference in overall survival (hazard ratio, 1.19; 95% CI, 0.82-1.72).

NSAIDS (Diclofenac)

Diclofenac (DCF) is a well-known and widely used non-steroidal anti-inflammatory drug (NSAID), with a range of actions of interest in an oncological context. (1028) There is considerable variation in COX-1/COX-2 selectivity between different NSAIDs, and some evidence that DCF binds to COX-2 via a different mechanism than other commonly used drugs.(1029) DCF was developed by Ciba-Geigy and is now available globally as a generic medication. Common trade names include Voltaren, Voltarol, Cataflam, Cambia, Zipsor, and Zorvolex. In some countries, low-dose formulations of oral DCF (typically 25 mg tablets) are available over the counter. In the U.S., DCF requires a prescription and is available as 25, 50, 75, and 100 mg delayed-release tablets.

DCF, which is a potent inhibitor of COX-2 and prostaglandin E2 synthesis, displays a range of effects on the immune system, the angiogenic cascade, chemo- and radio-sensitivity, and tumor metabolism. PGE2 are found in a range of different cancer types and are associated with the chronic inflammation that is found in a pro-tumor microenvironment. (1030)

Anticancer pathways and mechanisms

There are multiple mechanisms of action postulated to explain the diverse anticancer effects of DCF. These include anti-angiogenic, immunomodulation, pro-apoptotic, effect on platelet function, effects on Myc and glucose metabolism, and increasing treatment sensitivity. In addition, NSAIDs are associated with phosphodiesterase (PDE) 5 inhibition and activation of cGMP signaling which are closely associated with its ability to induce apoptosis of tumor cells. (1031)

Experimental models demonstrate DCF decrease in tumor angiogenesis, which was associated with a reduction of PGE2 synthesis. (1032) One mechanistic explanation is that PGE2 upregulates the production of VEGF. (1033) In experimental models, DCF decreased the expression of both VGEF and monocyte chemoattractant protein (MCP-1). (1034) PGE2 has been shown to induce the differentiation of bone marrow stem cells into MDSCs in a number of animal models of cancer. Decreases in PGE2 break the positive feedback loop of PGE2-MDSC expansion. (1035) It has been shown in autochthonous tumor models that blockade of PGE2 synthesis results in the downregulation of ARG1 expression and ROS production by MDSCs, followed by improved antitumor T-cell function and cancer chemoprevention. (1036, 1037)

Fujita and colleagues showed that in a mouse model of glioma, COX-2 blockade inhibited PGE2 production and delayed tumor progression. (1038) This was associated with reduced accumulation of MDSCs and an increased presence of cytotoxic T lymphocytes. Reduction of tumor-induced PGE2 using both selective and non-selective COX inhibitors has been shown to reduce T-reg populations and activity. (1039) DCF was able to reduce the intra-tumoral accumulation and activation of T-regs in a murine glioblastoma model. (1040) In addition to modulation of angiogenesis and immune suppression, there is some evidence for a pro-apoptotic mechanism of action for DCF in cancer. (1028, 1041) There is also some evidence that DCF has an impact on tumor metabolism that is independent of its action as a COX-inhibitor. Gottfried and colleagues showed that DCF downregulated Myc gene expression and glucose metabolism in a number of leukemia, prostate cancer, and melanoma cell lines in vitro and in an in vivo melanoma model. (1042)

Dysregulation of Wnt β-catenin/Tcf signaling pathway contributes to tumor progression. Sareddy et al demonstrated that diclofenac and celecoxib are potential therapeutic agents against glioblastoma cells by suppressing the activation of Wntβ-catenin/Tcf signaling. (1043) It is likely that DCF act synergistically with convention chemotherapeutic agents as well as with other adjunctive therapies. Indeed, Gerhofer demonstrated synergistic anti-migratory and anti-proliferative effects of the combined treatment with metformin and diclofenac on brain tumor initiating cells. (1044)

Clinical studies

In contrast to the wide range of in vitro and in vivo results, there is a relative paucity of clinical data with respect to the use of DCF as an anticancer agent. Forget and colleagues reported on a retrospective analysis of breast cancer patients treated with conservative surgery, with and without intraoperative NSAIDs (DCF or ketorolac). (446) Patients treated pre-incisionally with ketorolac (20 mg -30 mg) or DCF (75 mg) showed improved disease-free survival (HR = 0.57, 95% CI: 0.37–0.89, *P* = 0.01) and an improved overall survival (HR = 0.35, CI: 0.17–0.70, *P* = 0.03), compared to patients not treated with NSAIDs. (447) The findings of this study were, however, not replicated in a prospective RCT. (448)

Types of cancers diclofenac may be beneficial for

While there is limited data, diclofenac may be effective against the following tumors; (1028) desmoid tumors, inflammatory myofibroblastic tumors, neuroblastoma, osteosarcoma, head and neck cancers, esophageal cancer, breast cancer, ovarian cancer and non-small cell lung cancer.

Dosing and cautions

A dose of 75 to 100 mg/day diclofenac is suggested. As a potent COX2 inhibitor, DCF can increase the risk of peptic ulcer disease. For this reason, we suggest that DCF be combined with cimetidine, which is used to treat/prevent peptic ulcers; this drug combination likely has synergistic anticancer properties. NSAIDs cause an increased risk of serious cardiovascular thrombotic events, including myocardial infarction and stroke, which can be fatal. Diclofenac is contraindicated in the setting of coronary artery bypass graft surgery. DCF should be used cautiously in patients with known coronary artery disease; however, interventions that manage metabolic syndrome (and optimize the TG/DHL ratio) may mitigate this risk.

25. Nigella sativa

Anticancer pathways and mechanisms

The primary bioactive substance in Nigella sativa, thymoquinone (TQ), has anti-inflammatory and chemotherapeutic properties and can limit cell proliferation, increase cancer cell death, prevent cell invasion and metastasis, and inhibit angiogenesis. TQ disrupts the phosphorylation and subsequent activation of a few upstream tyrosine kinases (such as MAPK, Akt, mTOR, and PIP3) implicated in signaling pathways for tumor cell growth. (1045-1047)

TQ's anticancer effects predominantly involve the nuclear factor (NF)-κB, phosphoinositide 3 kinases (PI3K)/Akt, Notch, transforming growth factor (TGF)-β, c-Jun N-terminal kinase (JNK), and p38 mitogen-activated protein kinase (MAPK) signaling pathways as well as the regulation of the cell cycle, matrix metallopeptidase (MMP)-9 expression, and pyruvate kinase isozyme type M2 (PKM2) activity. (1045, 1046, 1048-1052) Additionally, TQ exhibits chemopreventive properties by upregulating cytoprotective enzymes (such as glutathione S-transferase, superoxide dismutase, and oxidoreductase), downregulating carcinogen metabolizing enzymes (such as CYP 1A2, CYP 3A4), and attenuating the production of pro-inflammatory mediators (e.g., cytokines, chemokines, and prostaglandins). (1046, 1048, 1053)

Clinical studies

Unfortunately, there are no published clinical studies that have investigated the effects of Nigella sativa in patients with cancer.

Types of cancers that Nigella sativa may be beneficial for

In vitro and in vivo experimental findings suggest that Nigella sativa may have anticancer action against a variety of malignancies, including ovarian, (1046, 1054, 1055) myeloblastic leukemia and other blood cancers, (1056) cervical, (1047, 1057, 1058) colon, (1047, 1053, 1059-1061) hepatic, (1053, 1062-1065) prostate, (1045, 1066) breast, (1045, 1059, 1061) renal, (1047, 1067) pancreatic, (1045, 1052, 1068) and lung carcinomas. (1045, 1059, 1069, 1070)

Dosing and cautions

Patients can be directed to take seeds (80 mg/kg once daily) or encapsulated oil (400 to 500 mg twice daily). The safety of Nigella sativa in pregnancy has not been established and it should probably be avoided.

26. Ganoderma lucidum (Reishi) and other medicinal mushrooms

More than 50 different types of mushrooms — such as Ganoderma lucidum (Reishi), G. tsugae, Sparassis crispa, Pleurotus tuberregium, P. rhinoceros, Trametes robiniophila Murill, Coriolus versicolor, Lentinus edodes, Grifola frondosa, Flammulina velutipes and others —have produced potential immunoceuticals with anticancer and immunomodulatory effects in vitro, in vivo, and in human malignancies. (1071)

The most research has been done on G. lucidum (Reishi). Beta-glucan polysaccharides and triterpenes are the bioactive compounds in Reishi mushroom. (1072)

Anticancer pathways and mechanisms

Antroquinonol, cordycepin, hispolon, lectin, krestin, polysaccharide, sulfated polysaccharide, lentinan, and Maitake D Fraction are the main anticancer compounds found in mushrooms. (1071) The therapeutic effects of these compounds include suppression of cancer cell growth, induction of autophagy and phagocytosis, improved immune system response, and induction of apoptotic cell death through upregulation of pro-apoptotic factors and downregulation of anti-apoptotic genes. (1073) The expression of caspase-3, -8, and -9, AKT, p27, p53, BAX, BCL2, NF-kB pathway, and mTOR (1074) were significantly implicated in these activities. (1073, 1075)

Bioactive substances derived from mushrooms stimulate and/or regulate the immune system by influencing the maturation, differentiation, and proliferation of immune cells, hence preventing the spread and growth of cancer cells. (1072) The strongest anticancer and immunomodulatory chemicals found in mushrooms are polysaccharides. (1072) By attaching to pathogen recognition receptors, chemicals produced from mushrooms stimulate immune cells to cause either cell-mediated or direct cytotoxicity in cancer cells. (1072, 1076, 1077) In addition, mushroom-derived compounds induce innate and adaptive immunity by enhancing immune surveillance against cancer by affecting monocytes, macrophages, NK cells, and B cells (1072, 1075-1080) which leads to cancer cell apoptosis, cell cycle arrest, and prevention of angiogenesis and metastasis. (1071) Consumption of mushroom compounds also boosts the secretion of antitumor cytokines by Directed Cytotoxic T Lymphocytes (CTLs) and activation of immune organs, thereby eliminating cancer cells and strengthening the weakened immune system. (1072, 1078)

By controlling a single molecule of a particular signaling pathway or by having many targets in the same or different signaling route(s), such as the PI3K/Akt, Wnt/-catenin, and MAPK pathways, mushroom compounds exhibit anticancer potential. Studies have demonstrated the effectiveness of components derived from mushrooms as standalone and adjunctive treatment agents in reversing multidrug resistance (MDR) by focusing on interactions between PD-1/PD-L1 and CTLA-4/CD80. (1072) Furthermore, the prebiotic benefits of medicinal mushrooms may help restore the gut microbiome. (1072)

A new, inflammatory type of programmed cell death called pyroptosis is defined by the executive protein gasdermin creating pores in the plasma membrane, which causes the cells to lyse and expel their contents. (1078, 1081) By activating caspase 3 and further cleaving the gasdermin E (GSDME) protein to create pores on the cell membrane, Ganoderma lucidum extract (GLE) causes pyroptosis, which releases many inflammatory factors into breast cancer cells. (1078) GLE blocks multi-steps of tumor metastasis including adhesion, migration, invasion, colonization, and angiogenesis. (1078)

Clinical studies

In a trial of patients with colorectal adenomas, a water-soluble Reishi extract (1.5 g/d, administered for 12 months) significantly reduced the number and overall size of adenomas in the intervention group as compared to the control group. (1082) G. lucidum (Reishi) at a dose of 5.4 g/day was demonstrated to have immuno-modulating properties in patients with advanced colorectal cancer. (1083) Patients with advanced-stage cancer who consumed a Reishi polysaccharide preparation showed increased natural killer cell activity. (1084) In a review of the literature, Huber et al reported that medicinal mushrooms improve the quality of life during and after conventional cancer therapy. (1085)

Types of cancers that Reishi and other medicinal mushrooms may be beneficial for

Noteworthy that mushroom extracts have the strongest anticancer effects against breast cancer. (1071, 1072, 1086) Mushrooms may also have activity against colorectal carcinoma, (1071, 1072, 1074, 1085, 1086) cervical, ovarian and endometrial cancers, (1071, 1085, 1086) lung cancer, (1071, 1085) astrocytoma, (1086) bladder cancer, (1071, 1086) esophageal cancer, (1086) fibrosarcoma, (1086) gastric cancer, (1071, 1086) glioblastoma, (1086) hepatocellular carcinoma, (1071, 1072, 1086) kidney cancer, (1086) laryngeal cancer, (1086) leukemia, (1071,

1086) melanoma, (1072, 1086) neuroblastoma, (1086) oral cancer, (1086) pancreatic cancer, (1086) prostate cancer, (1071, 1086) sarcoma, (1086) and skin epidermoid cancer. (1086)

Dosing and cautions
It is suggested that 6 to 12 g of Reishi extract be taken daily. (1087) Reishi has antiplatelet properties; hence it may increase the risk of bleeding, especially when taken in conjunction with anticoagulants.

27. Dipyridamole

Anticancer pathways and mechanisms
Dipyridamole is a vasodilator and antithrombotic drug. Its major effects involve the blocking of nucleoside uptake and phosphodiesterase inhibition, leading to increased levels of intracellular cAMP. Dipyridamole is a non-selective phosphodiesterase 5 inhibitor. (896) Several studies have shown that, in vitro, dipyridamole can significantly increase the cytotoxic and antitumor activities of a variety of chemotherapeutic agents. (1088) Furthermore, there is evidence for a contribution of platelets in metastasis formation with platelets interacting with tumor cells to form aggregates. The interaction of cancer cells with platelets leads to platelet activation and the pro-metastatic activities of platelets. (1089) Consequently, agents that interfere with platelet aggregation could prevent tumor metastases. (1090)

In a murine triple negative breast cancer model dipyridamole significantly reduced primary tumor growth and metastasis formation. (1088) In this study dipyridamole effects were mediated by Wnt, ERK1/2-MAPK and NF-kB pathways. Moreover, dipyridamole significantly decreased the infiltration of tumor-associated macrophages (TAM) and myeloid-derived suppressor cells (MDSC) in the primary tumors. Molecular chaperone HSP90 has been considered a promising target for anticancer drug development. Dipyridamole inhibits the growth and proliferation of human cancer cells by downregulating cell cycle regulators and upregulating apoptotic cell signaling, which are mediated by the binding of dipyridamole to HSP90 and phosphodiesterase. (1091)

Clinical studies
Dipyridamole has been used in combination with cytotoxic drugs in a number of small clinical trials. (1092-1095) The benefit or lack thereof of dipyridamole in these studies is difficult to ascertain.

28. High-dose Intravenous Vitamin C

The use of high-dose vitamin C for the treatment of cancer dates back to the 1970s, largely due to the work of Nobel laureate Linus Pauling. (1096) In the early 1970s, Cameron and Pauling published a thesis claiming that ascorbic acid is able to potentiate the intrinsic production of serum physiological hyaluronidase inhibitor, thereby protecting against the spreading of cancer cells. (1097) In 1976, these authors published the results of an observational case-control study in which 100 terminal cancer patients were given supplemental ascorbate (10 g IV for 10 days then 10 g orally) as a part of their routine management and were compared to 1,000 matched controls. (1098) The study showed that the mean survival time was more than four times longer for the ascorbate-treated subjects. In response to the data obtained by Cameron and Pauling, Creagan et al conducted in 1979 a randomized, controlled double-blind trial to evaluate the effect of vitamin C (10 g daily by oral route) on the severity of symptoms and survival rate in 123 patients with advanced and preterminal cancer. (1099) The study proved a lack of vitamin C effect, with no difference in survival time between ascorbate and control groups. Similarly, Moertel et al. in a double-blind placebo-controlled study with 100 advanced colorectal cancer patients failed to demonstrate a benefit of vitamin C (10 g orally). (1100)

The studies by Creagen et al and Moertel et al essentially ended the use of vitamin C for cancer at that time. It should, however, be appreciated that these studies used oral vitamin C and therefore did not replicate the work of Cameron and Pauling. It has subsequently been established that vitamin C is absorbed by the gut through vitamin C transporters that are saturated at a dose of about 500 mg.

In 2004 Padayatty et al demonstrated that 1.25 g vitamin C given orally produced a peak concentration of 180 umol/l where the same dose given IV resulted in a peak plasma concentration of about 1,000 umol/l. (1101) In this study, 50 g of vitamin C given intravenously produced a peak serum concentration of 12 mmol/l. It has subsequently been demonstrated that millimolar concentrations of vitamin C are toxic to cancer cells and that such concentrations can only be achieved through intravenous administration. (1102-1105)

Vitamin C has potent antioxidant effects when given orally, however, the millimolar concentration achieved with intravenous vitamin C has pro-oxidant effects, which are largely responsible for the cytotoxic effects on cancer cells. (441) While liposomal vitamin C is widely touted to produce serum levels similar to intravenous use, this contention is false, with liposomal formulations producing serum levels almost identical to that of regular vitamin C given orally. (1106-1109)

Animal and in vitro studies have indicated that free radicals such as reactive oxygen species can cause cellular damage and lead to cancer by altering cellular regulatory pathways. Vitamin C is an antioxidant that can prevent ROS-induced cellular damage. However, the efficacy of vitamin C supplements for prevention of cancer is controversial. Lee et al performed a meta-analysis of RCTs to investigate the efficacy of vitamin C supplements for prevention of cancer. (1110) Seven trials which enrolled 62,619 participants were included in this analysis. The demonstrated no association between vitamin C supplementation and cancer (relative risk, 1.00; 95% confidence intervals, 0.95–1.05). Similarly, subgroup meta-analysis by dose of vitamin C administered singly or in combination with other supplements demonstrated no reduction in the risk of cancer.

Anticancer pathways and mechanisms

Benade et al were the first to propose that the main cytotoxic mechanism of ascorbate was connected with intracellular generation of hydrogen peroxide (H_2O_2) produced upon oxidation of vitamin C. (1111) This occurs because cancer cells selectively take up more ascorbate compared to normal cells through the facilitated transport with participation of glucose transporters (GLUTs) due to an increased metabolic need for glucose. Catalase decomposes H_2O_2 to oxygen and water. Catalase activity in cancer cells is 10- to 100-fold lower than in normal cells, making them over-sensitive to ascorbate. (1111)

Yun et al reported that cultured human colorectal cancer cells with KRAS or BRAF mutations were selectively killed when exposed to high concentrations of vitamin C, and that effect resulted from an increased dehydroascorbate (DHA) uptake via the GLUT1 glucose transporter.(1112) Inside the cell, DHA is reduced by GSH, NADH, and NADPH-dependent enzymes leading to the depletion of glutathione, thioredoxin, and NADPH, thus increasing the intracellular oxidative stress. ROS accumulation inside cells inactivates glyceraldehyde 3-phosphate dehydrogenase (GAPDH), which leads to a decreased formation of glycolytic adenosine 5'-triphosphate (ATP) and pyruvate, causing an energetic crisis that triggers cell death. (1112) In experimental rodents after parenteral administration of vitamin C, not only the increased production of H2O2 was observed, but also the altered expression of genes involved in protein synthesis, cell cycle progression and angiogenesis, and reduced levels of HIF-1 and VEGF. (1096)

Clinical studies

While case reports of complete cancer remission or reduction in metastatic lesions have been reported, (1113-1115) case series which have administered high-dose IVC as a single anticancer treatment have not demonstrated beneficial results. (1096, 1116, 1117)

In vitro and animal studies have demonstrated that concomitant administration of vitamin C with many chemotherapeutic agents and radiotherapy works synergistically, resulting in a decreased tumor size and increased survival. (1118) These findings have not been reproduced in the small clinical trials conducted to date. (1096, 1119, 1120) In a phase III RCT, high-dose vitamin C plus chemotherapy failed to show superior progression-free survival compared with chemotherapy in patients with metastatic colorectal cancer as first-line treatment. (1121) In summary, high-dose intravenous vitamin C represents a promising and inexpensive anticancer therapeutic option that currently has limited supportive clinical data but should be further explored in clinical trials.

Dosing and cautions

High-dose IV vitamin C is considered to have a relatively good safety profile providing that appropriate precautions are taken, although it also can cause serious side effects in some patients. (1096) Vitamin C in gram doses is contraindicated in patients with glucose-6-phosphate dehydrogenase (G6PD) deficiency, due to a risk of developing intravascular hemolysis.

29. Dichloroacetate (DCA)

The Warburg effect is mediated in part by cancer cells inactivating a key enzyme complex called the pyruvate dehydrogenase complex (PDC), which acts as the control point for the entry of pyruvate into the mitochondria. Pyruvate is derived from glucose (glycolysis) and is the main fuel for mitochondrial oxidative phosphorylation. The mitochondrial PDC irreversibly decarboxylates pyruvate to acetyl coenzyme A, thereby linking glycolysis to the tricarboxylic acid cycle and a defining step in cellular bioenergetics. (1122) Cancer cells turn off PDC by upregulating pyruvate dehydrogenase kinase (PDK). Inhibition of PDC in the cancer cell is the key step in metabolic reprogramming.

The glycolysis inhibitor dichloroacetate (DCA) inhibits PDK. The inhibition of PDK by DCA results in diminished glycolysis in the cancer cell, forcing the cancer cell to use oxidative phosphorylation in the mitochondria as the main source of ATP. (1122, 1123) DCA has other anticancer effects, including the induction of protective autophagy, reduction of hypoxia-inducible factor (HIF-1) and angiogenesis, and eradication of cancer stem cells. (1122) Metformin, curcumin, fenbendazole, ivermectin, and doxycycline act synergistically to increase the efficacy of DCA. (727, 1124) Both thiamine and alpha lipoic acid are cofactors for PDC and are routinely recommended with DCA.

Clinical studies

A phase II study of dichloroacetate in combination with chemoradiotherapy for unresected, locally advanced head and neck squamous cell carcinoma reported an end-of-treatment complete response rate that was significantly higher in the DCA group compared to placebo (71.4% vs 37.5%, p=0.03); however, survival outcomes were not significantly different between groups. (1125) Case reports have demonstrated "long-term stabilization" of patients with metastatic melanoma, colon cancer, and non-Hodgkin's lymphoma treated with DCA. (1126-1128)

Types of cancers dichloroacetate may be beneficial for

Non-Hodgkin's lymphoma, colorectal cancer, endometrial cancer, breast cancer, glioblastoma, lung cancer, pancreatic cancer, gastric cancer, hepatocellular cancer, and multiple myeloma.

Dosing and cautions

An oral dose of 1,000 mg daily or 500 mg three times daily has been recommended. Neurotoxicity is a well-known reversible adverse effect of DCA, with peripheral neuropathy the most common symptom. Severe encephalopathy has also been described, (1129) suggesting that patients being treated with DCA be closely monitored.

DCA is available as a dietary supplement, though its use as a compounded medication has been discontinued by the FDA based upon a review in which it determined that there was insufficient evidence for its use in cancer. The Agency expressed the view that the evidence of benefit and concerns about potential toxicity if not properly dosed, did not outweigh the evidence favoring the use of approved chemotherapies or other agents for cancer.

30. Sulforaphane

Anticancer pathways and mechanisms

Epidemiologic studies suggest that cruciferous vegetable intake may lower overall cancer risk, including colon and prostate cancer. Sulforaphane (SFN) is an isothiocyanate found in cruciferous vegetables and is especially high in broccoli and broccoli sprouts.

The three major anti-cancer properties of sulforaphane include anti-angiogenesis, anti-metastatic and activation of protective autophagy. (1130) Sulforaphane inhibits HIF-1, NF-KB and proto-oncogene myc, resulting in the downregulation of key angiogenic and metastatic regulators, vascular endothelial growth factor (VEGF) and matrix metallopeptidase 9 (MMP-9) and thus the reduction of angiogenic and metastatic potential. (1130) *In vitro* experiments with sulforaphane indicate a pronounced role for cell cycle arrest in its anticancer properties. (1131) Sulforaphane and its metabolites act as histone deacetylase (HDAC) inhibitors.(1131)

In a breast cancer mouse model sulforaphane was shown to be highly potent for the elimination of cancer stem cells. (1132, 1133) Sulforaphane was demonstrated to inhibit pancreatic cancer stem cells by inhibition of the sonic hedgehog pathway. (1134) In preclinical in vitro and in vivo studies sulforaphane has shown activity against various cancer stem cells, including, triple negative breast cancer stem cells, lung, gastric and chronic leukemia stem cells.(1135-1137) Sulforaphane has synergistic anti-cancer activity with quercetin and EGCG.(1138, 1139)

Clinical studies

While the anticancer activity of sulforaphane has been established in many experimental models, clinical studies evaluating efficacy are limited. Cipolla performed a double-blind RCT in 78 males with rising PSA after radical prostatectomy for prostate cancer.(1140) Treatment consisted of 60 mg sulforaphane for 6 months over which time the sulforaphane group had a mean increase in PSA of 0.01 ng/ml compared to a 0.62 ng/ml increase for placebo. PSA doubling time in the sulforaphane group was 28.9 months compared to 15.5 months for the placebo group. Sulforaphane prolonged PSA doubling time, thus delaying "biochemical recurrence". These findings were not replicated in men with metastatic prostate cancer.(1141)

Dosing

The pharmacology and optimal dosing of sulforaphane are complex. Sulforaphane itself is unstable. The supplement should contain the two precursors, *glucoraphanin* and *myrosinase*, which react when the supplement is consumed. Broccoli "extracts" are produced in a way that completely destroys the activity of the myrosinase enzyme. As such, these extracts are incapable of producing sulforaphane when consumed in a supplement or food. (1142, 1143) We recommend a 100% whole broccoli sprout powder, which maximally retains both glucoraphanin and myrosinase whilst, at the same time, deactivating the inhibitors.

31. Artemisinin

Anticancer pathways and mechanisms

Artesunate (ART) is a derivative of artemisinin, the active principle of the Chinese herb Artemisia annua L. Artesunate is approved for the treatment of multidrug-resistant malaria and has an excellent safety profile. It has been shown that Artesunate, apart from its anti-malarial activity, has cytotoxic effects on a number of human cancer cell lines, including leukemia, colon cancer and melanoma. Artemisinin and its derivatives have been reported effective against 55 cancer cell lines with inhibitory effects against pancreatic cancer, osteosarcoma, lung cancer, colon, melanoma, breast, ovarian, prostate, central nervous system, lymphoma, leukemia and renal cancer cells. In addition, artesunate potentiates the effects of common chemotherapy drugs. (1144) A number of compounds such as resveratrol, pterostilbene, curcumin and high dose IV vitamin C have synergistic activity with artemisinin. (1145-1147)

The molecular mechanism by which artemisinin compounds serve as effective anti-cancer agents can be found in a feature of its molecular structure, the endoperoxide bridge, which reacts with the iron molecule producing a Fenton reaction, in which reactive oxygen species are generated. (146) These endogenously formed reactive species attack proteins, RNA and DNA, inducing oxidative DNA lesions such as 8-oxo-guanine and DNA double-strand breaks (DSBs). The rapid metabolic rate and rapid proliferation of cancer cells requires a large amount of iron.(1148) Cancer cells express high levels of transferrin receptors needed for internalization.(1144)The more aggressive the tumor, the greater the number of transferrin receptors.(1149) The higher iron content of cancer cells as compared to normal cells results in selective killing of cancer cells.

Artemisinin enters the cancer cell lysosome, which already contains iron as a degradation product from ferritin. The endoperoxide oxygen bridge in artemisinin with iron causing a "Fenton Reaction" producing hydroxyl radicals.(1150) Artemisinin enters cancers cells along with iron loaded ferritin. Both enter the lysosome, which then triggers ROS in mitochondria and caspase-3 programmed cell death. Artemisinin arrests the cell cycle and induce not only iron-dependent cell death (ferroptosis) but also other modes of cell death such as apoptosis. (1151) The cell death mode of ferroptosis is completely different from cell necrosis, autophagy, and apoptosis in terms of cell morphology, genetics, and biology. Artesunate is also an inducer of autophagy. Artesunate exerts antiproliferative effects by activating the ROS-triggered AMPK-mTOR axis.

Clinical studies

Artesunate administered at a dose of 200 mg per day orally was reported in a case series of 12 patients with glioblastoma.(1151) In this case series 4 patients showed a median survival of 46 months. A number of small phase I/II studies and case reports have been reported in patients with metastatic breast cancer as well as other solid tumors.(1152-1155) In a small single center, randomized, double-blind, placebo-controlled trial patients planned for curative resection of biopsy confirmed single primary site colorectal cancer were randomized (n = 23) to receive preoperatively either 14 daily doses of oral artesunate (200 mg) or placebo.(1156) The primary outcome measure was the proportion of tumour cells undergoing apoptosis. Apoptosis of greater than 7% was seen in 67% and 55% of patients in artesunate and placebo groups. During a median follow up of 42 months 1 patient in the artesunate and 6 patients in the placebo group developed recurrent CRC.

Dosing and Drug Availability

Generally, a dose of 200 mg orally daily is suggested. Anecdotal cases of hepatotoxicity, bone marrow suppression and cerebellar dysfunction have been reported; patients should be monitored for these side effects. The use of oral artemisinin-based monotherapies is considered to be a major factor contributing to the development of malarial resistance to artemisinin derivatives. The WHO has therefore urged the regulatory authorities to halt the production and marketing of oral monotherapy. Oral medication may therefore be scarce. Although IV artesunate 60 mg vials are widely used as first line malaria treatment in third world areas, inside the us this drug is neither DFA approved nor commercially available.(146)

32. Cannabinoids

Cannabis has been used as a healing herb since ancient times and is currently approved in many countries for recreational and medicinal use. There has been extraordinary public interest in the use of cannabis and cannabinoids for the treatment of cancer and cancer-related side effects. The prevalence of cannabis use in patients with a variety of malignant diagnoses ranges from 18% to 40% in surveys conducted in the U.S., Canada, and Israel. (1157) Despite the public enthusiasm for the efficacy of cannabinoids in treating cancer, the evidence supporting the use of cannabinoids is contradictory and controversial. (1158)

The *Cannabis sativa* plant contains over 400 different chemical compounds. Over 100 of these are 21-carbon terpenophenolic cannabinoids. Delta-9-tetrahydrocannabinol (THC), the main psychoactive component, is found in the highest concentration in the resin exuded from the flowers of the female plant. Dronabinol and nabilone are delta-9-THC medications that have been licensed and approved for the treatment of chemotherapy-induced nausea and vomiting since 1986.

Two cannabinoid receptors have been identified in the human body — CB1 and CB2. These are 7-transmembrane domain G-protein coupled receptors. (1157) The CB1 receptor is one of the most densely populated receptors in the human brain. The CB2 receptor was initially detected in macrophages and the marginal zone of the spleen, with a high concentration in B lymphocytes and natural killer cells. The receptors have been identified in all animal species. Animals have these receptors not because they were meant to use cannabis, but because, like endogenous opioids, endogenous cannabinoids also exist. It has been suggested that the reason for the existence of the system of endocannabinoids and cannabinoid receptors is to facilitate the modulation of pain.

Orally ingested cannabis has low (6–20%) and variable bioavailability. (1158) When inhaled, cannabinoids are rapidly absorbed into the bloodstream (with a peak concentration of about 2 to 10 minutes, declining rapidly for 30 minutes) and minimally generate the psychoactive 11-OH metabolite. Smoking remains the most common and fastest route of administration and is especially helpful for the treatment of acute symptoms. There are many medications based on natural or synthetic cannabinoids or cannabinoid analogs. (1158) Dronabinol (Marinol®, Mariette GA) is a 9-tetrahydrocannabinol (THC), used as an appetite stimulant, antiemetic, and analgesic. Nabilone (Cesamet®, Aliso Viejo CA) is a synthetic THC analog in oral form that is 10 times more potent than natural THC, approved in 2006 for chemotherapy-induced nausea and vomiting, and which has been used off-label for pain. Nabiximols is a mixture in an oro-mucosal spray form of THC and cannabidiol (CBD).

Cannabis maintains its U.S. federal status as a Schedule I substance with high potential for abuse and limited medical indications. Cannabinoids have demonstrated efficacy in the treatment of chemotherapy-induced nausea and vomiting in adults and in appetite stimulation in adults. (10) Delta-8-THC was reported to be an effective anti-emetic in children receiving chemotherapy. (1159) A Cochrane Review published in 2015 that included 23 randomized controlled trials concluded that cannabis-based medicines may be useful in treating refractory chemotherapy-induced nausea and vomiting. (1160) Most of the anti-emetic research that was conducted compared medical cannabis treatment to placebo or various neuroleptic drugs. However, these studies did not compare cannabinoids with the anti-emetogenic new medicines, as the potential role of smoked marijuana in treating chemotherapy-induced nausea and vomiting. Thus, cannabis should be prescribed as an anti-emetic drug only when conventional anti-emetogenic treatment has failed. (1158) Indeed, the American Society of Clinical Oncology convened an Expert Panel that concluded that "evidence remains insufficient for a recommendation regarding medical marijuana for the prevention of nausea and vomiting in patients with cancer receiving chemotherapy or radiation therapy." (1161)

A randomized, placebo-controlled trial that included 177 patients with cancer pain who experienced inadequate analgesia despite chronic opioid dosing showed statistically significant pain reduction with THC/CBD compared with placebo, while the THC group showed a non-significant improvement. (524) Twice as many patients taking THC/CBD showed a reduction of more than 30% from baseline pain numerical rating scale (NRS) score when compared with placebo. The long-term use of the THC/CBD spray is generally well-tolerated, with no evidence of a loss of effect for the relief of cancer-related pain with long-term use. (523) In a randomized, double-blind, placebo-controlled, graded-dose study, patients with advanced cancer and opioid-refractory pain nabiximols at a low dose (1–4 sprays/day) proved effective for pain control. (1162) However, in two double-blind, randomized, placebo-controlled phase 3 studies, nabiximols (Sativex®) did not demonstrate superiority to placebo in reducing self-reported pain numerical rating scale (NRS) scores in advanced cancer patients with chronic pain unalleviated by optimized opioid therapy. (1163)

There is evidence from in vitro studies and animal models that cannabis and cannabinoids may have anti-tumoral activity that has not yet been convincingly translated into benefit in humans.

(1157) Cannabinoids have direct tumor-killing effects by complexing with the CB1 receptor. This interaction leads to autophagy and increased apoptosis. In addition, cannabinoids have been demonstrated to inhibit vascular endothelial growth factor, thereby impairing angiogenesis, and decreasing tumor viability. In vitro studies also reveal that cannabinoids inhibit matrix mettaloproteinase-2, which allows cancer cells to become invasive and metastasize. Hence, pre-clinical evidence suggests that cannabinoids may inhibit tumor growth and proliferation by way of several mechanisms.

Nearly 40% of patients with cancer using cannabis believe it will treat their cancer, with numerous anecdotal reports shared online through social media platforms. Case reports have been published in peer-reviewed journals, but often lack key clinical information to validate anticancer claims. Guggisberg et al reviewed case reports published in peer-reviewed journals and appraised them as weak, moderate, or strong based on the quality of evidence provided supporting an anticancer effect. (1164) A total of 77 unique case reports described patients with various cancers (breast, central nervous system, gynecological, leukemia, lung, prostate, and pancreatic) using cannabis. These authors' appraisal showed 14% of the case reports were considered strong, 5% moderate, and the remaining 81% were weak. They concluded that the review of clinical data suggests most published, peer-reviewed case reports provide insufficient data to support the claim for cannabis as an anticancer agent. However, Likar et al described a case series of 9 patients with glioblastoma who received CBD in a daily dose of 400 mg concomitantly to the standard therapeutic procedure of maximal resection followed by radio-chemotherapy. (1165) By the end of follow-up, all but one patient was alive with a mean survival time of 22.3 months as compared to the median expected survival of 14 to 16 months.

Guzman et al performed a pilot phase I trial in which nine patients with recurrent glioblastoma multiforme were administered THC intratumorally. (1166) Median survival of the cohort from the beginning of cannabinoid administration was 24 weeks. D9-Tetrahydrocannabinol inhibited tumor-cell proliferation in vitro and decreased tumor cell immunostaining when administered to two patients. In a phase 1b RCT, Twelves et al studied nabiximols oro-mucosal cannabinoid spray plus dose-intense temozolomide in patients with first recurrence of GBM. (1167) Survival at 1 year was 83% for nabiximols and 44% for placebo-treated patients ($p = 0.042$).

In summary, while the clinical data is contradictory, cannabinoids may prolong survival in patients with cancer, particularly those with GBM. Therefore, with the current state of evidence, the widespread use of cannabis cannot be recommended. (1158) However, the use of the THC/CBD spray may be helpful in patients with advanced cancer and opioid-refractory pain. Cannabinoids may also be useful in patients with refractory chemotherapy-induced nausea and vomiting.

33. Fenofibrate

Since its clinical introduction as a third-generation fibrate in 1975, fenofibrate has been widely used in the treatment of hypercholesterolemia and hyperlipidemia. The lipid-lowering effect of fenofibrate is believed to be mediated through its stimulation of peroxisome proliferator-activated receptor α (PPARα). More recently, PPARα-specific agonists were reported to have anticancer effects in human cancer including acute myeloid leukemia, chronic lymphocytic leukemia, and solid tumors, including those of the liver, ovary, breast, skin, and lungs. (1168) Fenofibrate may exert anticancer effects *via* a variety of pathways involved in apoptosis, cell-cycle arrest, invasion, and migration. Fenofibrate exerted antitumor effects in several human cancer cell lines, such as breast, liver, glioma, prostate, pancreas, and lung cancer cell lines. Fenofibrate was found to inhibit the proliferation of breast cancer MDA-MB-231 cell lines by inducing apoptosis and cell-cycle arrest. Fenofibrate increased the expression of Bad, but decreased that of Bcl-xL and Survivin, and activated caspase-3. (1169) Fenofibrate also induced cell-cycle arrest at the G0/G1 phase by upregulation of p21, p27/Kip1, and downregulation of cyclin D1 and Cdk4. Activation of NF-κB pathway played an important role in the induction of apoptosis by fenofibrate.

Fenofibrate has been established to decrease the viability of human Hepatocellular carcinoma HepG2 cells partly by necrotic cell death. (1170) Fenofibrate can also lead to cell-cycle arrest in liver cancer cells. Fenofibrate significantly inhibited cell proliferation and induced apoptosis in human glioblastoma cell lines. (1171) Furthermore, the drug obviously reduced glioma stem cells (GSC) invasion probably through decreasing the expression of CD133. Fenofibrate can also inhibit cell growth through its impact on Fork-head box (Fox) family. (1172) FOX is a family of transcription factors that plays important roles in the regulation of the expression of genes involved in cell growth, proliferation, differentiation, and longevity. Low concentrations of fenofibrate induced cell-cycle arrest and apoptosis in the androgen-dependent prostate cancer cell line. (1173)

Despite the experimental data supporting the anticancer effects of fenofibrate there is no clinical data to support the use of this agent.

34. Niclosamide

Anticancer pathways and mechanisms

Niclosamide is an antiparasitic drug that was FDA approved for the treatment of tapeworm in 1982. Niclosamide has a broader clinical application including cancer, bacterial and viral infection and metabolic diseases such as type II diabetes and nonalcoholic steatohepatitis (NASH), endometriosis, rheumatoid arthritis and systemic sclerosis.(1174)

Niclosamide is a remarkable repurposed anti-cancer drug, achieving therapeutic levels at doses commonly used for treating parasites with no toxicity. The major anti-cancer mechanisms are mitochondrial uncoupling, which serves as an oxidative phosphorylation inhibitor which triggers protective autophagy, (1175, 1176) and inhibition of the Wnt/β catenin pathway. (1177, 1178) Niclosamide targets multiple additional signaling pathways including NF-KB, Notch, ROS, mTORC1 and Stat3. (1179-1181) Niclosamide was reported to target ovarian cancer stem cells in vitro and in vivo.(1182)

In cancer cells, antegrade trafficking or movement of lysosomes to the cell periphery near the cell membrane is associated with aggressive behavior and tumor cell invasion. The opposite, called perinuclear clustering is associated with a more benign state, with inhibition of tumor invasion.(1183) In a prostate cancer cell line Circu et al demonstrated that niclosamide caused antegrade lysosome trafficking inhibition (i.e. perinuclear clustering).(1184) This effect is related to loss of lysosomal acidity.

Clinical studies

Inspired by the promising results from the pre-clinical studies, several clinical trials are ongoing to assess the therapeutic effect of niclosamide in cancer patients. There are, however, currently no published case reports or clinical series which have reported the use of niclosamide in patients with cancer.

35. Pao Pereira

Pao extract is the extract of the bark of a tree that grows in the Amazon rain forest, *Geissospermum vellosii* Allemao (familiarly known as Pao Pereira), which has been used as a medicine by South American Indian tribes. In the 1990s, Mirko Beljanski reported that Pao extract had anticancer effects against melanoma and glioblastoma cells in vitro. (1185, 1186) Francois Mitterrand, the former President of France, was apparently treated somewhat successfully with Pao extract for metastatic prostate cancer. (6)

Pao extract has subsequently been evaluated against several cancer cell lines. Chang et al demonstrated that Pao extract suppressed castration-resistant prostate cancer (CRPC) cell growth in a dose- and time-dependent manner, through induction of apoptosis and cell cycle arrest. (1187) Furthermore, Pao extract induced the upregulation of pro-apoptotic Bax, reduction of anti-apoptotic Bcl-2, Bcl-xL, and XIAP expression, which were associated with the cleavage of PARP protein. Moreover, Pao extract treatment blocked CRPC cell migration and invasion.

Chen et al investigated two plant extracts from the medicinal plants Pao Pereira (Pao) and *Rauwolfia vomitoria* (Rau) each for their activities against ovarian cancer stem cells. (1188) Both Pao and Rau inhibited overall proliferation of human ovarian cancer cell lines and had limited cytotoxicity to normal epithelial cells. Furthermore, both Pao and Rau treatment significantly reduced the ovarian cancer stem cell population. Nuclear β-catenin levels were decreased, suggesting suppression of Wnt/β-catenin signaling pathway. Similarly, Dong et al demonstrated that an extract of Pao inhibited proliferation of human pancreatic cancer cell lines and had limited cytotoxicity to normal epithelial cells. (1189)

Bemis et al demonstrated that Pao Pereira extract significantly suppressed cell growth of a human prostate cancer cell line (LnCaP) in a dose-dependent fashion and induced apoptosis. (1190) **Furthermore, immunodeficient mice heterotopically xenografted with LNCaP cells were gavaged daily** with Pao Pereira extract or vehicle control over 6 weeks. Tumor growth was suppressed by up to 80% compared with tumors in vehicle-treated mice

Yu et al demonstrated that Pao Pereira selectively inhibited ovarian cancer cell growth. (1191) Pao induced apoptosis in a dose- and time-dependent manner. Pao greatly enhanced carboplatin cytotoxicity. Furthermore, when Pao was combined with carboplatin, tumor inhibition reached 97% and ascites were completely eradicated. Similarly, these authors demonstrated activity against a pancreatic cell line with synergy when combined with gemcitabine. (1192)

Despite the in vitro and animal model data, there is no human data to support the safety and efficacy of Pao Pereira in patients.

36. Dandelion Extract

Dandelion (Taraxacum genus), named "Pugongying" in China, is a perennial plant belonging to the Asteraceae family. In Asia, the Taraxacum genus is widely cultivated and also found wild in most parts of China, North Korea, Mongolia, and Russia. (1193) It grows in temperate regions globally, including on lawns, on roadsides, on disturbed banks and shores of waterways, and in other areas with moist soils.

As an edible medicinal herb and vegetable, dandelion has long been utilized for centuries in traditional medicine, folk remedies, and substitution therapies in many countries to treat diverse diseases. Dandelion extract has anti-inflammatory, antibacterial, immune enhancing, anti-oxidative, anti-depressant, and anti-cancer properties. Dandelion extract contains multiple bioactive compounds including sesquiterpenoids, phenolic compounds, essential oils, saccharides, flavonoids, sphingolipids, triterpenoids, sterols and coumarins. (1193)

Li et al demonstrated that dandelion seed extract significantly inhibited the growth, proliferation, migration, invasion, and angiogenesis and induced the apoptosis in human esophageal squamous carcinoma (ESCC) cells. (1194) In this study dandelion seed extract reduced survival rate and suppressed proliferation of ESCC cells by inhibiting the PI3K/Akt pathway and by down-regulation of MMP2, MMP9 and VEGF. In addition, dandelion seed extract induced apoptosis of human ESCC cells via regulating the expression of survivin, the ratio of Bcl-2 and Bax, and the levels of caspase3 and caspase9 proteins. Ovadje et al demonstrated that dandelion root extract affects colorectal cancer proliferation and survival through the activation of multiple death signaling pathways. (1195) In this study dandelion extract induced programmed cell death selectively in > 95% of colon cancer cells, irrespective of their p53 status, by 48 hours of treatment. The anti-cancer efficacy of this extract was confirmed in in-vivo studies, as the oral administration of DRE retarded the growth of human colon xenograft models by more than 90%. The induction of apoptosis was dependent on caspase-8 activation. Zhu et al demonstrated that that dandelion root extract specifically and effectively suppresses proliferation and migration in human gastric cells without inducing toxicity in noncancerous cells. (1196)

Deng et al demonstrated that dandelion may serve as a promising therapeutic strategy for breast cancer by modulating the tumor immune microenvironment. (1197) These authors demonstrated that dandelion extract inhibited the malignant property of triple negative breast cancer cells (TNBC) induced by tumor associated macrophages. In this study dandelion extract exerted inhibition on STAT3 and PD-L1 in TNBC cells under tumor associated macrophage microenvironment. Furthermore, in M2 macrophages, dandelion extract promoted the expression of M1-like marker TNF-α, IL-8, and iNOS, but reduced M2-like marker IL-10, CD206, Arginase-1, and TGF-β, indicative of macrophage repolarization. Similarly, Wang et al demonstrated the antitumor effects of dandelion extract against TNBC cells in vitro and demonstrated that dandelion extract could interfere with glycerophospholipids and unsaturated fatty acids metabolism via downregulating the CHKA (Choline kinase alpha) expression and inhibiting PI3K/AKT/SREBP/FADS2 axis. (1198) Lin et al demonstrated that dandelion exerted cytotoxic effects against breast cancer cell lines (including TNBC) by induction of apoptosis, the reduction of cell proliferation and the disruption of the mitochondrial membrane potential. (1199)

Despite the in vivo and in vitro data demonstrating the anti-cancer activity of dandelion extract there are no clinical studies to support the use of this botanical.

CHAPTER 10: TIER FOUR REPURPOSED DRUGS – RECOMMEND AGAINST

37. B Complex vitamins and antioxidants

B complex vitamins containing folate (folic acid) and vitamin B12 should be avoided in patients with cancer as they increase the risk of tumor progression and metastases. Indeed, these vitamins act as growth factor for the tumor. This observation is supported by the fact that anti-metabolites which block folate metabolism are effective anti-cancer chemotherapeutic agents.

Folic acid (Vitamin B9) is a water-soluble B vitamin found in leafy greens, legumes and cereals. In the US folate supplementation of flour is mandated. Even in well-nourished Western societies, routine supplementation of pregnant women with folate significantly reduces the risk of neural tube defects. Observational studies in the 1980 s suggested that a low-folate diet increased the risk of heart disease and colorectal cancer. (58) The enthusiasm for B vitamin supplementation led to studies to determine if it could reduce these diseases. Unfortunately, these studies proved harmful.

In observational studies, lower homocysteine levels are associated with lower rates of coronary heart disease and stroke. Folic acid and vitamins B6 and B12 lower homocysteine levels. In 2006 the HOPE2 study assessed whether supplementation with these vitamins reduced the risk of major cardiovascular events in patients with vascular disease. (1200) The HOPE2 found that supplementation with folate, vitamin B6 and B12 failed to reduce heart disease. However, the study demonstrated a worrisome 36% increased risk of colon cancer (not statistically significant) and a 21% increased risk of prostate cancer. The Aspirin/Folate prevention of large bowel polyps clinical trial found that six years of folate supplementation increased the risk of advanced cancer by 67%. (1201)

In the Cooperative Group Clinical Trial (SWOG S0221) patients with breast cancer randomly assigned to an intergroup metronomic trial of cyclophosphamide, doxorubicin, and paclitaxel were queried on their use of supplements at registration and during treatment. (439) In this study the use of any antioxidant supplement (vitamins A, C, and E; carotenoids; coenzyme Q10) both before and during treatment was associated with an increased hazard of recurrence (HR 1.41; 95% CI, 0.98 to 2.04; P = .06) Furthermore, vitamin B12 use both before and during chemotherapy was significantly associated with poorer disease-free survival (HR, 1.83; 95% CI, 1.15 to 2.92; P , .01) and overall survival (HR, 2.04; 95% CI, 1.22 to 3.40; P,.01).

Two large trials, the Norwegian Vitamin (NORVIT) trial and the Western Norway B intervention trial (WENBIT) confirmed that high dose B vitamin supplements did not reduce heart disease. (1202, 1203) It should be noted that folate supplementation of grains and other produce is not performed in Norway. Ebbing et al performed a combined analysis and extended follow-up of participants from these two studies focusing on the risk of cancer. (1204) After a mean follow-up of 77 months, participants who received folic acid plus vitamin B12 vs placebo had an increased risk of cancer (HR, 1.21; 95% CI 1.03-1.41; *P*=.02). and an increased death from cancer (HR, 1.38; 95% CI, 1.07-1.79; *P*=.01). Vitamin B6 treatment was not associated with any significant effects.

It should be noted that in the Selenium and Vitamin E Cancer Prevention Trial (SELECT) vitamin E was associated with a significant increased risk of prostate cancer (HR 1.17, 99% CI 1.004-1.36, p=.008). (1205)

Antioxidant supplements (vitamins A, C, and E; coenzyme Q10, and N-acetyl cysteine) should be avoided in patients with cancer. In an experimental model, Wang et al demonstrated that vitamin C, vitamin E and n-acetylcysteine (NAC) increased tumor angiogenesis by BACH1 mechanism (redox-sensitive transcription factor BTB and CNC homology 1). (438)

38. Colchicine

Colchicine, the main alkaloid of the poisonous plant meadow saffron (Colchicum autumnale L.), is a classical drug used for the treatment of gout and familial Mediterranean fever. (1206-1208)

Colchicine exerts antiproliferative effects through the inhibition of microtubule formation by blocking the cell cycle at the G2/M phase and triggering apoptosis. (1208) Due to its toxicity colchicine is rarely used to treat cancer. However, numerous analogues of colchicine have been synthesized in the hope of developing novel, useful drugs with more favorable pharmacological profiles. (1206, 1207, 1209) Several colchicine semisynthetics are less toxic than colchicine and research is being carried out on effective, less toxic colchicine semisynthetic formulations with potential drug-delivery strategies directly targeting multiple solid cancers.

Anticancer pathways and mechanisms
Colchicine, a well-known anti-mitotic drug, keeps mitotic cells from progressing into the metaphase. (1206) Colchicine forms the tubulin-colchicine (TC) complex by attaching to the ends of microtubules. This prevents the production and polymerization of microtubules by interfering with the dynamics of the tubulin lattice. (1206, 1210-1212) Colchicine interferes with numerous cellular activities, including cell migration, cell division, ion channel regulation and cell shape which are dependent on microtubule function. (1206, 1213) Colchicine has anti-inflammatory characteristics, which are mostly brought on by the disruption of leukocytes and microtubule downstream cellular functions. (1206) Colchicine inhibits angiogenesis and suppresses cell invasion, cell migration, and adhesion via MMP9 and FAK/SRC reduced expression. (1206, 1214, 1215) Colchicine promoted caspase-3-mediated apoptosis through the suppression of the PI3K/Akt/mTOR signaling pathway in NCI-N87 cells. (1206, 1216-1219) The pro-apoptotic protein p21 has also been activated in cells by derivatives of colchicine. (1206, 1220)

Clinical studies
The majority of clinical investigations are in vitro or vivo, and data indicated that colchicine may be a viable adjunctive treatment for hypopharyngeal, gastric, breast, and other cancers,

prostate, colon, liver, leukemia, and pancreatic cancers. (1206, 1221-1224) Kuo et al reported that colchicine use was linked to a lower incidence of incident all-cause malignancies, especially in prostate and colorectal cancers, among male Taiwanese patients with gout, according to findings from a 12-year cohort research. (1225)

Safety of colchicine
Colchicine has a narrow therapeutic index, with no clear-cut distinction between nontoxic, toxic, and lethal doses, causing substantial safety concerns with this drug. (1208, 1226) Furthermore, drug accumulation and high dosages can be associated with severe, often fatal, consequences. (1227) Although colchicine poisoning is sometimes intentional, unintentional toxicity is common and often associated with a poor outcome. (1227)

Gastrointestinal effects, including nausea, vomiting, and diarrhea, are the most common side effects associated with colchicine therapy. (1208) However, colchicine can cause myelosuppression, leukopenia, granulocytopenia, thrombocytopenia, pancytopenia, and aplastic anemia, which can be life-threatening or fatal. In addition, colchicine is associated with neuromuscular and hepatic toxicity and rhabdomyolysis. Due to its narrow therapeutic index and toxicity, colchicine is not recommended for routine use in patients with cancer.

39. Shark Cartilage

Since the publication of W Lane's '*Sharks Don't Get Cancer*' in 1992, shark cartilage was touted as the new "cancer cure" of the 1990s. In 1995, the annual world market for shark cartilage products exceeded US $30 million, and dozens of products, usually as food supplements, are on the market. (1228)

The promotion of crude shark cartilage extracts as a cure for cancer has contributed to at least two significant negative outcomes: a dramatic decline in shark populations and a diversion of patients from effective cancer treatments. (1229)

An alleged lack of cancer in sharks constitutes a key justification for its use. (1229) The proponents of this therapy assume that since the largest part of sharks' bulk is cartilage, something in shark cartilage must account for the rarity of cancer in this animal. Therefore, the argument goes, if patients simply ingest an arbitrary quantity of this cartilage (which presumably has been ground up and made into pills), cancer will regress. The explanation is simple and superficially appealing and offers hope that a nontoxic substance can eliminate cancer. Unfortunately, the claims for the benefits of shark cartilage are completely unsubstantiated by any objective data from controlled clinical trials.

The proposed mechanisms of antitumor action of shark cartilage includes direct or indirect inhibition of angiogenesis. Two glycoproteins, sphyrnastatin 1 and 2, have been isolated from cartilage of the hammerhead shark and reported to have strong antiangiogenic activity and to inhibit tumor neovascularization. (1230)

Miller et al performed a phase I/II clinical trial evaluating the safety and efficacy of shark cartilage in the treatment of advanced cancer. (1231) Sixty patients were treated with shark cartilage at a dose of 1 g/kg daily orally in three divided doses. Five patients were taken off the study because of gastrointestinal toxicity or intolerance to shark cartilage. Progressive disease at 12 weeks occurred in 27 patients. No complete (CRs) or partial responses (PRs) were noted. Median time to tumor progression in the entire study population was 7+/-9.7 weeks. It was concluded that in patients with advanced-stage cancer, shark cartilage had no salutary effect on quality of life. The 16.7% rate of stable disease was similar to results in patients with advanced cancer treated with supportive care alone.

The North Central Cancer Treatment Group trial studied patients with breast or colorectal carcinoma receiving the standard care and who were randomized to receive a shark cartilage product or an identical-appearing and smelling placebo 3 to 4 times each day. (1232) Data on a total of 83 evaluable patients were analyzed. There was no difference in overall survival between patients receiving standard care plus a shark cartilage product versus standard care plus placebo. Likewise, there was no suggestion of improvement in quality of life for patients receiving shark cartilage, compared with those receiving placebo.

40. Laetrile (amygdalin)

The use of Laetrile for the treatment of cancer is highly controversial, with claims of an organized coverup to suppress in-vitro efficacy data as well as conspiracy theories. In summary, while laetrile does have some in-vitro anti-cancer activity, reliable reproducible animal model data is lacking with no credible anti-cancer efficacy in patients. Furthermore, the potential of significant toxicity exists.

Amygdalin is a natural cyanogenic glycoside occurring in the seeds of some edible plants, such as bitter almonds and peaches. Bitter almonds have been used since ancient times to treat fevers, headache (via their purging activity) and as a diuretic. (1233) Amygdalin is composed of two molecules of glucose, plus one molecule each of benzaldehyde and hydrogen cyanide. The anticancer activity of amygdalin is thought to be related to the cytotoxic effects of enzymatically released HCN and non-hydrolyzed cyanogenic glycosides.

In 1952, Ernst Theodore Krebs, Jr. synthesized a less harmful amygdalin derivative of amygdalin with one subunit of glucose, which he called Laetrile. The mixture of amygdalin and its modified form was described by Krebs as "vitamin B17", although in the literal sense neither amygdalin nor Laetrile are vitamins. (1233) In 1977, the U.S. FDA issued a statement indicating that there was no evidence of the safety and efficacy of Laetrile. It is forbidden to sell amygdalin and Laetrile in the U.S. and Europe.

Laetrile, which is derived from amygdalin, has been used as an alternative natural medicine in the treatment of cancer for over 30 years. The use of Laetrile/amygdalin in the treatment of cancer is controversial; on the one hand, this compound has in vitro anticancer activity;

however, it can be toxic via enzymatic degradation and production of hydrogen cyanide. (1233) Furthermore, despite studies demonstrating anti-cancer activity on cancer cell lines, the clinical evidence for the anticancer activity of amygdalin has not been established. Moreover, high dose exposures to amygdalin can produce cyanide toxicity. (1233)

In vitro cell culture studies show several amygdalin activities that would be beneficial in cancer treatment.(1234, 1235) For example, amygdalin has the capacity to control apoptotic proteins and signaling molecules, which may be an explanation for a decrease in tumor proliferation. Amygdalin treatment increased expression of Bax, decreased expression of Bcl-2 and induced caspase-3 activation in human DU145 and LNCaP prostate cancer cells, (1236) induced apoptosis of HeLa cervical cancer cells mediated by endogenous mitochondrial pathway, (1237) and reduced adhesion and migration of UMUC-3 and RT112 bladder cancer cells through activation of focal adhesion kinase (FAK) and modulation of β1 integrin. (1238)

Laetrile was studied in a mouse model By Dr Konematsu Suguira at Sloan Kettering Cancer institute during the 1970's. This research was never published in a peer reviewed paper but was promoted in the media by Ralf Moss a science writer originally employed by Sloan Kettering. In a series of 6 experiments with CD8F1 mice with spontaneous mammary adenocarcinomas Sugiura noted by macrovisual observation with some histology an overall average of 21% of mice with lung metastases when treated with 1,000--2,000 mg/kg/day of amygdalin compared with 90% of the control mice. (1239) The significance attributed to these early observations is challenged by the negative findings of 3 independent investigators, by 2 out of 3 negative cooperative experiments in which Sugiura participated, and particularly by the blind experiment in which he and others under blind readings found no anticancer activity. (1239) Control animals often lived longer than those treated with various doses and schedules of amygdalin.(1240) However, the accuracy of these negative findings has been questioned and a "coverup" has been suggested. In a documentary entitled *"Second Opinion: Laetrile at Sloan-Kettering"* Mr. Moss claims that "laetrile stopped the spread of cancer, yet they lied to us about it" http://www.secondopinionfilm.com/. The true findings of Dr Suguira's research are unclear as his data was never published nor has his work been reproduced by other investigators. However, the lack of proven clinical efficacy of laetrile (as outlined below) raises serious questions as to the validity of his findings.

In 1978 the National Cancer Institute (NCI) published a special report on Laetrile based on a national retrospective analysis. (1241) Cases thought to have shown objective benefit from Laetrile were solicited by mail request to 385,000 physicians and 70,000 other health professionals in the US. Although it is estimated that at least 70,000 Americans used Laetrile, only 93 cases were submitted for evaluation. Twenty-six of these Laetrile cases had to be eliminated because of insufficient documentation. an equal number of conventionally treated cases selected from the institute's files were added to the records to be analyzed. A panel of 12 oncologists, who had no knowledge of the actual treatments given, was then asked to evaluate the results of 160 courses of treatment (68 Laetrile, 68 chemotherapy, 24 "no treatment") in the abstracted records from 93 patients. The panel judged six Laetrile courses to have produced a response (two complete and four partial). These results allow no definite conclusions supporting the anti-cancer activity of Laetrile.

In 1982, a clinical trial of 178 patients with cancer who were treated with Laetrile was published in the *New England Journal of Medicine*. (1242) No substantive benefit was observed in terms of cure, improvement, or stabilization of cancer, improvement of symptoms related to cancer, or extension of life span. The hazards of amygdalin therapy were evidenced in several patients by symptoms of cyanide toxicity. The paper concluded with this statement: "Amygdalin (Laetrile) is a toxic drug that is not effective as a cancer treatment." Fatal and nonfatal toxicities from orally ingested cyanogenic glycosides have been reported worldwide.(1240) A systematic review published in 2007 included 36 studies, none of which "proved the effectiveness of laetrile." (1237) A Cochrane systematic review published in 2015 failed to identify any studies that met their inclusion criteria. (1243) The authors of this review concluded that "the claims that laetrile or amygdalin have beneficial effects for cancer patients are not currently supported by sound clinical data." Based on the "best available" data the use of laetrile cannot be recommended.

CHAPTER 11: POTENTIAL ADJUNCTIVE THERAPIES

TUMOR TREATING FIELDS

Tumor treating fields (TTF) are a non-invasive antimitotic therapy that delivers alternating electric fields via the Optune® system. (1244) TTF are 100 – 400 kHz alternating current (AC) electric fields transmitted transdermally to tumors using two orthogonal sets of transducer arrays. Transducer arrays are activated sequentially each second, effecting a direction change of the incident field on the target. (1245) TTF mechanism of action involves polarizable intra-cellular structures and mitotic disruption. TTF induces mitotic spindle assembly checkpoint arrest leading to a cell-cycle arrest, followed by mitotic slippage, and subsequent cell death or senescence. (1245) In addition, TTF promotes autophagy by inducing AMPK, miR29b and other drivers of autophagy. TTF has immunological effects including activation of the STING pathway, increased expression of MHC II, CD80, and CD40 on dendritic cells and M1 macrophage polarization. (1245) TTF has been shown to suppress the migration and invasion of LN-18 glioma cells in experimental models. TTF do not have a systemic half-life like oral or intravenous therapies and exert their therapeutic effect while the electric fields are being applied only on actively dividing cancer cells but not on healthy cells. Thus, compliance with treatment is critical to maximize effectiveness. (1244)

TTF has been studied most extensively in patients with glioblastoma multiforme (GBM). TTF is currently undergoing evaluation as adjunctive treatment in patients with NSCLC, pancreatic and ovarian cancer. (1245) In patients with GBM, TTF is delivered to the region of the tumor via transducer arrays placed on the patient's scalp. The Phase III EF-14 RCT (n=695) in newly diagnosed GBM patients demonstrated significantly improved progression-free survival (HR, 0.63; 95%CI, 0.52-0.76; *P* < .001) and overall survival (HR, 0.63; 95%CI, 0.53-0.76; *P* < .001) when TTF were used together with maintenance temozolomide (TMZ) compared with TMZ alone. (1246, 1247) The National Comprehensive Cancer Network (NCCN) recommends TTF in combination with TMZ for the treatment of patients with both newly diagnosed and recurrent glioblastoma. (1248) Based on this information patients with GBM should consider TTF, when feasible, as an adjunctive treatment option. (1249)

PHOTODYNAMIC THERAPY

Photodynamic therapy (PDT) is a treatment approach that causes tissue destruction by visible light in the presence of a photosensitizer and oxygen. (1250) When sensitizer molecules are exposed to light energy, electrons at low-energy singlet states jump to high-energy singlet states, and some spontaneously convert to excited triplet states. The excited triplet state interacts with oxygen-producing reactive oxygen species. Reactive oxygen species cause cell death locally through a complex interplay of apoptosis, necrosis, and autophagy-associated cell death. (1251)

Light has been known to provide a therapeutic potential for several thousands of years. Over 3,000 years ago, since the ancient Indian and Chinese civilizations, it has been used for the treatment of various diseases mainly in combination with reactive chemicals, for example, to treat conditions like vitiligo, psoriasis, and skin cancer. Sunshine has enormous therapeutic effects both due to ultraviolet-B (UVB) and the synthesis of vitamin D in the skin and near infrared (NIR) radiation (about 40% of solar radiation), which has enormous health benefits including mitochondrial melatonin synthesis. (1252, 1253) Due to our modern lifestyle, modern man has a profound deficiency of NIR exposure. (1253)

Of all the wavelengths of sunlight, NIR-A radiation has the deepest penetration into tissues, up to 23 cm. During the 1918 influenza pandemic, "open-air treatment of influenzae" (sunshine) appears to have been the most effective treatment for seriously ill patients. (413) A more recent prospective study demonstrated that avoiding sun exposure is a risk factor for all-cause mortality. (414) In this study, the mortality rate amongst avoiders of sun exposure was approximately twofold higher compared with the highest sun exposure group.

Dermatologists commonly use PDT with a topical photosensitizing agent for the treatment of actinic keratoses and early nonmelanoma skin cancers, but the potential applications for PDT are far broader, including solid tumors. (1250) When PDT is utilized to treat malignant and premalignant tumors, a patient is administered a sensitizer agent that preferentially accumulates in neoplastic lesions and is activated by light to produce cell death. (1251)

PDT for cutaneous indications commonly utilizes a topical photosensitizer, such as 5-aminolevulinic acid or methyl aminolevulinate, which are precursors of protoporphyrin IX. (1250) Treatment of visceral tumors requires an intravenous or oral photosensitizer, and the most commonly used photosensitizing agent for this indication is porfimer sodium. Porfimer sodium absorbs light at 630 nm (red light). PDT has been performed with various light sources including lasers, incandescent light, laser-emitting diodes, transcutaneous fiberoptic devices, and daylight. (1254)

While the efficacy of PDT in killing cancer cells has been demonstrated in experimental models, (1255) clinical studies demonstrating the benefit of this modality in patients with non-cutaneous malignancies is limited. (1254, 1256-1258) The role of PDT and photobiomodulation in patients with non-cutaneous cancer requires further evaluation. However, to improve mitochondrial function we suggest that all patients expose themselves to about 30 minutes of midday sunshine whenever possible (at least 3 times a week); this is best achieved with a brisk midday walk.

HYPERBARIC OXYGEN THERAPY

Hypoxia is a critical hallmark of solid tumors and involves enhanced cell survival, angiogenesis, glycolytic metabolism, and metastasis. Hyperbaric oxygen treatment (HBOT) has for centuries been used to improve or cure disorders involving hypoxia and ischemia, by enhancing the amount of dissolved oxygen in the plasma and thereby increasing O2 delivery to the tissue. (1259)

HBOT leads to hyperoxia and elevated levels of reactive oxygen species (ROS), which overwhelm the cancer cells' antioxidant defense and lead to cell death. (1260, 1261) The molecular mechanisms behind hyperoxia-induced cell death involve a complex signaling system including protein kinases and receptors such as RAGE, CXCR2, TLR3, and TLR4. (1262) Furthermore, contrary to what would be expected, HBOT has been shown to induce an antiangiogenic effect in tumor models. (1260, 1263)

While HBOT appears to have limited effects on cancer growth, it may potentiate the effects of other treatment modalities. Hoff et al demonstrated that a ketogenic diet combined with HBO had significant anticancer effects in a natural model of systemic metastatic cancer. (1264) Hypoxia has been described as an important factor for chemotherapeutic resistance. (1259) Studies on HBOT as a chemotherapeutic adjuvant have shown augmented effects both in vitro and in vivo. (1259) However, it is important to emphasize Mayer et al. list five chemotherapeutic agents (doxorubicin, bleomycin, disulfiram, cisplatin, and mafenide acetate) which are strongly contradictory in combination with HBOT due to potential potentiation of toxicity. Radiotherapy in combination with HBOT has been used clinically in two different applications: (a) as a therapeutic agent for treating late radiation injury and (b) as a radiosensitizer, aiming to increase the effect of radiotherapy. (1259) An updated Cochrane systematic review concluded that "there is some evidence that HBOT improves local tumor control and mortality in tumors of the head and neck; however, the outcomes seem to be related to the use of unusual fractionation schemes, and thereby conclude that the benefits of HBOT should be interpreted with caution." (1265) While HBOT may have promise as an anticancer intervention, especially when combined with other treatment modalities, the clinical data to support this intervention is limited at this time.

METRONOMIC DOSING

Metronomic therapy is a new type of chemotherapy in which anti-cancer drugs are administered in a lower dose than the maximum tolerated dose repetitively over a long period to treat cancers with fewer side effects. (1266) Metronomic therapy is shown to affect both tumor microenvironment and tumor cells to achieve its therapeutic effects. Metronomic therapy is also cost-effective as a lower dose is used compared to conventional chemotherapy. Metronomic dosing will avoid side effects by administering low doses continuously, and efficacy should be seen as prolonged progression free survival and overall survival, rather than in rapid tumor responses. (1267) Metronomic chemotherapy has been most commonly used in patients with metastatic breast cancer, non-small cell lung cancer, and glioblastoma. (1267) A meta-analysis of 22 clinical trials reported promising results in patients with advanced breast cancer. (1268)

THE BASICS OF CHEMOTHERAPY

Despite the introduction of a significant number of new cancer therapeutics that target specific molecular pathways within malignant cells, the use of DNA damaging cytotoxic chemotherapy currently remains the mainstay in the management of most malignancies. (1269) Chemotherapy drugs typically kill cancer cells by interrupting DNA synthesis in all cells but will most significantly inhibit cells that are multiplying the fastest. Most chemotherapy drugs act by altering the structure/function of DNA thereby preventing cell division. (1270-1272) The mitotic spindle inhibitors modify the function/formation of spindle microtubules leading to mitotic arrest and cell death. Chemotherapy drugs cause cell death by apoptosis, either by directly interfering with DNA, or by targeting the key proteins required for cell division. (1273)

Unfortunately, they can also be 'cytotoxic' to normal dividing cells, particularly those with a high turnover, such as the bone marrow and mucous membranes. Chemotherapy agents in general act by killing rapidly dividing cells. Therefore, these agents act on the rapidly proliferating population of cancer cells. As the tumor increases in size the degree of cellular heterogeneity increases. The greater the degree of heterogeneity the less likely will be the response to chemotherapy. Chemotherapy is often poorly effective with metastatic disease because of the large tumor burden, the cell population is highly heterogenous, with a population of cancer stem cells which divide very slowly. Further as already discussed, rather than killing cancer stem cells, chemotherapy may potentiate the growth and dissemination of cancer stem cells. Excluding germ cell tumors and lymphomas, most patients with solid tumors diagnosed with metastatic disease are not curable and treatment is with palliative intent (see Table 7). (1272) From their introduction in the 1940s there are now over 50 licensed drugs for the management of malignant disease. (1272) Chemotherapy drugs can be divided into two classes depending on their origin. They can be either plant derived or of synthetic origin. (1270, 1271) Depending on their mechanism of action, they can be divided into alkylating agents, antimetabolites, topoisomerase inhibitors, mitotic spindle inhibitors and others (see Figure 11). (1270, 1271, 1273) Most chemotherapy regimens in clinical practice consist of several agents from different classes used in combination. (1272, 1273) Disadvantages of many cytotoxic agents include bone marrow suppression, gastrointestinal tract lesions, hair loss, nausea, and the development of clinical resistance. These side effects occur because cytotoxic agents act on both tumor cells and healthy cells. (1271)

The duration of the cell cycle is similar in tumors and healthy tissues, but tumors present a higher proportion of cells undergoing mitosis. Metastases commonly have a growth rate almost twice that of the primary tumor. At any one time less than 10% of cancer cells from solid tumors are actively dividing. (1274) Chemotherapeutic agents that work at certain points in the cell cycle are called cell cycle specific agents and need the cancer cells to be actively dividing to be maximally effective. Cell cycle specific chemotherapeutic drugs include Taxol, etoposide, vincristine, bleomycin and the antimetabolite drugs methotrexate and 5-fluorouracil. Some of the more common chemotherapeutic drugs that are not cell cycle specific include cyclophosphamide, cisplatin, and doxorubicin.

Individualized decisions regarding chemotherapy should be based on the expected response of the tumor (curability), the stage and extent of the disease (tumor bulk), the presence of metastases and the patients' comorbidities counterbalanced by the toxicity of the chemotherapy. The curability of various cancers in response to chemotherapy is listed in Table 4. (11, 213) Patients with metastatic solid tumors generally have incurable disease. The sites of metastases of common tumors are listed in Table 8. Patients with local disease may be cured with surgery (see Table 9). (11) The standard full chemotherapy protocol is suggested in patients with "chemotherapy curable tumors" and treatment should be initiated as soon as possible. The curability of "chemotherapy curable malignancies" may be related to the natural apoptotic sensitivity of the cancer stem cells of these tumors. (213, 1275, 1276) Repurposed drugs and metabolic therapy should be strongly considered in all cancer types (curability), adapted to the patients' individual preferences (see Figure 12). The contrasting effect of conventional chemotherapy and repurposed anti-cancer drugs are illustrated in Table 10.

Traditional chemotherapy often fails for solid tumors for the following reasons:

- Solid tumors are composed of heterogeneous population of cells many of which are slowly growing.
- Most of the tumor cells are in the rest phase of the cell cycle.
- Chemotherapy does not correct the cancer microenvironment (which promotes cancer cell proliferation) and likely makes it worse.
- Chemotherapy enhances rather than kills cancer stem cells.
- Cancer cells become resistant to the chemotherapeutic agent. (1270)

Cancer Curable	Improves Survival	Palliation Only (metastatic)
Choriocarcinoma	Breast cancer	Colorectal, gallbladder
Acute lymphatic leukemia	Ovarian Cancer	Pancreatic, stomach
Chronic lymphatic leukemia	ALL in adults	Esophageal, liver
Acute promyelocytic leukemia	AML	Prostate, bladder, kidney
Testicular cancer	Thyroid Cancer	Endometrial and cervical
Ovarian germ cell tumor	Small cell lung cancer	NSCLC (lung cancer)
Hodgkin's lymphoma	Multiple myeloma	Brain, adrenal, melanoma
High Grade non-Hodgkin's lymphoma	Osteosarcoma	Adenocarcinoma primary unknown
Rare childhood malignancies	Wilms tumor	H&N cancer

Table 7. Tumor stratification according to response to chemotherapy.

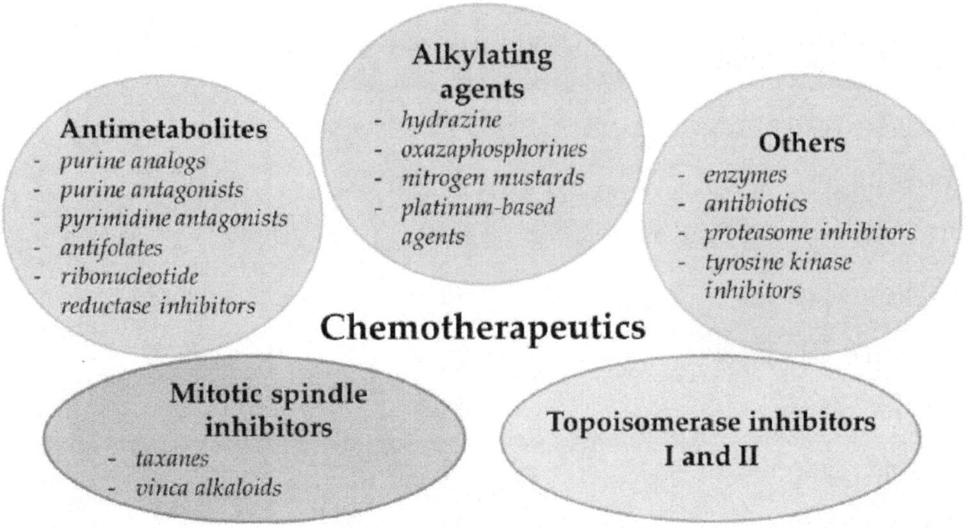

Cancer	Major Site of Metastases
Bladder	Regional lymph nodes, bone, lung, liver
Breast	Bone, brain, liver, lung
Colorectal	Regional lymph nodes, liver, lung, peritoneal cavity
Kidney	Adrenal gland, bone, brain, liver, lung
Leukemia	Lymph nodes, spleen, major blood vessels, central nervous system
Liver	Lung, portal vein, portal lymph nodes
Lung	Adrenal gland, bone, brain, liver, other lung
Melanoma	Other areas of skin, subcutaneous tissue, bone, brain, liver, lung
Head and Neck	Lymph noes neck, salivary glands, lung
Ovary	Peritoneal cavity, omentum, fallopian tube
Pancreas	Liver, peritoneal cavity, lung, bone, stomach, intestine
Prostate	Bone, lung, liver, adrenal gland
Stomach	Liver, lung, peritoneal cavity
Thyroid	Regional lymph node, lung, bone, spine
Uterus and cervix	Vagina, peritoneal cavity, pelvic lymph nodes

Table 8. Some common cancers and sites of metastases. (1277)

Cancer	5-year Survival (%)
Breast	99
Prostate	99
Thyroid	99
Melanoma of skin	99
Endometrial cancer	95
Kidney cancer	93
Ovarian cancer	92
Uterine Cervix	93
Colorectal	91

Table 9. Surgically "Curable" cancers: Five-year survival for local disease with surgical removal.(11) Local disease- An invasive malignant cancer confined entirely to the organ of origin.

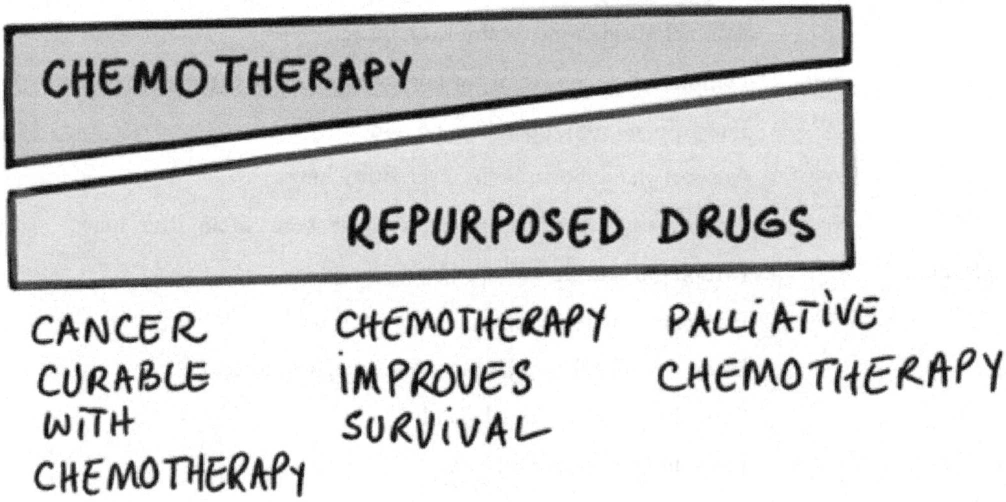

Figure 12. Role of chemotherapy and repurposed drugs according to "chemotherapy curability" [Source: Dr. Mobeen Syed].

The kinetics of tumor growth are crucial in determining the prognosis and are also factors in determining response to chemotherapy. The doubling time is the time that it takes for tumor cells to double. The faster the doubling time, the more likely the cancer will respond to chemotherapy but also the quicker (if no therapy is given) the cancer will kill the person. It is generally believed that once a tumor has reached the size of clinical detectability (1 cm size) has already undergone approximately 30 doublings to reach 10^9 cells (See figure 13). Only 10 further doubling cycles are required to produce a tumor burden of approximately 1 kg (2.2 pounds), which is usually lethal. The average doubling time for breast tumors has been reported to be 180 days while that for small cell lung cancer (SCLC) averages 86 days. (1278-1281)

	Chemotherapy	Repurposed Drugs
Tumor Cell population	Actively dividing cells only (~ 10% of cells)	All malignant cells
Tumor selectivity	++	+++
Tumor Stem Cells	Enhances	Suppresses/kills
Effect on adaptive immunity	Suppressive	Enhances
Effect on Tumor Microenvironment	Negative effect	Improves/enhances
Myelotoxic	Yes	No
Severe systemic side effects	Yes	No
Tumor cell resistance develops	Yes	No
Cost	+++++	+

Table 10. Contrasting effects of conventional chemotherapy versus metabolic treatment and repurposed drugs for cancer treatment.

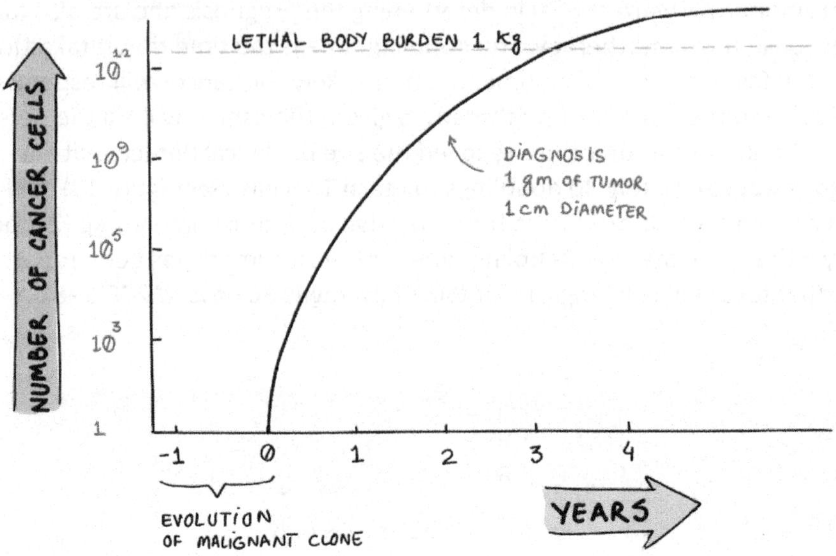

Figure 13. Tumor burden and tumor growth kinetics [Source: Dr. Mobeen Syed].

INTEGRATIVE APPROACHES TO THE TREATMENT OF CHEMOTHERAPY-RELATED ADVERSE EVENTS

Oral Mucositis/Xerostomia/Altered taste

Oral mucositis is an inflammatory mucosal destruction characterized by erythema and/or ulceration of oral mucosa as a result of chemotherapy (30-76%) and/or radiation therapy (over 50%) for the treatment of cancer all over the body. (1282) The most common features of oral mucositis include oedema, erythema, ulcerations, bleeding, and pain, problems in swallowing, eating, drinking, talking and taste changes appearing in different levels of severity. In severe cases (grade 3, 4) it can impair patients' quality of life.

In recent years, various natural agents in plants have been studied in mucositis, which can improve oral mucositis symptoms via different interventions, e.g., their antioxidant and anti-inflammatory properties. (1282) These natural treatments include: (1282, 1283)

- Honey application (1284, 1285)
- Topical application of aloe vera (1286-1288)
- Topical chamomile (1289, 1290)
- Turmeric mouthwash (1291, 1292)
- Sage tea (1293, 1294)
- Indigo wood root (1283)

- Milk thistle (1295)
- Sage tea-thyme-peppermint solution (1296)
- Propolis, aloe vera, calendula, and chamomile solution (1297)
- Carob, Sage, Tahini mix

Chemo induced nausea and vomiting

- Ginger root extract, tea, etc. (1298-1303)
- Chamomile (1302, 1303)
- Cannabinoids (1160, 1304, 1305)
- Lemon extract/juice

Chemo/cancer fatigue

- Ginseng (1306-1309)
- Ashwagandha (879, 880, 1310)
- Mistletoe (867, 873, 876)
- Nigella sativa
- Wheatgrass

Chemo/cancer anxiety/stress

- Ashwagandha (395, 400, 1311)
- Chamomile
- Mistletoe (867, 873, 1312, 1313)
- Lavender (1314)
- Peppermint

APPENDICES

APPENDIX 1. Hierarchy of evidence for the stratification of repurposed drugs/nutraceuticals

It is critically important that the highest level of scientific evidence be used to justify a clinical intervention. If an observation is scientifically valid it is reproducible, over and over again. Traditionally a meta-analysis of randomized controlled trials (RCT's) is considered the highest level of evidence. However, RCTs have many limitations including the fact that they don't reflect real world medicine and they can generally only test a single intervention (e.g., drug A vs placebo). Furthermore, RCT's are very expensive to perform and hence most are funded by Big Pharma who have inherent conflicts of interest. Nevertheless, emerging data suggests that the results of well conducted prospective longitudinal studies produce results quantitatively similar to those of RCTs. (434) For this monograph we therefore consider prospective observational studies and meta-analyses of these studies to be equivalent to RCTs in the hierarchy of evidence.

While *in vitro* and *in vivo* experimental studies are essential starting points to prove that a repurposed drug or nutraceutical has anti-cancer, it is essential that this data be supplemented by clinical data which demonstrates the SAFETY and EFFECTIVENESS of the compound in humans with the disease of interest. Furthermore, *in vitro* and *in vivo* studies are critical in evaluating the synergy between different interventions and the effects of these interventions on the tumor micro-environment. However, this data is insufficient to extrapolate the effects to patients. The failure of Laetrile to improve the outcome of patients with cancer despite encouraging experimental data, is an example of this issue. Furthermore, while case studies can provide useful information (especially safety data), in general they have too many confounding variables that can provide alternative explanations for the observed results. For these reasons well reported case series, retrospective observational studies, prospective longitudinal studies, epidemiological studies or RCTs are the preferred level of evidence to support any particular intervention.

Hierarchy of Evidence

1. Meta analysis of observational and/or randomized controlled trials (RCTs).
2. Prospective RCTs and/or observational studies.
3. Epidemiological data demonstrating that the agent reduces the risk of cancer and/or improves survival in those with cancer.
4. Case series (≥ 3 cases).
5. Individual case reports (at least 2).
6. *In Vivo* model demonstrating favorable effect on tumor microenvironment.
7. *In Vivo*/*In Vitro* model demonstrating synergistic/additive cancer cell killing in presence of cancer chemotherapeutic agent(s).
8. *In Vivo* model demonstrating killing of tumor cells and/or cancer stem cells.
9. *In Vitro* model (cell culture) demonstrating killing of cancer cells.

APPENDIX 2. Other potential agents with limited evidence of anti-cancer activity

These listed drugs/nutraceuticals/botanicals* have *in-vitro, in-vivo,* and in some cases limited human data demonstrating anti-cancer activity. This list is adapted from the ReDO database. (5)

In order for a "medication" to be recommended for clinical use it requires *in vitro* data demonstrating that the compound kills cancer cells (apoptosis) and that this killing is enhanced in the presence of chemotherapeutic drugs, that the agent kills/inhibits cancer stem cells (CSC), that the compound kills cancer cells in animal models (*in vivo*) and that in these models the agent favorably alters the tumor microenvironment. Furthermore, to be recommended in humans there needs to be *sufficient scientific evidence* that the agent is both "safe and effective". This *does not* require the "gold standard" RCT, but *sufficient and reproducible* data from case reports, case series, and observational studies. This is an evolving process and when sufficient evidence accumulates the medication can then be included in the list of recommended agents.

It should be noted that while "anecdotes" are important in the totality of evidence, anecdotes do not represent objective scientific evidence and are not listed in Chapter 7 and 8. If a practitioner claims to have *"cured hundreds of patients"* with a particular intervention, it should be relatively simple to publish this data in a peer-reviewed medical journal.

Acetaminophen
Allopurinol
Alpha-Lipoic Acid
Allium Sativum (Garlic)
Aminophylline
Amiodarone
Annona muricata (soursop, graviola or guanabana)
Aprotinin
Atovaquone
Atrial Natriuretic Peptide
Azithromycin
Bosentan
Bromocriptine
Caffeine
Carvedilol
Chloroquine
Clarithromycin
Clopidogrel
Cyproheptadine
Dapagliflozin
Deferoxamine
Digoxin
Enalapril

Enoxaparin
Esomeprazole
Famotidine
Fenofibrate
Finasteride
Gallic Acid (tea other plants)
Ganciclovir
Hydroxychloroquine
Imipramine
Irbesartan
Ketoconazole
Levofloxacin
Licorice root
Loratadine
Losartan
Meclizine
Metoclopramide
Miconazole
Nicardipine
Nifedipine
Nitroglycerine
Omeprazole
Pentoxifylline
Phenytoin
Propranolol
Propolis (honeybee extract)
Pyridoxine (Vitamin B6)
Spironolactone
Sulfasalazine
Valproic Acid

* Nutraceuticals/Botanicals indicated by *italics.*

APPENDIX 3. Footnote for Figure 10

Cell Cycle. p21: Protein 21, p16: Protein 16, p53: Protein 53, EZH2: Enhancer of Zeste Homolog 2, Cyclin A: Cyclin A, Cyclin B1: Cyclin B1, Cyclin D1: Cyclin D1, Cyclin E: Cyclin. **Apoptosis.** Cleaved caspase-3, 7, 9: Cleaved caspase-3, 7, 9, Cleaved PARP: Cleaved Poly (ADP-ribose) polymerase, Caspase 3: Caspase-3, miR-15a: microRNA-15a, miR-16: microRNA-16, TAZ: Transcriptional coactivator with PDZ-binding motif, YAP: Yes-associated protein, EZH2: Enhancer of Zeste Homolog 2. **Transcription Factors.** ERE: Estrogen Response Element, PPAR-gamma: Peroxisome Proliferator-Activated Receptor Gamma, Nrf-2: Nuclear factor erythroid 2-related factor 2, p21: Protein 21, p53: Protein 53, FOX03: Forkhead box O3, Beta-catenin: Beta-catenin, STAT-1: Signal Transducer and Activator of Transcription 1, STAT-3: Signal Transducer and Activator of Transcription 3, STATE-4: Signal Transducer and Activator of Transcription 4, STAT-4: Signal Transducer and Activator of Transcription 4, CREB-BP: cAMP Response Element-Binding Protein Binding Protein, AP-1: Activator Protein 1, Notch-1: Notch receptor 1, HIF-1: Hypoxia-Inducible Factor 1. **Signaling Pathways.** AKT: Protein Kinase B (also known as Akt), AXL: AXL Receptor Tyrosine Kinase, Beta-catenin: Beta-catenin, Slug: Snail Family Transcriptional Repressor 2, Vimentin: Vimentin (an intermediate filament protein), STAT3: Signal Transducer and Activator of Transcription 3, NF-kB: Nuclear Factor-kappa B, **Receptors.** DR-5: Death Receptor 5, Fas-L: Fas Ligand, IR: Insulin Receptor, Fas: Fas Receptor, R: Receptor, H2R: Histamine H2 Receptor, HER-2: Human Epidermal Growth Factor Receptor 2, IL-8: Interleukin-8, CXCR4: C-X-C chemokine receptor type 4, AHR: Aryl Hydrocarbon Receptor, AR: Androgen Receptor, ER-alpha: Estrogen Receptor-alpha, EGFR: Epidermal Growth Factor Receptor, EPCR: Endothelial Protein C Receptor. **Growth Factors.** DR-5: Death Receptor 5, Fas-L: Fas Ligand, CTGF: Connective Tissue Growth Factor, FGF: Fibroblast Growth Factor, HGF: Hepatocyte Growth Factor, TF: Transcription Factor, NGF: Nerve Growth Factor, EGF: Epidermal Growth Factor, PDGF: Platelet-Derived Growth Factor, TGF-Beta 1: Transforming Growth Factor-Beta 1, VEGF: Vascular Endothelial Growth Factor. **Protein Kinases.** JNK: c-Jun N-terminal Kinase, AMPK: AMP-activated Protein Kinase, ASK1: Apoptosis Signal-regulating Kinase 1, FAK: Focal Adhesion Kinase, EGFR-K: Epidermal Growth Factor Receptor-Kinase, Pp60C-tk: Protein Tyrosine Kinase p60c-src, JAK2: Janus Kinase 2, PI3K: Phosphoinositide 3-Kinase, PGK1: Phosphoglycerate Kinase 1, PAK: p21-Activated Kinase, PKA: Protein Kinase A, PKB: Protein Kinase B (Akt), PTK: Protein Tyrosine Kinase, MAPK: Mitogen-Activated Protein Kinase. **Enzymes.** Telomerase: Telomerase, Desaturase: Desaturase, GCL: Glutamate-Cysteine Ligase, MMP: Matrix Metalloproteinase, GICL: Glutathione Induced Cancer-like Protein, iNOS: Inducible Nitric Oxide Synthase, NQO-1: NAD(P)H Quinone Dehydrogenase 1, FPT: Farnesyl Protein Transferase, Src-2: Steroid Receptor Coactivator 2, DNA pol: DNA Polymerase, TMMP-3: Tissue Matrix Metalloproteinase-3, GST: Glutathione S-transferase, ODC: Ornithine Decarboxylase, PhP: Phosphohexose Isomerase, D: D-aminopeptidase, 5-LOX: 5-Lipoxygenase, COX-2: Cyclooxygenase-2, ATPase: Adenosine Triphosphatase, ATFase: Adenosine Triphosphatase (ATPase) Activator, AATF-1: Apoptosis Antagonizing Transcription Factor 1. **Inflammatory Cytokines.** IL-1: Interleukin-1, IL-2: Interleukin-2, IL-6: Interleukin-6, IL-8: Interleukin-8, IL-12: Interleukin-12, IL-18: Interleukin-18, MCP: Monocyte Chemoattractant Protein, MIP: Macrophage Inflammatory Protein, MaIP: Macrophage-activating Inflammatory Protein, TNF-alpha: Tumor Necrosis Factor-alpha. **Endoplasmic Reticulum Stress Markers.** XBP-1: X-Box

Binding Protein 1, IRE1: Inositol-Requiring Enzyme 1, GADD153: Growth Arrest and DNA Damage-Inducible Protein 153, CHOP: C/EBP Homologous Protein, ATF6: Activating, Transcription Factor 6, GRP78: Glucose-Regulated Protein 78. **Adhesion Molecules.** ICAM-1: Intercellular Adhesion Molecule-1, VCAM-1: Vascular Cell Adhesion Molecule-1, ELAM-1: Endothelial Leukocyte Adhesion Molecule-1.

REFERENCES

1. Marik PE, Khangoora V, Rivera R, Hooper MH, Catravas J. Hydrocortisone, Vitamin C and Thiamine for the treatment of severe sepsis and septic shock: A retrospective before-after study. Chest. 2017;151:1229-38.
2. Wittich CM, Burkle CM, Lanier WL. Ten common questions (and their answers) about off-label drug use. Mayo Clin. Proc. 2012;87:982-90.
3. Halma MT, Plothe C, Marik P, Lawrie T. Strategies for the management of spike protein-related pathology. Microorganisms. 2023.
4. McLelland J. How to starve cancer... and then kill it with ferroptosis. 2nd Edition ed. Central Books, United Kingdom: Agenor Publishing; 2021.
5. Pantziarka P, Verbaanderd C, Sukhatme V, Rica C, I, Crispino S, Gyawali B, et al. ReDO_DB: the repurposing drugs in oncology database. Ecancermedicalscience. 2018;12:886.
6. Beljanski S. Winning the war against cancer. New York: Beljanski Foundation; 2018.
7. Christofferson T. Tripping over the truth. Charlston, SC: CreateSpace; 2014.
8. Vapiwala N, Mick R, Hampshire MK, Metz JM, DeNittis AS. Patient initiation of complementary and alternative medical therapies (CAM) following cancer diagnosis. Cancer J. 2006;12(6):467-74.
9. Yates JS, Mustian KM, Morrow GR, Gillies LJ, Padmanaban D, Atkins JN, et al. Prevalence of complementary and alternative medicine use in cancer patients during treatment. Support Care Cancer. 2005;13(10):806-11.
10. Diorio C, Kelly KM, Afungchwi GM, Ladas EJ, Marjerrison S. Nutritional traditional and complementary medicine strategies in pediatric cancer: A narrative review. Pediatr Blood Cancer. 2020;67 Suppl 3:e28324.
11. Cancer Facts & Figures 2023. Atlanta; 2023.
12. Winters N, Kelley JH. The Metabolic Approach to Cancer: Integrating Deep Nutrition, the Ketogenic Diet, and Nontoxic Bio-Individualized Therapies. White river Junction, VT: Chelsea Green Publishing; 2017.
13. Hope JR. Surviving Cancer, COVID-19 & Disease. The repurposed drug revolution. Redding, CA: Hope Pressworks International; 2020.
14. Wulaningsih W, Garmo H, Holmberg L, Hammar N, Jungner I, Walldius G, et al. Serum Lipids and the Risk of Gastrointestinal Malignancies in the Swedish AMORIS Study. J Cancer Epidemiol. 2012;2012:792034.
15. Ten Trends Transforming The Business of Oncology. https://www.obroncology.com/blog/ten-trends-transforming-the-business-of-oncology-2: OBR Oncology; 2011.
16. Abrams HR, Durbin S, Huang CX, Johnson SF, Nayak RK, Zahner GJ, et al. Financial toxicity in cancer care: origins, impact, and solutions. Transl Behav Med. 2021;11(11):2043-54.
17. Jemal A, Siegel R, Ward E, Hao Y, Xu J, Murray T, et al. Cancer Statistics, 2008. CA Cancer J. Clin. 2008;58:71-96.
18. Morgan G, Ward R, Barton M. The contribution of cytotoxic chemotherapy to 5-year survival in adult malignancies. Clinical Oncology. 2004;16:549-60.
19. Ladanie A, Schmitt AM, Speich B, Naudet F, Agarwal A, Pereira TV, et al. Clinical Trial Evidence Supporting US Food and Drug Administration Approval of Novel Cancer Therapies Between 2000 and 2016. JAMA Netw Open. 2020;3(11):e2024406.
20. Del Paggio JC, Berry JS, Hopman WM, Eisenhauer EA, Prasad V, Gyawali B, et al. Evolution of the Randomized Clinical Trial in the Era of Precision Oncology. JAMA Oncol. 2021;7(5):728-34.
21. Hanahan D, Weinberg RA. The hallmarks of cancer. Cell. 2000;100(1):57-70.

22. Hanahan D, Weinberg RA. Hallmarks of cancer: The next generation. Cell. 2011;144:646-74.
23. Warburg O, Wind F, Negelein E. The metabolism of tumors in the body. J. Gen. Physiol. 1927;6:519-30.
24. Warburg O. On the origin of cancer cells. Science. 1956;123:309.
25. Wang Z, Jensen MA, Zenklusen JC. A Practical Guide to The Cancer Genome Atlas (TCGA). Methods Mol. Biol. 2016;1418:111-41.
26. Alexandrov LB, Kim J, Haradhvala NJ, Huang MN, Tian Ng AW, Wu Y, et al. The repertoire of mutational signatures in human cancer. Nature. 2020;578(7793):94-101.
27. Blum A, Wang P, Zenklusen JC. SnapShot: TCGA-Analyzed Tumors. Cell. 2018;173(2):530.
28. Watson J. To Fight Cancer, Know the Enemy. https://www.nytimes.com/2009/08/06/opinion/06watson.html. Op-Ed Contribution ed: New York Times; 2009.
29. Szent-Gyorgyi A. The living state and cancer. Proc. Natl. Acad. Sci. U. S. A. 1977;74:2844-7.
30. Seyfried TN, Shelton LM. Cancer as a metabolic disease. Nutrition & Metabolism. 2010;7:7.
31. Seyfried TN. Cancer as a metabolic disease. On the origin, management, and prevenion of cancer. Hoboken, New Jersey: Wiley; 2012.
32. Vander Heiden MG, Cantley LC, Thompson CB. Understanding the Warburg effect: The metabolic requirements of cell proliferation. Science. 2009;324:1029-33.
33. Galluzzi L, Morselli E, Kepp O, Vitale I, Rigoni A, Vacchelli E, et al. Mitochondrial gateways to cancer. Molecular Aspects of Medicine. 2010;31:1-20.
34. John AP. Dysfunctional mitochondria, not oxygen insufficiency, cause cancer cells to produce inordinate amounts of lactic acid: the impact of this on the treatment of cancer. Medical Hypotheses. 2001;57:429-31.
35. Guezva JM, Krajewska M, de Heredia ML, Krajewski S, Santamaria G, Kim H, et al. The bioenergetic signature of cancer; a marker of tumor progression. Cancer Res. 2002;15:6674-81.
36. Kiebish MA, Han X, Cheng H, Chuang JH, Seyfried TN. Cardiolipin and electron transport chain abnormalities in mouse brain tumor mitochondria: lipidomic evidence supporting the Warburg theory of cancer. J. Lipid Res. 2008;49:2545-56.
37. Ramanathan A, Wang C, Schreiber SL. Perturbational profiling of a cell-line model of tumorigenesis by using metabolic measurements. PNAS. 2005;102:5992-7.
38. Chen Y, Cairns R, Papandreou I, Koong A, Denko NC. Oxygen consumption can regulate the growth of tumors, a new perspective on the Warburg effect. PloS ONE. 2009;4:e7033.
39. Lengauer C, Kinzler KW, Vogelstein B. Genetic instabilities in human cancers. Nature. 1998;396:643-9.
40. Roskelley RC, Mayer N, Horwitt BN, Salter WT. Studies in cancer. VII. Enzyme deficiency in human and experimental cancer. J. Clin. Invest. 1943;22:743-51.
41. Nowell PC. Tumor progression: a brief historical perspective. Seminars in Cancer Biology. 2002;12:261-6.
42. Yokota J. Tumor progression and metastasis. Carcinogenesis. 2000;21:497-503.
43. Delsite R, Kachhap S, Anbazhagan R, Gabrielson E, Singh KK. Nucelar genes involved in mitochondria-to-nuceus communication in breast cancer cells. Molecular Cancer. 2002;1:6.
44. Israel BA, schaeffer WI. Cytoplasmic suppression of malignancy. In Vitro Cell Dev. Biol. 1987;23:627-32.
45. Howell AN, Sagar R. Tumorigenicity and its suppression in cybrids of mouse and Chinese hamster cell lines. Proc. Natl. Acad. Sci. U. S. A. 1978;75:2358-62.
46. Singh KK, Kulawiec M, Still I, Desouki MM, Geradts J, Matsui SI. Inter-genomic cross talk between mitochondria and the nucleus plays an important role in tumorigenesis. Gene. 2005;354:140-6.

47. Li L, Connelly MC, Wetmore C, Curran T, Morgan JI. Mouse embryos cloned from brain tumors. 63. 2003(2733):2736.
48. Hochedlinger K, Blelloch R, Brennan C, Yamada Y, Kim M, Chin L, et al. Reprogramming of a melanoma genome by nuclear transplantation. Gene & Development. 2004;18:1875-85.
49. Koike K. Hepatitis B virus X gene is implicated in liver carcinogenesis. Cancer Letters. 2009;286:60-8.
50. D'Agostino DM, Bernardi P, Chieco-Bianchi L, Ciminale V. Mitochondria as functional targets of proteins coded by human tumor viruses. 94. 2005(87):142.
51. Clippinger AJ, Bouchard MJ. Hepatitis B virus Hbx protein localizes to mitochondria in primary rat hepatocytes and modulates mitochondrial membrane potential. J. Virol. 2008;82:6798-811.
52. Seyfried TN, Arismendi-Morillo G, Mukherjee P, Chinopoulos C. On the Origin of ATP Synthesis in Cancer. iScience. 2020;23(11):101761.
53. Chinopoulos C, Seyfried TN. Mitochondrial Substrate-Level Phosphorylation as Energy Source for Glioblastoma: Review and Hypothesis. ASN Neuro. 2018;10:1759091418818261.
54. Mukherjee P, Augur ZM, Li M, Hill C, Greenwood B, Domin MA, et al. Therapeutic benefit of combining calorie-restricted ketogenic diet and glutamine targeting in late-stage experimental glioblastoma. Commun Biol. 2019;2:200.
55. Seyfried TN, Kiebish MA, Marsh J, Shelton LM, Huysentruyt LC, Mukherjee P. Metabolic management of brain cancer. Biochim Biophys Acta. 2011;1807(6):577-94.
56. Oizel K, Chauvin C, Oliver L, Gratas C, Geraldo F, Jarry U, et al. Efficient Mitochondrial Glutamine Targeting Prevails Over Glioblastoma Metabolic Plasticity. Clin Cancer Res. 2017;23(20):6292-304.
57. Chen Q, Kirk K, Shurubor YI, Zhao D, Arreguin AJ, Shahi I, et al. Rewiring of Glutamine Metabolism Is a Bioenergetic Adaptation of Human Cells with Mitochondrial DNA Mutations. Cell Metab. 2018;27(5):1007-25.e5.
58. Fung J. The Cancer Code. New York, NY: Harper Collins; 2020.
59. Yuan C, Bao Y, Sato K, Nimptsch K, Song M, Brand-Miller JC, et al. Influence of dietary insulin scores on survival in colorectal cancer patients. Br J Cancer. 2017;117(7):1079-87.
60. Meyerhardt JA, Sato K, Niedzwiecki D, Ye C, Saltz LB, Mayer RJ, et al. Dietary glycemic load and cancer recurrence and survival in patients with stage III colon cancer: findings from CALGB 89803. J Natl Cancer Inst. 2012;104(22):1702-11.
61. Goldman S, Bron D, Tousseyn T, Vierasu I, Dewispelaere L, Heimann P, et al. Rapid Progression of Angioimmunoblastic T Cell Lymphoma Following BNT162b2 mRNA Vaccine Booster Shot: A Case Report. Front Med (Lausanne). 2021;8:798095.
62. Mizutani M, Mitsui H, Amano T, Ogawa Y, Deguchi N, Shimada S, et al. Two cases of axillary lymphadenopathy diagnosed as diffuse large B-cell lymphoma developed shortly after BNT162b2 COVID-19 vaccination. J Eur Acad Dermatol Venereol. 2022;36(8):e613-e5.
63. Sekizawa A, Hashimoto K, Kobayashi S, Kozono S, Kobayashi T, Kawamura Y, et al. Rapid progression of marginal zone B-cell lymphoma after COVID-19 vaccination (BNT162b2): A case report. Front Med (Lausanne). 2022;9:963393.
64. Costanzo M, De Giglio MAR, Roviello GN. Deciphering the Relationship between SARS-CoV-2 and Cancer. Int. J Mol. Sci. 2023;24(9).
65. Department of Defence;Pageshttps://www.health.mil/Military-Health-Topics/Health-Readiness/AFHSD/Data-Management-and-Technical-Support/Defense-Medical-Epidemiology-Database.
66. Paardekooper C. Cancer and COVID vaccines. Medrxiv. 2023.
67. Alegria C, Wiseman DM, Nunes Y. US - Death Trends for Neoplasms ICD codes: C00-D48, Ages 15-44. Research Gate. 2024.

68. Alegria C, Nunes Y. UK - Death and Disability Trends for Malignant Neoplasms, Ages 15-44. Research Gate. 2024.
69. Gibo M, Kojima S, fujisawa A, Kikuchi T, Fukushima M. Increased Age-Adjusted Cancer Mortality After the Third mRNA-Lipid Nanoparticle Vaccine Dose During the COVID-19 Pandemic in Japan. Cureus. 2024;16:e57860.
70. Johnston TS, Li SH, Painter MM, Atkinson RK, Douek NR, Reeg DB, et al. Immunological imprinting shapes the specificity of human antibody responses against SARS-CoV-2 variants. Immunity. 2024;57(4):912-25.e4.
71. Vatti A, Monsalve DM, Pacheco Y, Chang C, Anaya JM, Gershwin ME. Original antigenic sin: A comprehensive review. J Autoimmun. 2017;83:12-21.
72. Parry PI, Lefringhausen A, Turni C, Neil CJ, Cosford R, Hudson NJ, et al. 'Spikeopathy': COVID-19 Spike Protein Is Pathogenic, from Both Virus and Vaccine mRNA. Biomedicines. 2023;11(8).
73. Goubran H, Stakiw J, Seghatchian J, Ragab G, Burnouf T. SARS-CoV-2 and cancer: the intriguing and informative cross-talk. Transfus. Apher. Sci. 2022;61(4):103488.
74. Valdes Angues R, Perea Bustos Y. SARS-CoV-2 Vaccination and the Multi-Hit Hypothesis of Oncogenesis. Cureus. 2023;15(12):e50703.
75. Clough E, Chean KT, Inigo J, Tubbesing KE, Chandra D, Chaves L. Mitochondrial dynamics in SARS-CoV-2 spike protein treated human microglia: Implications for neuro-COVID. Journal of Neuroimmune Pharmacology. 2021;16:770-84.
76. Diaz-Resendiz KJ, Benitez-Trinidad AB, Covantes-Rosales CE, Toledo-Ibarra GA. Loss of mitochondrial membrane potential in leucocytes as post-COVID-19 sequelae. J. Leukoc. Biol. 2022.
77. Medini H, Zirmman A, Mishmar D. Immune system cells from COVID-19 patients display compromised mitochondrial-nuclear expression co-regulation and rewiring toward glycolysis. iScience. 2021;24:103471.
78. Pliss A, Kuzmin AN, Prasad PN, Mahajan SD. Michochondrial dysfunction: A prelude to neuropathogenesis of SARS-COV-2. ACS Chem. Neurosci. 2022;13:308-12.
79. Mortezaee K, Majidpoor J. CD8(+) T Cells in SARS-CoV-2 Induced Disease and Cancer-Clinical Perspectives. Front Immunol. 2022;13:864298.
80. Bhardwaj K, Liu P, Leibowitz JL, Kao CC. The coronavirus endoribonuclease Nsp15 interacts with retinoblastoma tumor suppressor protein. J Virol. 2012;86(8):4294-304.
81. Sheng Y, Laister RC, Lemak A, Wu B, Tai E, Duan S, et al. Molecular basis of Pirh2-mediated p53 ubiquitylation. Nat Struct Mol Biol. 2008;15(12):1334-42.
82. Tan X, Cai K, Li J, Yuan Z, Chen R, Xiao H, et al. Coronavirus subverts ER-phagy by hijacking FAM134B and ATL3 into p62 condensates to facilitate viral replication. Cell Rep. 2023;42(4):112286.
83. Jiang H, Mei YF. SARS-CoV-2 Spike Impairs DNA Damage Repair and Inhibits V(D)J Recombination In Vitro. Viruses. 2021;13(10).
84. Seneff S, Nigh G, Kyriakopoulos AM, McCullough PA. Innate immune suppression by SARS-C-V-2 mRNA vaccinations: The role of G-quadruplexes, exosomes and microRNAs. Food & Chemical Toxicology. 2022;164:113008.
85. Musella M, Manic G, De Maria R, Vitale I, Sistigu A. Type-I-interferons in infection and cancer: Unanticipated dynamics with therapeutic implications. Oncoimmunology. 2017;6(5):e1314424.
86. Vilchez RA, Madden CR, Kozinetz CA, Halvorson SJ, White ZS, Jorgensen JL, et al. Association between simian virus 40 and non-Hodgkin lymphoma. Lancet. 2002;359(9309):817-23.
87. Uversky VN, Redwan EM, Makis W, Rubio-Casillas A. IgG4 Antibodies Induced by Repeated Vaccination May Generate Immune Tolerance to the SARS-CoV-2 Spike Protein. Vaccines (Basel). 2023;11(5).

88. Irrgang P, Gerling J, Kocher K, Lapuente D, Steininger P, Wytopil M. Class switch towards non-inflammatory, spike-specific IgG4 antibodies after repeated SARS-CoV-2 mRNA vaccination. Science Immunology. 2022.
89. Wang H, Xu Q, Zhao C, Zhu Z, Zhu X, Zhou J, et al. An immune evasion mechanism with IgG4 playing an essential role in cancer and implication for immunotherapy. J Immunother Cancer. 2020;8(2).
90. Crescioli S, Correa I, Karagiannis P, Davies AM, Sutton BJ, Nestle FO, et al. IgG4 Characteristics and Functions in Cancer Immunity. Curr Allergy Asthma Rep. 2016;16(1):7.
91. Halma MT, Tuszynski J, Marik P. David vs Goliath: Low-cost approaches to treating and preventing cancer. Public Health Reviews. 2023.
92. Spatial, temporal, and demographic patterns in prevalence of smoking tobacco use and attributable disease burden in 204 countries and territories, 1990-2019: a systematic analysis from the Global Burden of Disease Study 2019. Lancet. 2021;397(10292):2337-60.
93. Pesch B, Kendzia B, Gustavsson P, Jöckel KH, Johnen G, Pohlabeln H, et al. Cigarette smoking and lung cancer--relative risk estimates for the major histological types from a pooled analysis of case-control studies. Int J Cancer. 2012;131(5):1210-9.
94. Cornelius ME, Loretan CG, Jamal A, Davis Lynn BC, Mayer M, Alcantara IC, et al. Tobacco Product Use Among Adults - United States, 2021. MMWR Morb Mortal Wkly Rep. 2023;72(18):475-83.
95. Benbrook CM. Impacts of Genetically Engineered Crops on Pesticide Use in the U.S. -- the First Sixteen Years. Environmental Sciences Europe. 2012;24:24.
96. Chang ET, Delzell E. Systematic review and meta-analysis of glyphosate exposure and risk of lymphohematopoietic cancers. J Environ Sci Health B. 2016;51(6):402-34.
97. Merhi M, Raynal H, Cahuzac E, Vinson F, Cravedi JP, Gamet-Payrastre L. Occupational exposure to pesticides and risk of hematopoietic cancers: meta-analysis of case-control studies. Cancer Causes Control. 2007;18(10):1209-26.
98. Martin P. Immigration and Farm Labor: Policy Options and Consequences. American Journal of Agricultural Economics. 2013;95:470-5.
99. Benbrook CM. Trends in glyphosate herbicide use in the United States and globally. Environ Sci Eur. 2016;28(1):3.
100. Bradbury KE, Balkwill A, Spencer EA, Roddam AW, Reeves GK, Green J, et al. Organic food consumption and the incidence of cancer in a large prospective study of women in the United Kingdom. Br J Cancer. 2014;110(9):2321-6.
101. Taylor KW, Troester MA, Herring AH, Engel LS, Nichols HB, Sandler DP, et al. Associations between Personal Care Product Use Patterns and Breast Cancer Risk among White and Black Women in the Sister Study. Environ Health Perspect. 2018;126(2):027011.
102. Yoo JJ, Kim HY. Use of Beauty Products among U.S. Adolescents: An Exploration of Media Influence. Journal of Global Fashion Marketing. 2010;1:172-81.
103. Schreder ED, Uding N, La Guardia MJ. Inhalation a significant exposure route for chlorinated organophosphate flame retardants. Chemosphere. 2016;150:499-504.
104. Hoffman K, Lorenzo A, Butt CM, Hammel SC, Henderson BB, Roman SA, et al. Exposure to flame retardant chemicals and occurrence and severity of papillary thyroid cancer: A case-control study. Environ Int. 2017;107:235-42.
105. Alaee M, Arias P, Sjödin A, Bergman A. An overview of commercially used brominated flame retardants, their applications, their use patterns in different countries/regions and possible modes of release. Environ Int. 2003;29(6):683-9.
106. van der Veen I, de Boer J. Phosphorus flame retardants: properties, production, environmental occurrence, toxicity and analysis. Chemosphere. 2012;88(10):1119-53.
107. Appleton JD. Radon: sources, health risks, and hazard mapping. Ambio. 2007;36(1):85-9.

108. Schmid K, Kuwert T, Drexler H. Radon in indoor spaces: an underestimated risk factor for lung cancer in environmental medicine. Dtsch Arztebl Int. 2010;107(11):181-6.
109. Ahlstrom LH, Sparr Eskilsson C, Bjorklund E. Determination of Banned Azo Dyes in Consumer Goods. TrAC trends in Analytical Chemistry. 2005;24:49-56.
110. Chequer FM, Dorta DJ, Oliveira DP. de Azo Dyes and Their Metabolites: Does the Discharge of the Azo Dye into Water Bodies Represent Human and Ecological Risks? Advances in Treating Textile Effluent; IntechOpen. 2011:704-8.
111. Browne AJ, Chipeta MG, Haines-Woodhouse G, Kumaran EPA, Hamadani BHK, Zaraa S, et al. Global antibiotic consumption and usage in humans, 2000-18: a spatial modelling study. Lancet Planet Health. 2021;5(12):e893-e904.
112. Kilkkinen A, Rissanen H, Klaukka T, Pukkala E, Heliövaara M, Huovinen P, et al. Antibiotic use predicts an increased risk of cancer. Int J Cancer. 2008;123(9):2152-5.
113. Urbinello D, Joseph W, Verloock L, Martens L, Röösli M. Temporal trends of radio-frequency electromagnetic field (RF-EMF) exposure in everyday environments across European cities. Environ Res. 2014;134:134-42.
114. Teepen JC, van Dijck JA. Impact of high electromagnetic field levels on childhood leukemia incidence. Int J Cancer. 2012;131(4):769-78.
115. Keadle SK, McKinnon R, Graubard BI, Troiano RP. Prevalence and trends in physical activity among older adults in the United States: A comparison across three national surveys. Prev Med. 2016;89:37-43.
116. Kvaavik E, Batty GD, Ursin G, Huxley R, Gale CR. Influence of individual and combined health behaviors on total and cause-specific mortality in men and women: the United Kingdom health and lifestyle survey. Arch Intern Med. 2010;170(8):711-8.
117. Bin YS, Marshall NS, Glozier N. Secular trends in adult sleep duration: a systematic review. Sleep Med Rev. 2012;16(3):223-30.
118. Hoyos C, Glozier N, Marshall NS. Recent Evidence on Worldwide Trends on Sleep Duration. Current Sleep Medicine Reports. 2015;1.
119. Wang X, Ma H, Gupta S, Heianza Y, Fonseca V, Qi L. The Joint Secular Trends of Sleep Quality and Diabetes Among US Adults, 2005-2018. J Clin Endocrinol Metab. 2022;107(11):3152-61.
120. Erren TC, Morfeld P, Foster RG, Reiter RJ, Groß JV, Westermann IK. Sleep and cancer: Synthesis of experimental data and meta-analyses of cancer incidence among some 1,500,000 study individuals in 13 countries. Chronobiol Int. 2016;33(4):325-50.
121. Liu Y, Wheaton AG, Chapman DP, Cunningham TJ, Lu H, Croft JB. Prevalence of Healthy Sleep Duration among Adults--United States, 2014. MMWR Morb Mortal Wkly Rep. 2016;65(6):137-41.
122. Rigó M, Dragano N, Wahrendorf M, Siegrist J, Lunau T. Work stress on rise? Comparative analysis of trends in work stressors using the European working conditions survey. Int Arch Occup Environ Health. 2021;94(3):459-74.
123. Yang T, Qiao Y, Xiang S, Li W, Gan Y, Chen Y. Work stress and the risk of cancer: A meta-analysis of observational studies. Int J Cancer. 2019;144(10):2390-400.
124. Wagan F, Memon GN. Changing trends of indications and rate of cesarean section: An audit. Medical Channel. 2011;17.
125. Ganeriwal SA, Ryan GA, Purandare NC, Purandare CN. Examining the role and relevance of the critical analysis and comparison of cesarean section rates in a changing world. Taiwan J Obstet Gynecol. 2021;60(1):20-3.
126. Han MA, Storman D, Al-Rammahy H, Tang S, Hao Q, Leung G, et al. Impact of maternal reproductive factors on cancer risks of offspring: A systematic review and meta-analysis of cohort studies. PLoS One. 2020;15(3):e0230721.

127. Betrán AP, Ye J, Moller AB, Zhang J, Gülmezoglu AM, Torloni MR. The Increasing Trend in Caesarean Section Rates: Global, Regional and National Estimates: 1990-2014. PLoS One. 2016;11(2):e0148343.
128. Chang ET, Montgomery SM, Richiardi L, Ehlin A, Ekbom A, Lambe M. Number of siblings and risk of Hodgkin's lymphoma. Cancer Epidemiol Biomarkers Prev. 2004;13(7):1236-43.
129. Altieri A, Castro F, Bermejo JL, Hemminki K. Number of siblings and the risk of lymphoma, leukemia, and myeloma by histopathology. Cancer Epidemiol Biomarkers Prev. 2006;15(7):1281-6.
130. Sobotka T. Post-transitional fertility: The role of childbearing postponment in fueling the shift to low and unstable fertility levels. J Biosoc Sci. 2017;49(S1):S20-s45.
131. Merrill RM, Fugal S, Novilla LB, Raphael MC. Cancer risk associated with early and late maternal age at first birth. Gynecol Oncol. 2005;96(3):583-93.
132. MacMahon B, Cole PE, Lin TM, Lowe CR, Mirra AP. Age at First Birth and Breast Cancer Risk. Bull World Health Organ. 1970;43:209-21.
133. Ramgopal S, Aronson PL, Marin JR. United States' Emergency Department Visits for Fever by Young Children 2007-2017. West J Emerg Med. 2020;21(6):146-51.
134. Albonico HU, Bräker HU, Hüsler J. Febrile infectious childhood diseases in the history of cancer patients and matched controls. Med Hypotheses. 1998;51(4):315-20.
135. Pasvol TJ, Macgregor EA, Rait G, Horsfall L. Time trends in contraceptive prescribing in UK primary care 2000-2018: a repeated cross-sectional study. BMJ Sex Reprod Health. 2022;48(3):193-8.
136. Daniels K, Mosher WD. Contraceptive methods women have ever used: United States, 1982-2010. Natl Health Stat Report. 2013(62):1-15.
137. Mørch LS, Skovlund CW, Hannaford PC, Iversen L, Fielding S, Lidegaard Ø. Contemporary Hormonal Contraception and the Risk of Breast Cancer. N Engl J Med. 2017;377(23):2228-39.
138. Daniels K, Daugherty J, Jones J, Mosher W. Current Contraceptive Use and Variation by Selected Characteristics Among Women Aged 15-44: United States, 2011-2013. Natl Health Stat Report. 2015(86):1-14.
139. Scoccianti C, Key TJ, Anderson AS, Armaroli P, Berrino F, Cecchini M, et al. European Code against Cancer 4th Edition: Breastfeeding and cancer. Cancer Epidemiol. 2015;39 Suppl 1:S101-6.
140. Martin RM, Middleton N, Gunnell D, Owen CG, Smith GD. Breast-feeding and cancer: the Boyd Orr cohort and a systematic review with meta-analysis. J Natl Cancer Inst. 2005;97(19):1446-57.
141. Babic A, Sasamoto N, Rosner BA, Tworoger SS, Jordan SJ, Risch HA, et al. Association Between Breastfeeding and Ovarian Cancer Risk. JAMA Oncol. 2020;6(6):e200421.
142. Bustamante E, Pedersen PL. High aerobic glycolysis of rat hepatoma cells in culture: role of mitochondrial hexokinase. Proc. Natl. Acad. Sci U. S. A. 1977;74(9):3735-9.
143. Ciscato F, Ferrone L, Masgras I, Laquatra C, Rasola A. Hexokinase 2 in Cancer: A Prima Donna Playing Multiple Characters. Int. J Mol. Sci. 2021;22(9).
144. Mathupala SP, Ko YH, Pedersen PL. Hexokinase-2 bound to mitochondria: cancer's stygian link to the "Warburg Effect" and a pivotal target for effective therapy. Semin. Cancer Biol. 2009;19(1):17-24.
145. Patra KC, Hay N. Hexokinase 2 as oncotarget. Oncotarget. 2013;4(11):1862-3.
146. Dach J. Cracking Cancer Toolkit: Using repurposed drugs for cancer treatment: Amazon digitial Services LLC- KDP Print US, 2020; 2020.
147. Harris SL, Levine AJ. The p53 pathway: positive and negative feedback loops. Oncogene. 2005;24:2899-908.

148. Liu S, Chen S, Zeng J. TGF-B signaling: A complex role in tumorigenesis. Molecular Medicine Reports. 2018;17:699-704.
149. Zhan T, Rindtorff N, Boutros M. Wnt signaling in cancer. Oncogene. 2017;36:1461-73.
150. Krishnamurthy N, Kurzrock R. Targeting the Wnt/beta-catenin pathway in cancer: Update on effectors and inhibitors. Cancer Treat Rev. 2018;62:50-60.
151. Nowell CS, Radtke F. Notch as a tumour suppressor. Nature Reviews Cancer. 2017;17:145-59.
152. Koduru S, Kumar R, Srinivasan S, Evers MB, Damodaran C. Notch-1 inhibition by Withaferin-A: a therapeutic target against colon carcinogenesis. Mol Cancer Ther. 2010;9(1):202-10.
153. Rascio F, Spadaccino F, Rocchetti MT, Castellano G, Stallone G, Netti GS, et al. The pathogenic role of PI3K/AKT pathway in cancer onset and drug resistance: An updated review. Cancers. 2021;13:3949.
154. Carballo GB, Honorato JR, de Lopes GPF, Spohr TCLS. A highlight on Sonic hedgehog pathway. Cell Commun. Signal. 2018;16(1):11.
155. Larsen AR, Bai RY, Chung JH, Borodovsky A, Rudin CM, Riggins GJ, et al. Repurposing the antihelmintic mebendazole as a hedgehog inhibitor. Mol. Cancer. Ther. 2015;14:3-13.
156. Awad RM, De Vlaeminck Y, Maebe J, Goyvaerts C, Breckpot K. Turn back the TIMEe: Targeting tumor infiltrating myeloid cells to revert cancer progression. Front. Immunol. 2023;9:1977.
157. Wang Q, Shao X, Zhang Y, Zhu M, Wang FXC, Mu J, et al. Role of tumor microenvironment in cancer progression and therapeutic strategy. Cancer Med. 2023;12:11149 - 65.
158. Braun S, Vogl FD, Naume B, Janni W, Osborne MP, Coombes RC, et al. A pooled analysis of bone marrow micrometastasis in breast cancer. N. Engl. J Med. 2005;353(8):793-802.
159. Cole K, Al-Kadhimi Z, Talmadge JE. Role of myeloid-derived suppressor cells in tumor recurrence. Cancer and Metastasis Reviews. 2023.
160. Ma T, Renz BW, Ilmer M, Koch D, Yang Y, Werner J, et al. Myeloid-Derived Suppressor Cells in Solid Tumors. Cells. 2022;11(2).
161. Noman MZ, Desantis G, Janji B, Hasmim M, Karray S, Dessen P, et al. PD-L1 is a novel direct target of HIF-1Î±, and its blockade under hypoxia enhanced MDSC-mediated T cell activation. J Exp Med. 2014;211(5):781-90.
162. Condamine T, Mastio J, Gabrilovich DI. Transcriptional regulation of myeloid-derived suppressor cells. J Leukoc. Biol. 2015;98(6):913-22.
163. Yan HH, Pickup M, Pang Y, Gorska AE, Li Z, Chytil A, et al. Gr-1+CD11b+ myeloid cells tip the balance of immune protection to tumor promotion in the premetastatic lung. Cancer Res. 2010;70(15):6139-49.
164. Law AMK, Valdes-Mora F, Gallego-Ortega D. Myeloid-Derived Suppressor Cells as a Therapeutic Target for Cancer. Cells. 2020;9(3).
165. Gallego-Ortega D, Ledger A, Roden DL, Law AM, Magenau A, Kikhytyak Z, et al. ELF5 drives lung metastasis in luminal breast cancer through recruitment of Gr1+ CD11b+ myeloid-derived suppressor cells. PLoS Biol. 2015;13:e1002330.
166. Zea AH, Rodriguez PC, Atkins MB, Hernandez C, Signoretti S, Zabaleta J, et al. Arginase-producing myeloid suppressor cells in renal cell carcinoma patients: a mechanism of tumor evasion. Cancer Res. 2005;65(8):3044-8.
167. Huang B, Pan PY, Li Q, Sato AI, Levy DE, Bromberg J, et al. Gr-1+CD115+ immature myeloid suppressor cells mediate the development of tumor-induced T regulatory cells and T-cell anergy in tumor-bearing host. Cancer Res. 2006;66(2):1123-31.
168. Pan PY, Ma G, Weber KJ, Ozao-Choy J, Wang G, Yin B, et al. Immune stimulatory receptor CD40 is required for T-cell suppression and T regulatory cell activation mediated by myeloid-derived suppressor cells in cancer. Cancer Res. 2010;70(1):99-108.

169. Sharabi A, tsokos MG, Ding Y, Malek TR, Klatzmann D, Tsokos GC. Regulatory T cells in the treatment of disease. Nature Reviews. 2018;17:823-44.
170. Li C, Jiang P, Wei S, Xu X, Wang J. Regulatory T cells in tumor microenvironment: new mechanisms, potential therapeutic strategies and future prospects. Mol. Cancer. 2020;19(1):116.
171. Raffin C, Vo LT, Bluestone JA. T(reg) cell-based therapies: challenges and perspectives. Nat. Rev Immunol. 2020;20(3):158-72.
172. Tie Y, Tang F, Wei YQ, Wei XW. Immunosuppressive cells in cancer: mechanisms and potential therapeutic targets. J Hematol. Oncol. 2022;15(1):61.
173. Ohue Y, Nishikawa H. Regulatory T (Treg) cells in cancer: Can Treg cells be a new therapeutic target? Cancer Sci. 2019;110(7):2080-9.
174. Wu T, Wu X, Wang HY, Chen L. Immune contexture defined by single cell technology for prognosis prediction and immunotherapy guidance in cancer. Cancer Commun. (Lond). 2019;39(1):21.
175. Becht E, Giraldo NA, Dieu-Nosjean MC, SautÃ¨s-Fridman C, Fridman WH. Cancer immune contexture and immunotherapy. Curr. Opin. Immunol. 2016;39:7-13.
176. Knochelmann HM, Dwyer CJ, Bailey SR, Amaya SM, Elston DM, Mazza-McCrann JM, et al. When worlds collide: Th17 and Treg cells in cancer and autoimmunity. Cell Mol. Immunol. 2018;15(5):458-69.
177. Giraldo NA, Becht E, Remark R, Damotte D, SautÃ¨s-Fridman C, Fridman WH. The immune contexture of primary and metastatic human tumours. Curr. Opin. Immunol. 2014;27:8-15.
178. Fridman WH, PagÃ¨s F, SautÃ¨s-Fridman C, Galon J. The immune contexture in human tumours: impact on clinical outcome. Nat. Rev Cancer. 2012;12(4):298-306.
179. Ino Y, Yamazaki-Itoh R, Shimada K, Iwasaki M, Kosuge T, Kanai Y, et al. Immune cell infiltration as an indicator of the immune microenvironment of pancreatic cancer. Br. J Cancer. 2013;108(4):914-23.
180. Cassetta L, Pollard JW. Tumor-associated macrophages. Curr. Biol. 2020;30(6):R246-R8.
181. Pan Y, Yu Y, Wang X, Zhang T. Tumor-Associated Macrophages in Tumor Immunity. Front Immunol. 2020;11:583084.
182. Kumari N, Choi SH. Tumor-associated macrophages in cancer: recent advancements in cancer nanoimmunotherapies. J Exp Clin. Cancer Res. 2022;41(1):68.
183. Heng Y, Zhu X, Lin H, Jingyu M, Ding X, Tao L, et al. CD206(+) tumor-associated macrophages interact with CD4(+) tumor-infiltrating lymphocytes and predict adverse patient outcome in human laryngeal squamous cell carcinoma. J Transl. Med. 2023;21(1):167.
184. Murray PJ, Wynn TA. Protective and pathogenic functions of macrophage subsets. Nat. Rev Immunol. 2011;11(11):723-37.
185. Bronte V, Brandau S, Chen SH, Colombo MP, Frey AB, Greten TF, et al. Recommendations for myeloid-derived suppressor cell nomenclature and characterization standards. Nat. Commun. 2016;7:12150.
186. Beury DW, Parker KH, Nyandjo M, Sinha P, Carter KA, Ostrand-Rosenberg S. Cross-talk among myeloid-derived suppressor cells, macrophages, and tumor cells impacts the inflammatory milieu of solid tumors. J Leukoc. Biol. 2014;96(6):1109-18.
187. Veglia F, Sanseviero E, Gabrilovich DI. Myeloid-derived suppressor cells in the era of increasing myeloid cell diversity. Nat. Rev Immunol. 2021;21(8):485-98.
188. Komohara Y, Jinushi M, Takeya M. Clinical significance of macrophage heterogeneity in human malignant tumors. Cancer Sci. 2014;105(1):1-8.
189. Liu W, Wang W, Wang X, Xu C, Zhang N, Di W. Cisplatin-stimulated macrophages promote ovarian cancer migration via the CCL20-CCR6 axis. Cancer Lett. 2020;472:59-69.

190. Li X, Liu R, Su X, Pan Y, Han X, Shao C, et al. Harnessing tumor-associated macrophages as aids for cancer immunotherapy. Mol. Cancer. 2019;18(1):177.
191. Ruffell B, Coussens LM. Macrophages and therapeutic resistance in cancer. Cancer Cell. 2015;27(4):462-72.
192. Zhao X, Qu J, Sun Y, Wang J, Liu x, Wang F, et al. Prognostic significance of tumor-associated macrophages in breast cancer: a meta-analysis of the literature. Oncotarget. 2017;8(18):30576-86.
193. Yuan X, Zhang J, Li D, Mao Y, Mo F, Du W, et al. Prognostic significance of tumor-associated macrophages in ovarian cancer: A meta-analysis. Gynecol. Oncol. 2017;147(1):181-7.
194. Komohara Y, Niino D, Ohnishi K, Ohshima K, Takeya M. Role of tumor-associated macrophages in hematological malignancies. Pathol. Int. 2015;65(4):170-6.
195. Kitano Y, Okabe H, Yamashita YI, Nakagawa S, Saito Y, Umezaki N, et al. Tumour-infiltrating inflammatory and immune cells in patients with extrahepatic cholangiocarcinoma. Br. J Cancer. 2018;118(2):171-80.
196. D'Errico G, Alonso-Nocelo M, Vallespinos M, Hermann PC, AlcalÃ¡ S, GarcÃ-a CP, et al. Tumor-associated macrophage-secreted 14-3-3 signals via AXL to promote pancreatic cancer chemoresistance. Oncogene. 2019;38(27):5469-85.
197. Gyori D, Lim EL, Grant FM, Spensberger D, Roychoudhuri R, Shuttleworth SJ, et al. Compensation between CSF1R+ macrophages and Foxp3+ Treg cells drives resistance to tumor immunotherapy. JCI Insight. 2018;3(11).
198. Seyfried TN, Huysentruyt LC. On the origin of cancer metastasis. Crit. Rev. Oncog. 2013;18:43-73.
199. Fan CS, Chen LL, Hsu TA, Chen CC, Chua KV, Li CP, et al. Endothelial-mesenchymal transition harnesses HSP90Î±-secreting M2-macrophages to exacerbate pancreatic ductal adenocarcinoma. J Hematol. Oncol. 2019;12(1):138.
200. Wang W, Liu Y, Guo J, He H, Mi X, Chen C, et al. miR-100 maintains phenotype of tumor-associated macrophages by targeting mTOR to promote tumor metastasis via Stat5a/IL-1ra pathway in mouse breast cancer. Oncogenesis. 2018;7(12):97.
201. Cassetta L, Fragkogianni S, Sims AH, Swierczak A, Forrester LM, Zhang H, et al. Human Tumor-Associated Macrophage and Monocyte Transcriptional Landscapes Reveal Cancer-Specific Reprogramming, Biomarkers, and Therapeutic Targets. Cancer Cell. 2019;35(4):588-602.
202. Debebe A, Medina V, Chen CY, Mahajan IM, Jia C, Fu D, et al. Wnt/b-catenin activation and macrophage induction during liver cancer development following steatosis. Oncogene. 2017;36(43):6020-9.
203. Chen Q, Zhang XH, Massagu J. Macrophage binding to receptor VCAM-1 transmits survival signals in breast cancer cells that invade the lungs. Cancer Cell. 2011;20(4):538-49.
204. Yin Z, Ma T, Huang B, Lin L, Zhou Y, Yan J, et al. Macrophage-derived exosomal microRNA-501-3p promotes progression of pancreatic ductal adenocarcinoma through the TGFBR3-mediated TGF-b signaling pathway. J Exp Clin. Cancer Res. 2019;38(1):310.
205. Klimp AH, Hollema H, Kempinga C, van der Zee AG, de Vries EG, Daemen T. Expression of cyclooxygenase-2 and inducible nitric oxide synthase in human ovarian tumors and tumor-associated macrophages. Cancer Res. 2001;61(19):7305-9.
206. Pan B, Ge L, Xun YQ, Chen YJ, Gao CY, Han X, et al. Exercise training modalities in patients with type 2 diabetes mellitus: a systematic review and network meta-analysis. Int. J Behav. Nutr. Phys. Act. 2018;15(1):72.
207. Majety M, Runza V, Lehmann C, Hoves S, Ries CH. A drug development perspective on targeting tumor-associated myeloid cells. FEBS J. 2018;285(4):763-76.

208. Labelle M, Begum S, Hynes RO. Direct signaling between platelets and cancer cells induces an epithelial-mesenchymal-like transition and promotes metastasis. Cancer Cell. 2011;20(5):576-90.
209. Labelle M, Begum S, Hynes RO. Platelets guide the formation of early metastatic niches. Proc. Natl. Acad. Sci U. S. A. 2014;111(30):E3053-E61.
210. McCarty OJ, Mousa SA, Bray PF, Konstantopoulos K. Immobilized platelets support human colon carcinoma cell tethering, rolling, and firm adhesion under dynamic flow conditions. Blood. 2000;96(5):1789-97.
211. Heinmoller E, Weinel RJ, Heidtmann HH, Salge U, Seitz R, Schmitz I, et al. Studies on tumor-cell-induced platelet aggregation in human lung cancer cell lines. J Cancer Res Clin. Oncol. 1996;122(12):735-44.
212. Grignani G, Pacchiarini L, Ricetti MM, Dionigi P, Jemos V, Zucchella M, et al. Mechanisms of platelet activation by cultured human cancer cells and cells freshly isolated from tumor tissues. Invasion Metastasis. 1989;9(5):298-309.
213. Savage P. Clinical observations on chemotherapy curable malignancies: unique genetic events, frozen development and enduring apoptotic potential. BMC Cancer. 2015;15:11.
214. Al-Hajj M, Clarke MF. Self-renewal and solid tumor stem cells. Oncogene. 2004;23(43):7274-82.
215. Butti R, Gunasekaran VP, Kumar TVS, Banerjee P, Kundu GC. Breast cancer stem cells: Biology and therapeutic implications. Int. J Biochem. Cell Biol. 2019;107:38-52.
216. Medema JP. Targeting the Colorectal Cancer Stem Cell. N Engl J Med. 2017;377(9):888-90.
217. Nassar D, Blanpain C. Cancer Stem Cells: Basic Concepts and Therapeutic Implications. Annu. Rev Pathol. 2016;11:47-76.
218. Huang Z, Wu T, Liu AY, Ouyang G. Differentiation and transdifferentiation potentials of cancer stem cells. Oncotarget. 2015;6(37):39550-63.
219. Singh VK, Saini A, Chandra R. The Implications and Future Perspectives of Nanomedicine for Cancer Stem Cell Targeted Therapies. Front Mol. Biosci. 2017;4:52.
220. Dionisio MR, Vieira AF, Carvalho R, Conde I, Oliveira M, Gomes M, et al. BR-BCSC Signature: The Cancer Stem Cell Profile Enriched in Brain Metastases that Predicts a Worse Prognosis in Lymph Node-Positive Breast Cancer. Cells. 2020;9(11).
221. Kurtova AV, Xiao J, Mo Q, Pazhanisamy S, Krasnow R, Lerner SP, et al. Blocking PGE2-induced tumour repopulation abrogates bladder cancer chemoresistance. Nature. 2015;517(7533):209-13.
222. Reiter RJ, Rosales-Corral SA, TTan DX, Acuna-Castroviejo D, Qin L, Yang SF, et al. Melatonin, a full service anti-cancer agent: Inhibition of initiation, progression and metastasis. Int. J. Mol. Sci. 2017;18:843.
223. Fong D, Christensen CT, Chan MM. Targeting Cancer Stem Cells with Repurposed Drugs to Improve Current Therapies. Recent Pat Anticancer Drug Discov. 2021;16(2):136-60.
224. Proietti S, Cucina A, D'Anselmi F, Dinicola S, Pasqualato A, Lisi E, et al. Melatonin and vitamin D3 synergistically down-regulate Akt and MDM2 leading to TGFÎ²-1-dependent growth inhibition of breast cancer cells. J Pineal Res. 2011;50(2):150-8.
225. Dominguez-Gomez G, Chavez-Blanco A, Medina-Franco JL, Saldivar-Gonzalez F, Flores-Torrontegui Y, Juarez M, et al. Ivermectin as an inhibitor of cancer stem-like cells. Mol. Med Rep. 2018;17(2):3397-403.
226. Puar YR, Shanmugam MK, Fan L, Arfuso F, Sethi G, Tergaonkar V. Evidence for the Involvement of the Master Transcription Factor NF-ÎºB in Cancer Initiation and Progression. Biomedicines. 2018;6(3).
227. Malcomson FC, Parra-Soto S, Ho FK, Lu L, Celis-Morales C, Sharp L, et al. Adherence to the 2018 World Cancer Research Fund (WCRF)/American Institute for Cancer Research (AICR) Cancer

Prevention Recommendations and risk of 14 lifestyle-related cancers in the UK Biobank prospective cohort study. BMC Med. 2023;21(1):407.
228. Farvid MS, Sidahmed E, Spence ND, Mante AK, Rosner BA, Barnett JB. Consumption of red meat and processed meat and cancer incidence: a systematic review and meta-analysis of prospective studies. Eur J Epidemiol. 2021;36(9):937-51.
229. Kim SR, Kim K, Lee SA, Kwon SO, Lee JK, Keum N, et al. Effect of Red, Processed, and White Meat Consumption on the Risk of Gastric Cancer: An Overall and Dose-Response Meta-Analysis. Nutrients. 2019;11(4).
230. Shams-White MM, Brockton NT, Mitrou P, Romaguera D, Brown S, Bender A, et al. Operationalizing the 2018 World Cancer Research Fund/American Institute for Cancer Research (WCRF/AICR) Cancer Prevention Recommendations: A Standardized Scoring System. Nutrients. 2019;11(7).
231. Bischoff-Ferrari HA, Vellas B, Rizzoli R, Kressig RW. Effect of Vitamin D supplementation, omega-3 fatty acid supplementation, or a strengh-training excercise program on clinical outcomes in older adults. the DO-HEALTH randomized clinical trial. JAMA. 2020;324:1855-68.
232. Bischoff-Ferrari HA, Willett WC, Manson JE, Dawson-Hughes B, Manz MG, Theller R, et al. Combined Vitamin D, omega-3 fatty acids, and a simple home exercise program may reduce cancer risk among active adults aged 70 and older: A randomized clinical trial. Front. Aging. 2022;3:852643.
233. Manson JE, Cook NR, Lee IM, Christen W, Bassuk SS, Mora S, et al. Vitamin D Supplements and Prevention of Cancer and Cardiovascular Disease. N. Engl. J Med. 2019;380(1):33-44.
234. Li XX, Liu C, Dong SL, Ou CS, Lu JL, Ye JH. Anticarcinogenic potentials of tea catechins. Front. Nutr. 2022;9:1060783.
235. Singh BN, Shankar S, Srivastava RK. Green tea catechin, epigallocatechin-3-gallate (EGCG): mechanisms, perspectives and clinical applications. Biochem. Pharmacol. 2011;82(12):1807-21.
236. Bannister CA, Holden SE, Jenkins-Jones S, Morgan CL, Halcox JP, Schernthaner G, et al. Can people with type 2 diabetes live longer than those without? A comparison of mortality in people initiated with metformin or sulphonylurea monotherapy and matched, non-diabetic controls. Diabetes Obes. Metab. 2014;16(11):1165-73.
237. Tseng CH. Metformin significantly reduces incident prostate cancer risk in Taiwanese men with type 2 diabetes mellitus. Eur J Cancer. 2014;50(16):2831-7.
238. Gandini S, Puntoni M, Heckman-Stoddard BM, Dunn BK, Ford L, DeCensi A, et al. Metformin and cancer risk and mortality: a systematic review and meta-analysis taking into account biases and confounders. Cancer Prev. Res (Phila). 2014;7(9):867-85.
239. Zhang P, Li H, Tan X, Chen L, Wang S. Association of metformin use with cancer incidence and mortality: a meta-analysis. Cancer Epidemiol. 2013;37(3):207-18.
240. Fiolet T, Srour B, Sellem L, Kesse-Guyot E, Allès B, Méjean C, et al. Consumption of ultra-processed foods and cancer risk: results from NutriNet-Santé prospective cohort. Bmj. 2018;360:k322.
241. Chazelas E, Srour B, Desmetz E, Kesse-Guyot E, Julia C, Deschamps V, et al. Sugary drink consumption and risk of cancer: results from NutriNet-Santé prospective cohort. Bmj. 2019;366:l2408.
242. Debras C, Chazelas E, Srour B, Kesse-Guyot E, Julia C, Zelek L, et al. Total and added sugar intakes, sugar types, and cancer risk: results from the prospective NutriNet-Santé cohort. Am J Clin Nutr. 2020;112(5):1267-79.
243. Kim TL, Jeong GH, Yang JW, Lee KH, Kronbichler A, van der Vliet HJ, et al. Tea Consumption and Risk of Cancer: An Umbrella Review and Meta-Analysis of Observational Studies. Adv Nutr. 2020;11(6):1437-52.

244. Sarma DN, Barrett ML, Chavez ML, Gardiner P, Ko R, Mahady GB, et al. Safety of green tea extracts. A systematic review by the US Pharmacopeia. Drug Safety. 2008;31:464-84.
245. Talib WH, Alsayed AR, Abuawad A, Daoud S, Mahmod AI. Melatonin in cancer treatment: Current knowledge and future opportunities. Molecules. 2021;26:2506.
246. Bower JE, Partridge AH, Wolff AC, Thorner ED, Irwin MR, Joffe H, et al. Targeting Depressive Symptoms in Younger Breast Cancer Survivors: The Pathways to Wellness Randomized Controlled Trial of Mindfulness Meditation and Survivorship Education. J Clin Oncol. 2021;39(31):3473-84.
247. Gok Metin Z, Karadas C, Izgu N, Ozdemir L, Demirci U. Effects of progressive muscle relaxation and mindfulness meditation on fatigue, coping styles, and quality of life in early breast cancer patients: An assessor blinded, three-arm, randomized controlled trial. Eur J Oncol Nurs. 2019;42:116-25.
248. Greenlee H, DuPont-Reyes MJ, Balneaves LG, Carlson LE, Cohen MR, Deng G, et al. Clinical practice guidelines on the evidence-based use of integrative therapies during and after breast cancer treatment. CA Cancer J Clin. 2017;67(3):194-232.
249. Büttner-Teleagă A, Kim YT, Osel T, Richter K. Sleep Disorders in Cancer-A Systematic Review. Int J Environ Res Public Health. 2021;18(21).
250. Chen Y, Tan F, Wei L, Li X, Lyu Z, Feng X, et al. Sleep duration and the risk of cancer: a systematic review and meta-analysis including dose-response relationship. BMC Cancer. 2018;18(1):1149.
251. Medysky ME, Temesi J, Culos-Reed SN, Millet GY. Exercise, sleep and cancer-related fatigue: Are they related? Neurophysiol Clin. 2017;47(2):111-22.
252. Williamson T, Bai RY, Staedtke V, Huso D, Riggins GJ. Mebendazole and a non-steroidal anti-inflammatory combine to reduce tumor initiation in a colon cancer preclinical model. Oncotarget. 2016;7:68571-84.
253. Chandrasekaran B, Pal D, Kolluru V, Tyagi A, Baby B, Dahiya NR, et al. The chemopreventive effect of withaferin A on spontaneous and inflammation-associated colon carcinogenesis models. Carcinogenesis. 2018;39(12):1537-47.
254. Huang W, Sundquist J, Sundquist K, Ji J. Use of Phosphodiesterase 5 Inhibitors Is Associated With Lower Risk of Colorectal Cancer in Men With Benign Colorectal Neoplasms. Gastroenterology. 2019;157(3):672-81.
255. Gorodetska I, Kozeretska I, Dubrovska A. BRCA Genes: The Role in Genome Stability, Cancer Stemness and Therapy Resistance. J Cancer. 2019;10(9):2109-27.
256. Kowalska E, Narod SA, Huzarski T, Zajaczek S, Huzarska J, Gorski B, et al. Increased rates of chromosome breakage in BRCA1 carriers are normalized by oral selenium supplementation. Cancer Epidemiol Biomarkers Prev. 2005;14(5):1302-6.
257. Agrawal S, Vamadevan P, Mazibuko N, Bannister R, Swery R, Wilson S. A new method for ethical and efficient evidence generation for off-label medication use in oncology (A case study in glioblastoma). Front. Pharmacol. 2019;10:681.
258. Mukherjee P, Sotnokov AV, Mangian HJ, Zhou JR, Visek WJ, Clinton SK. Energy intake and prostate tumor growth, angiogenesis, and vascular endothelial growth factor expression. J. Natl. Cancer Inst. 1999;91:512-23.
259. Mavropoulos JC, Buschemeyer WC, Tewari AK, Rokheld D, Pollak M, Zhao Y. The effects of varying dietary carbohydrate and fat content on survival in a murine LNCap prostate coancer Zenograft model. Cancer Prev. Pre. 2009;2:557-65.
260. Hursting SD, Smith SM, Lashinger LM, Harvey AE, Perkins SN. Calories and carcinogenesis: lessons learnt form 30 years of calorie restriction research. Carcinogenesis. 2010;31:83-9.
261. Kari FW, Dunn SE, French JE, Barrett JC. Roles for insulin-like growth factor-1 in mediating the anti-carcinogenic effects of caloric restriction. J. Nutr. Health Aging. 1999;3:92-101.

262. Bonorden MJ, Rogozina OP, Kluczny CM, Grossmann ME, Grambsch PL, Grande JP, et al. Intermittent calorie restriction delays prostate tumor detection and increases survival time in TRAMP mice. Nutr. Cancer. 2009;61:265-75.
263. Thompson HJ, Jiang W, Zhu Z. Mechanisms by which energy restriction inhibits carcinogenesis. Adv. Exp. Med. Biol. 1999;470:77-84.
264. Zhou W, Mukherjee P, Kiebish MA, Markis WT, Mantis JG, Seyfried TN. The calorically restricted ketogenic diet, an effective alternative therapy for malignant brain cancer. Nutrition & Metabolism. 2007;4:5.
265. Morales-Oyarvide V, Yuan C, Babic A, Zhang S, Niedzwiecki D, Brand-Miller JC, et al. Dietary Insulin Load and Cancer Recurrence and Survival in Patients With Stage III Colon Cancer: Findings From CALGB 89803 (Alliance). J Natl Cancer Inst. 2019;111(2):170-9.
266. Hur J, Otegbeye E, Joh HK, Nimptsch K, Ng K, Ogino S, et al. Sugar-sweetened beverage intake in adulthood and adolescence and risk of early-onset colorectal cancer among women. Gut. 2021;70(12):2330-6.
267. Hodge AM, Bassett JK, Milne RL, English DR, Giles GG. Consumption of sugar-sweetened and artificially sweetened soft drinks and risk of obesity-related cancers. Public Health Nutr. 2018;21(9):1618-26.
268. Laguna JC, Alegret M, Cofán M, Sánchez-Tainta A, Díaz-López A, Martínez-González MA, et al. Simple sugar intake and cancer incidence, cancer mortality and all-cause mortality: A cohort study from the PREDIMED trial. Clin Nutr. 2021;40(10):5269-77.
269. Goncalves MD, Lu C, Tutnauer J, Hartman TE, Hwang SK, Murphy CJ, et al. High-fructose corn syrup enhances intestinal tumor growth in mice. Science. 2019;363(6433):1345-9.
270. Jiang Y, Pan Y, Rhea PR, Tan L, Gagea M, Cohen L, et al. A Sucrose-Enriched Diet Promotes Tumorigenesis in Mammary Gland in Part through the 12-Lipoxygenase Pathway. Cancer Res. 2016;76(1):24-9.
271. McGirt MJ, Chaichana KL, Gathinji M, Attenello F, Than K, Ruiz AJ, et al. Persistent outpatient hyperglycemia is independently associated with decreased survival after primary resection of malignant brain astrocytomas. Neurosurgery. 2008;63:286-91.
272. Meynet O, Ricci JE. Caloric restriction and cancer: molecular mechanisms and clinical implications. Trends in Molecular Medicine. 2014;20:419-27.
273. Godsland IF. Insulin resistance and hyperinsulinaemia in the development and progression of cancer. Clin Sci (Lond). 2009;118(5):315-32.
274. Currie CJ, Poole CD, Gale EA. The influence of glucose-lowering therapies on cancer risk in type 2 diabetes. Diabetologia. 2009;52(9):1766-77.
275. Wilder RM. The effects of ketonemia on the course of episepsy. Mayo Clin Proc. 1921;2:307-8.
276. Weber DD, Aminzadeh-Gohari S, Tulipan J, Catalano L, Feichtinger RG, Kofler B. Ketogenic diet in the treatment of cancer - Where do we stand? Mol Metab. 2020;33:102-21.
277. Lewis NE, Abdel-Haleem AM. The evolution of genome-scale models of cancer metabolism. Front Physiol. 2013;4:237.
278. Weber DD, Aminzadeh-Gohari S, Thapa M, Redtenbacher AS, Catalano L, Capelôa T, et al. Ketogenic diets slow melanoma growth in vivo regardless of tumor genetics and metabolic plasticity. Cancer Metab. 2022;10(1):12.
279. Woolf EC, Syed N, Scheck AC. Tumor Metabolism, the Ketogenic Diet and β-Hydroxybutyrate: Novel Approaches to Adjuvant Brain Tumor Therapy. Front Mol Neurosci. 2016;9:122.
280. Woolf EC, Curley KL, Liu Q, Turner GH, Charlton JA, Preul MC, et al. The Ketogenic Diet Alters the Hypoxic Response and Affects Expression of Proteins Associated with Angiogenesis, Invasive Potential and Vascular Permeability in a Mouse Glioma Model. PLoS One. 2015;10(6):e0130357.

281. Lussier DM, Woolf EC, Johnson JL, Brooks KS, Blattman JN, Scheck AC. Enhanced immunity in a mouse model of malignant glioma is mediated by a therapeutic ketogenic diet. BMC Cancer. 2016;16:310.
282. Li J, Zhang H, Dai Z. Cancer Treatment With the Ketogenic Diet: A Systematic Review and Meta-analysis of Animal Studies. Front Nutr. 2021;8:594408.
283. Abdelwahab MG, Fenton KE, Preul MC, Rho JM, Lynch A, Stafford P, et al. The ketogenic diet is an effective adjuvant to radiation therapy for the treatment of malignant glioma. PLoS One. 2012;7(5):e36197.
284. Puchalska P, Crawford PA. Multi-dimensional roles of ketone bodies to fuel metabolism, signaling, and therapeutics. Cell Metabolism. 2017;25:262-84.
285. Hwang CY, Choe W, Yoon KS, Ha J, Kim SS, Yeo EJ, et al. Molecular mechanisms for ketone body metabolism, signaling functions, and therapeutic potential in cancer. Nutrients. 2022;14:4932.
286. Newman JC, Verdin E. Ketone bodies as signaling metabolites. Trends in Endocrinology and Metabolism. 2014;25:42-52.
287. Shimazu T, Hirschey MD, Newman J, He W, Shirakawa K, Le Moan N, et al. Suppression of oxidative stress by B-hydroxybutyrate, and endogenous histone deacetylase inhibitor. Science. 2013;339:211-4.
288. Mulrooney TJ, Marsh J, Urits I, Seyfried TN, Mukherjee P. Influence of caloric restriction on constitutive expression of NFkB in an experimental mouse astrocytoma. PloS ONE. 2011;6(3):e18085.
289. Chi JT, Lin PH, Tolstikov V, Howard L, Chen EY, Bussberg V, et al. Serum metabolomic analysis of men on a low-carbohydrate diet for biochemically recurrent prostate cancer reveals the potential role of ketogenesis to slow tumor growth: a secondary analysis of the CAPS2 diet trial. Prostate Cancer Prostatic. Dis. 2022;25(4):770-7.
290. Freedland SJ, Allen J, Jarman A, Oyekunle T, Armstrong AJ, Moul JW, et al. A Randomized Controlled Trial of a 6-Month Low-Carbohydrate Intervention on Disease Progression in Men with Recurrent Prostate Cancer: Carbohydrate and Prostate Study 2 (CAPS2). Clin Cancer Res. 2020;26(12):3035-43.
291. Cohen CW, Fontaine KR, Arend RC, Soleymani T, Gower BA. Favorable Effects of a Ketogenic Diet on Physical Function, Perceived Energy, and Food Cravings in Women with Ovarian or Endometrial Cancer: A Randomized, Controlled Trial. Nutrients. 2018;10(9).
292. Cohen CW, Fontaine KR, Arend RC, Alvarez RD, Leath CA, III, Huh WK, et al. A Ketogenic Diet Reduces Central Obesity and Serum Insulin in Women with Ovarian or Endometrial Cancer. J Nutr. 2018;148(8):1253-60.
293. Khodabakhshi A, Akbari ME, Mirzaei HR, Mehrad-Majd H, Kalamian M, Davoodi SH. Feasibility, Safety, and Beneficial Effects of MCT-Based Ketogenic Diet for Breast Cancer Treatment: A Randomized Controlled Trial Study. Nutr Cancer. 2020;72(4):627-34.
294. Evangeliou AE, Spilioti MG, Vassilakou D, Goutsaridou F, Seyfried TN. Restricted Ketogenic Diet Therapy for Primary Lung Cancer With Metastasis to the Brain: A Case Report. Cureus. 2022;14(8):e27603.
295. Seyfried TN, Shivane AG, Kalamian M, Maroon JC, Mukherjee P, Zuccoli G. Ketogenic Metabolic Therapy, Without Chemo or Radiation, for the Long-Term Management of IDH1-Mutant Glioblastoma: An 80-Month Follow-Up Case Report. Front Nutr. 2021;8:682243.
296. Meidenbauer JJ, Mukherjee P, Seyfried TN. The glucose ketone index calculator: a simple tool to monitor therapeutic efficacy for metabolic management of brain cancer. Nutr. Metab (Lond). 2015;12:12.

297. Augustin K, Khabbush A, Williams S, Eaton S, Orford M, Cross JH, et al. Mechanisms of action for the medium-chain triglyceride ketogenic diet in neurological and metabolic disorders. Lancet Neurol. 2018;17(1):84-93.
298. Shukla SK, Gebregiworgis T, Purohit V, Chaika NV, Gunda V, Radhakrishnan P, et al. Metabolic reprogramming induced by ketone bodies diminishes pancreatic cancer cachexia. Cancer Metab. 2014;2:18.
299. Miyata Y, Shida Y, Hakariya T, Sakai H. Anti-cancer effects of green tea polyphenols against prostate cancer. Molecules. 2019;24:193.
300. Yang C, Sudderth J, Dang T, Bachoo RG, McDonald JG, Deberardinis RJ. Glioblastoma cells require glutamate dehydrogenase to survive impairements of glucose metabolism or Akt signaling. Cancer Res. 2009;69:7986-93.
301. Li M, Li C, Allen A, Stanley CA, Smith TJ. The structure and allosteric regulaion of mammalian glutamate dehydrogenase. Arch. Biochem. Biophys. 2012;519:69-80.
302. Li C, Allen A, Kwagh J, Doliba NM, Qin W, Najafi H, et al. Green tea polyphenols modulate insulin secretion by inhibiting glutamate dehydrogenase. J. Blol. Chem. 2006;281:10214-21.
303. Bettuzzi S, Brausi M, Rizzi F, Castagnetti G, Peracchia G, Corti A. Chemoprevention of human prostate cancer by oral administration of green tea catechins in volunteers with high-grade prostate intraepithelial neoplasia: A preliminary report from a one-year proof-of-principle study. Cancer Res. 2006;66:1234-40.
304. Mukherjee P, Greenwood B, Henao J, Kiebish MA, Seyfried TN. Ketogenic diet as a metabolic vehicle for enhancing the therapeutic efficacy of mebendazole and devimistat in preclinical pediatric glioma. bioRxiv. 2023.
305. Ifland J, Marcus MT, Preuss HG. Processed Food Addiction. Foundations, Assessment, and Recovery. Boca Rotan, FL: CRC Press; 2018.
306. Kliemann N, Rauber F, Bertazzi Levy R, Viallon V, Vamos EP, Cordova R, et al. Food processing and cancer risk in Europe: results from the prospective EPIC cohort study. Lancet Planet Health. 2023;7(3):e219-e32.
307. Cheng WY, Wu CY, Yu J. The role of gut microbiota in cancer treatment: friend or foe? Gut. 2020;69(10):1867-76.
308. Lee KA, Luong MK, Shaw H, Nathan P, Bataille V, Spector TD. The gut microbiome: what the oncologist ought to know. Br J Cancer. 2021;125(9):1197-209.
309. Sadrekarimi H, Gardanova ZR, Bakhshesh M, Ebrahimzadeh F, Yaseri AF, Thangavelu L, et al. Emerging role of human microbiome in cancer development and response to therapy: special focus on intestinal microflora. J Transl Med. 2022;20(1):301.
310. Zitvogel L, Galluzzi L, Viaud S, Vétizou M, Daillère R, Merad M, et al. Cancer and the gut microbiota: an unexpected link. Sci Transl Med. 2015;7(271):271ps1.
311. Boursi B, Mamtani R, Haynes K, Yang YX. Recurrent antibiotic exposure may promote cancer formation--Another step in understanding the role of the human microbiota? Eur J Cancer. 2015;51(17):2655-64.
312. Cao Y, Wu K, Mehta R, Drew DA, Song M, Lochhead P, et al. Long-term use of antibiotics and risk of colorectal adenoma. Gut. 2018;67(4):672-8.
313. Banting W. Letter on Corpulence, Addressed to the Public. 3rd ed. London, UK: Harrison; 1864.
314. Creed SA. The Real Meal Revolution. The Radical, Sustainable Approach to Healthy Eating. London, UK: Robinson; 2015.
315. Meadows W. The Banting Diet: Letter on Corpulence: FCD Publising; 2015.
316. Muscaritoli M, Lucia S, Farcomeni A, Lorusso V, Saracino V, Barone C, et al. Prevalence of malnutrition in patients at first medical oncology visit: the PreMiO study. Oncotarget. 2017;8(45):79884-96.

317. Baracos VE, Martin L, Korc M, Guttridge DC, Fearon KCH. Cancer-associated cachexia. Nat Rev Dis Primers. 2018;4:17105.
318. Nishikawa H, Goto M, Fukunishi S, Asai A, Nishiguchi S, Higuchi K. Cancer Cachexia: Its Mechanism and Clinical Significance. Int J Mol Sci. 2021;22(16).
319. Fearon K, Strasser F, Anker SD, Bosaeus I, Bruera E, Fainsinger RL, et al. Definition and classification of cancer cachexia: an international consensus. Lancet Oncol. 2011;12(5):489-95.
320. Baldwin C, Spiro A, McGough C, Norman AR, Gillbanks A, Thomas K, et al. Simple nutritional intervention in patients with advanced cancers of the gastrointestinal tract, non-small cell lung cancers or mesothelioma and weight loss receiving chemotherapy: a randomised controlled trial. J Hum Nutr Diet. 2011;24(5):431-40.
321. Bourdel-Marchasson I, Blanc-Bisson C, Doussau A, Germain C, Blanc JF, Dauba J, et al. Nutritional advice in older patients at risk of malnutrition during treatment for chemotherapy: a two-year randomized controlled trial. PLoS One. 2014;9(9):e108687.
322. Advani SM, Advani PG, VonVille HM, Jafri SH. Pharmacological management of cachexia in adult cancer patients: a systematic review of clinical trials. BMC Cancer. 2018;18(1):1174.
323. Temel JS, Abernethy AP, Currow DC, Friend J, Duus EM, Yan Y, et al. Anamorelin in patients with non-small-cell lung cancer and cachexia (ROMANA 1 and ROMANA 2): results from two randomised, double-blind, phase 3 trials. Lancet Oncol. 2016;17(4):519-31.
324. Antoni R, Johnston KL, Collins AL, Robertson MD. Effects of intermittent fasting on glucose and lipid metabolism. Proc. Nutr. Soc. 2017;76(3):361-8.
325. Cheng CW, Adams GB, Perin L, Wei M, Zhou X, Lam BS. Prolonged fasting reduces IGF-1/PKA to promote hematopoietic-stem-cell-based regeneration and reverse immunosppression. Cell Stem Cell. 2014;14:810-23.
326. de Cabo R, Mattson MP. Effects of intermittent fasting on health, aging, and disease. N. Engl. J. Med. 2019;381:2541-51.
327. Mattson MP, Longo VD, Harvie M. Impact of intermittent fasting on health and disease processes. Ageing Res. Rev. 2017;39:46-58.
328. Vasim I, Majeed CN, DeBoer MD. Intermittent fasting and metabolic health. Nutrients. 2022;14:631.
329. Takeshige K, Baba M, Tsuboi S, Noda T, Ohsumi Y. Autophagy in yeast demonstrated with proteinase-deficient mutants and conditions for its induction. J. Cell. Biol. 1992;119:301-11.
330. Tsukada M, Ohsumi Y. Isolation and characterization of autophagy-defective mutants of *Saccharomyces cerevisiae*. FEBS. 1993;333:169-74.
331. Antures F, Erustes AG, Costa AJ, Nascimento AC, Bincoletto C, Ureshino RP, et al. Autophagy and intermittent fasting: the connection for cancer therapy? Clinics. 2018;73 (Suppl 1):e814S.
332. A.P. C, Massari JR, Berdiel MJ, Olalde J, Gonzalez MJ. Intermittent fasting and cancer. Journal of Restorative Medicine. 2022.
333. Fung J, Moore J. The complete guide to fasting: Victory Belt Publishing; 2016.
334. Whittaker DS, Akhmetova L, Carlin D, Romero H, Welsh DK, Colwell CS, et al. Circadian modulation by time-restricted feeding rescues brain pathology and improves memory in mouse models of Alzheimer's disease. Cell Metab. 2023.
335. Munoz A, Grant WB. Vitamin D and Cancer: An Historical Overview of the Epidemiology and Mechanisms. Nutrients. 2022;14(7).
336. Das M, Ellies LG, Kumar D, Sauceda C, Oberg A, Gross E, et al. Time-restricted feeding normalizes hyperinsulinemia to inhibit breast cancer in obese postmenopausal mouse models. Nature Communications. 2021;12:565.

337. Buschemeyer WC, Klink JC, Mavropoulos JC, Poulton SH, Hursting SD. Effectof intermittent fasting with or without caloric restriction on prostate cancer growth and survival in SCID mice. Prostate. 2010;70:1037-43.
338. Sundaram S, Yan L. Time-restricted feeding mitigates high fat diet enhanced mammary tumorigenesis in MMTV-PyMT mice. Nutrition Research. 2018;59:72-9.
339. Yan L, Sundaram S, Mehus AA, Picklo MJ. Time-restricted feeding attenuates high-fat diet-enhanced spontaneous metastasis of Lewis lung carcinoma in mice. Anticancer Research. 2019;39:1739-48.
340. Sun P, Wang H, He Z, Chen X, Wu Q, Chen W, et al. Fasting inhibits colorectal cancer growth by reducing M2 polarization of tumor-assocaited macrophages. Oncotarget. 2017;8:74649-60.
341. Lee C, Raffaghello L, Brandhorst S, Safdie FM, Bianchi G, Pistoria V, et al. Fasting cycles retard growth of tumors and sensitize a range of cancer cell types to chemotherapy. Science Translational Medicine. 2012;4:124ra27.
342. Marinac CR, Nelson SH, Breen CI, Hartman SJ, Natarajan L, Pierce JP, et al. Prolonged Nightly Fasting and Breast Cancer Prognosis. JAMA Oncol. 2016;2(8):1049-55.
343. Agrawal S, Wozniak M, Luc M, Makuch S, Pielka E, Agrawal AK, et al. Insulin enhancement of the antitumor activity of chemotherapeutic agents in colorectal cancer is linked with downregulating PIK3CA and GRB2. Sci Rep. 2019;9(1):16647.
344. Sissung TM, Schmidt KT, Figg WD. Insulin potentiation therapy for cancer? Lancet Oncol. 2019;20(2):191-2.
345. Ayre SG, Bellon DP, Garcia DP, Jr. Insulin, chemotherapy, and the mechanisms of malignancy: the design and the demise of cancer. Med Hypotheses. 2000;55(4):330-4.
346. Lasalvia-Prisco E, Cucchi S, VÃ¡zquez J, Lasalvia-Galante E, Golomar W, Gordon W. Insulin-induced enhancement of antitumoral response to methotrexate in breast cancer patients. Cancer Chemother. Pharmacol. 2004;53(3):220-4.
347. Teicholz N. The Big FAT Suprise. Why butter, meat and cheese belong in a healthy diet. New York: Simon & Schuster; 2014.
348. Dehghan M, Mente A, Zhang X, Swaminathan S. Associations of fats and carbohydrate intake with cardiovascular disease and mortality in 18 countries from five continents (PURE): a prospective cohort study. Lancet. 2017;390:2050-62.
349. Inchauspe J. Glucose Revolution. New York: Simon & Schuster; 2022.
350. Barclay AW, Augustin LS, Brighenti F, Delport E, Henry CJ, Sievenpiper JL, et al. Dietary glycaemic index labelling: A global perspective. Nutrients. 2021;13:3244.
351. Matthan NR, Ausman LM, Meng H, Tighiouart H, Lichtenstein AH. Estimating the reliability of glycemic index values and potential sources of methodological and biological variability. Am. J. Clin. Nutr. 2016;104:1004-13.
352. Lustig RH. Metabolical. The lure and lies of processed food, Nutrition and Modern Medicine: Harper; 2021.
353. Corkey BE. Banting lecture 2011: hyperinsulinemia: cause or consequence? Diabetes. 2012;61(1):4-13.
354. Santos HO, de Moraes WM, da Silva GA, restes J, Schoenfeld BJ. Vinegar (acetic acid) intake on glucose metabolism: A narrative review. Clinical Nutrition ESPEN. 2019;32:1-7.
355. Shishehbor F, Mansoori A, Shirani F. Vinegar consumption can attenuate postproandial glucose and insulin responses: a systematic review and meta-analysis of clinical trials. Diabetes Research and Clinical Practice. 2017;127:1-9.
356. Siddiqui FJ, Assam PN, de Souza NN, Sultana R, Dalan r, Chan ES. Diabetes control: Is vinegar a promising candidate to help achieve targets?? Journal of Evidence-Based Integrative Medicine. 2018;23:1-12.

357. Petsiou EI, Mitrou PI, Raptis SA, Dimitriadis GD. Effect and mechanisms of action of vinegar on glucose metabolism,lipid profile, and body weight. Nutrition Reviews. 2014;72:651-61.
358. Little JP, Gillen JB, Percival ME, Safdar A, Tarnopolsky MA, Punthakee Z, et al. Low-volume high-intensity interval training reduces hyperglycemia and increases muscle mitochondrial capacity in patients with type 2 diabetes. Journal of Applied Physiology. 2011;111(6):1554-60.
359. Praet SF, Manders RJ, Lieverse AG, Kuipers H, Stehouwer CD, Keizer HA. Influence of acute excercise on hyperglycemia in insulin-treated type-2 diabets. Medicine & Science in Sports & Exercise. 2006(2037):2044.
360. Dipla K, Zafeiridis A, Mintziori G, Boutou AK, Goulis DG, Hackney AC. Exercise as a therapeutic intervention in gestational diabetes mellitus. Endocrines. 2021;2:65-78.
361. Halilton MT, Hamilton D, Zderic TW. A potent physiological method to magnify and sustain soleus oxidative metabolism improves glucose and lipid regulation. iScience. 2022;25:104869.
362. Yu EW, Gao L, Stastka P, Cheney MC, Soto MT, Ford CB, et al. Fecal microbiota transplantation for the improvement of metabolism in obesity: The FMT-TRIM double-blind placebo-controlled pilot trial. PloS ONE. 2020;17:e1003051.
363. Pedersen HK, Gudmundsdottir V, Nielsen HB, Hyotylainen T, Nielsen T, Jensen BA, et al. Human gut microbes impact host serum metabolome and insulin sensitivity. Nature. 2016;535:376-81.
364. Sung MM, Kim TT, Denou E, Soltys CL, Hamza SM, Byrne NJ, et al. Improved glucose homeostasis in obese mice treated with resveratrol is associated with alterations in the gut microbiome. Diabetes. 2017;66:418-25.
365. Nieuwdorp M, Gilijamse PW, Pai N, Kaplan LM. Role of the microbiome in energy regulation and metabolism. Gastroenterology. 2014;146:1525-33.
366. Rebello CJ, Burton J, Heiman M, Greenway FL. Gastrointestinal microbiome modulator improves glucose tolerance in overweight and obese subjects: A randomized controlled pilto trial. J. Diabetes Complications. 2015;29:1272-6.
367. Maruvada P, Leone V, Kaplan LM, Chang EB. The human microbiome and obesity: Moving beyond associations. Cell Host & Microbe. 2017;22:589-99.
368. Vallianou NG, Stratigou T, Tsagarakis S. Microbiome and diabetes: Where are we now? Diabetes Research and Clinical Practice. 2018;146:111-8.
369. Wastyk HC, Fragiadakis GK, Perelman D, Dahan D, Merrill BD, Yu FB, et al. Gut-microbiota-targeted diets modulate human immune status. Cell. 2021;184(16):4137-53.e14.
370. Teicholz N. A short history of saturated fat: the making and unmaking of a scientific consensus. Curr. Opin. Endo. Diab. Obesity. 2023;30:65-71.
371. Astrup A, Teicholz N, Magkos F, Bier DM, Brenna JT, King JC, et al. Dietary saturated fats and health: Are the U.S. Guidelines evidence-based? Nutrients. 2021;13:3305.
372. Keys A, Mienotti A, Karvonen MJ, Aravanis C, Blackburn H, Buzina R, et al. The diet and 15-year death rate in the seven countries study. Am. J. Epidemiol. 1986;124:903-15.
373. Page IH, Allen EV, Chamberlain FL, Keys A, Stamler J, Stare FJ. Dietary fat and its relation to heart attacks and strokes. Circulation. 1961;23:133-6.
374. Dayton S, Pearce ML, Hashimoto S, Fakler LJ, Hiscock E, Dixon WJ. A controlled clinical trial of a diet high in unsaturated fat. Preliminary observations. N. Engl. J. Med. 1962;266:1017-23.
375. Ramsden CE, Zamora D, Faurot KR, Broste SK, Frantz RP, Davis JM, et al. Re-evaluation of the traditional diet-heart hypothesis: analysis of recovered data form the Minnesota Coronary Experiment (1968-1973). BMJ. 2016;353:i1246.
376. Ramsden CE, Zamora D, Faurot KR, Ringel A, Davis JM, Hibbeln JR. Use of dietary linoleic acid for secondary prevenion of heart disease and death: evaluation of recovered data form the Sydney Diet Heart Study and updated meta-analysis. BMJ. 2013;346:e8707.

377. Hamer J, Warner E. Lifestyle modifications for patients with breast cancer to improve prognosis and optimize overall health. Cmaj. 2017;189(7):E268-e74.
378. Montagnese C, Porciello G, Vitale S, Palumbo E, Crispo A, Grimaldi M, et al. Quality of Life in Women Diagnosed with Breast Cancer after a 12-Month Treatment of Lifestyle Modifications. Nutrients. 2020;13(1).
379. Berrino F, Villarini A, Traina A, Bonanni B, Panico S, Mano MP, et al. Metabolic syndrome and breast cancer prognosis. Breast Cancer Res Treat. 2014;147(1):159-65.
380. Ligibel JA, Bohlke K, May AM, Clinton SK, Demark-Wahnefried W, Gilchrist SC, et al. Exercise, Diet, and Weight Management During Cancer Treatment: ASCO Guideline. J Clin. Oncol. 2022;40(22):2491-507.
381. Oberoi S, Robinson PD, Cataudella D, Culos-Reed SN, Davis H, Duong N, et al. Physical activity reduces fatigue in patients with cancer and hematopoietic stem cell transplant recipients: A systematic review and meta-analysis of randomized trials. Crit Rev Oncol. Hematol. 2018;122:52-9.
382. Scott JM, Zabor EC, Schwitzer E, Koelwyn GJ, Adams SC, Nilsen TS, et al. Efficacy of Exercise Therapy on Cardiorespiratory Fitness in Patients With Cancer: A Systematic Review and Meta-Analysis. J Clin. Oncol. 2018;36(22):2297-305.
383. Garcia DO, Thomson CA. Physical activity and cancer survivorship. Nutr. Clin. Pract. 2014;29(6):768-79.
384. Aydin M, Kose E, Odabas I, Meric BB, Demirci D, Aydin Z. The Effect of Exercise on Life Quality and Depression Levels of Breast Cancer Patients. Asian Pac. J Cancer Prev. 2021;22(3):725-32.
385. Kenfield SA, Stampfer MJ, Giovannucci E, Chan JM. Physical activity and survival after prostate cancer diagnosis in the health professionals follow-up study. J Clin Oncol. 2011;29(6):726-32.
386. Lopez P, Galvao DA, Taaffe DR, Newton RU, Souza G, Trajano GS, et al. Resistance training in breast cancer patients undergoing primary treatment: a systematic review and meta-regression of exercise dosage. Breast Cancer. 2021;28(1):16-24.
387. An KY, Morielli AR, Kang DW, Friedenreich CM, McKenzie DC, Gelmon K, et al. Effects of exercise dose and type during breast cancer chemotherapy on longer-term patient-reported outcomes and health-related fitness: A randomized controlled trial. Int. J Cancer. 2020;146(1):150-60.
388. Lahart IM, Metsios GS, Nevill AM, Carmichael AR. Physical activity, risk of death and recurrence in breast cancer survivors: A systematic review and meta-analysis of epidemiological studies. Acta Oncol. 2015;54(5):635-54.
389. Beasley JM, Kwan ML, Chen WY, Weltzien EK, Kroenke CH, Lu W, et al. Meeting the physical activity guidelines and survival after breast cancer: findings from the after breast cancer pooling project. Breast Cancer Res Treat. 2012;131(2):637-43.
390. Chen X, Lu W, Zheng W, Gu K, Matthews CE, Chen Z, et al. Exercise after diagnosis of breast cancer in association with survival. Cancer Prev Res (Phila). 2011;4(9):1409-18.
391. Kelly P, Williamson C, Niven AG, Hunter R, Mutrie N, Richards J. Walking on sunshine: scoping review of the evidence for walking and mental health. Br J Sports Med. 2018;52(12):800-6.
392. Lee IM, Buchner DM. The importance of walking to public health. Med Sci Sports Exerc. 2008;40(7 Suppl):S512-8.
393. Chida Y, Hamer M, Wardle J, Steptoe A. Do stress-related psychosocial factors contribute to cancer incidence and survival? Nat Clin Pract Oncol. 2008;5(8):466-75.
394. Lundt A, Jentschke E. Long-Term Changes of Symptoms of Anxiety, Depression, and Fatigue in Cancer Patients 6 Months After the End of Yoga Therapy. Integr Cancer Ther. 2019;18:1534735418822096.

395. Lopresti AL, Smith SJ, Malvi H, Kodgule R. An investigation into the stress-relieving and pharmacological actions of an ashwagandha (Withania somnifera) extract: A randomized, double-blind, placebo-controlled study. Medicine (Baltimore). 2019;98(37):e17186.
396. Salve J, Pate S, Debnath K, Langade D. Adaptogenic and Anxiolytic Effects of Ashwagandha Root Extract in Healthy Adults: A Double-blind, Randomized, Placebo-controlled Clinical Study. Cureus. 2019;11(12):e6466.
397. Gopukumar K, Thanawala S, Somepalli V, Rao TSS, Thamatam VB, Chauhan S. Efficacy and Safety of Ashwagandha Root Extract on Cognitive Functions in Healthy, Stressed Adults: A Randomized, Double-Blind, Placebo-Controlled Study. Evid Based Complement Alternat Med. 2021;2021:8254344.
398. Chandrasekhar K, Kapoor J, Anishetty S. A prospective, randomized double-blind, placebo-controlled study of safety and efficacy of a high-concentration full-spectrum extract of ashwagandha root in reducing stress and anxiety in adults. Indian J Psychol Med. 2012;34(3):255-62.
399. Langade D, Thakare V, Kanchi S, Kelgane S. Clinical evaluation of the pharmacological impact of ashwagandha root extract on sleep in healthy volunteers and insomnia patients: A double-blind, randomized, parallel-group, placebo-controlled study. J Ethnopharmacol. 2021;264:113276.
400. Akhgarjand C, Asoudeh F, Bagheri A, Kalantar Z, Vahabi Z, Shab-Bidar S, et al. Does Ashwagandha supplementation have a beneficial effect on the management of anxiety and stress? A systematic review and meta-analysis of randomized controlled trials. Phytother Res. 2022;36(11):4115-24.
401. Vyazovskiy VV, Delogu A. NREM and REM Sleep: Complementary Roles in Recovery after Wakefulness. Neuroscientist. 2014;20(3):203-19.
402. Hirshkowitz M, Whiton K, Albert SM, Alessi C, Bruni O, DonCarlos L, et al. National Sleep Foundation's sleep time duration recommendations: methodology and results summary. Sleep Health. 2015;1(1):40-3.
403. Ohayon M, Wickwire EM, Hirshkowitz M, Albert SM, Avidan A, Daly FJ, et al. National Sleep Foundation's sleep quality recommendations: first report. Sleep Health. 2017;3(1):6-19.
404. Cheah KL, Norhayati MN, Husniati Yaacob L, Abdul Rahman R. Effect of Ashwagandha (Withania somnifera) extract on sleep: A systematic review and meta-analysis. PLoS One. 2021;16(9):e0257843.
405. Itani O, Jike M, Watanabe N, Kaneita Y. Short sleep duration and health outcomes: a systematic review, meta-analysis, and meta-regression. Sleep Med. 2017;32:246-56.
406. Biswal BM, Sulaiman SA, Ismail HC, Zakaria H, Musa KI. Effect of Withania somnifera (Ashwagandha) on the development of chemotherapy-induced fatigue and quality of life in breast cancer patients. Integr Cancer Ther. 2013;12(4):312-22.
407. Andersen BL, Yang HC, Farrar WB, Golden-Kreutz DM, Emery CF, Thornton LM, et al. Psychologic intervention improves survival for breast cancer patients: a randomized clinical trial. Cancer. 2008;113(12):3450-8.
408. Andersen BL, Farrar WB, Golden-Kreutz DM, Glaser R, Emery CF, Crespin TR, et al. Psychological, behavioral, and immune changes after a psychological intervention: a clinical trial. J Clin Oncol. 2004;22(17):3570-80.
409. Andersen BL, Shelby RA, Golden-Kreutz DM. RCT of a psychological intervention for patients with cancer: I. mechanisms of change. J Consult Clin Psychol. 2007;75(6):927-38.
410. Andersen BL, Farrar WB, Golden-Kreutz D, Emery CF, Glaser R, Crespin T, et al. Distress reduction from a psychological intervention contributes to improved health for cancer patients. Brain Behav Immun. 2007;21(7):953-61.

411. Andersen BL, Thornton LM, Shapiro CL, Farrar WB, Mundy BL, Yang HC, et al. Biobehavioral, immune, and health benefits following recurrence for psychological intervention participants. Clin Cancer Res. 2010;16(12):3270-8.
412. Heiskanen V, Pfiffner M, Partonen T. Sunlight and health; shifting the focus from vitamin D3 to photobiomodulation by red and near-infrared light. Ageing Research Reviews. 2022;61:101089.
413. Hobday RA, Cason JW. The open-air treatment of pandemic influenza. Am. J. Public Health. 2022;99 Suppl.2:S236-S42.
414. Lindqvist PG, Epstein E, Landin-Olsson M, Ingvar C, Nielsen K, stenbeck M, et al. Avoidance of sun exposure is a risk factor for all-cause mortality: results form the Melanoma in Southern Sweden cohort. Journal of Internal Medicine. 2014;276:77-86.
415. Garland CF, Gorham ED, Mohr SB, Garland FC. Vitamin D for cancer prevention: global perspective. Ann Epidemiol. 2009;19(7):468-83.
416. Grant WB. Cancer Incidence Rates in the US in 2016–2020 with Respect to Solar UVB Doses, Diabetes and Obesity Prevalence, Lung Cancer Incidence Rates, and Alcohol Consumption: An Ecological Study. Nutrients. 2024;16:1450.
417. Hamblin MR. Mechanisms and application of the anti-inflammatory effects of photobiomodulation. AIMS Biophys. 2017;4:337-61.
418. Gordon R. Skin cancer: an overview of epidemiology and risk factors. Semin Oncol Nurs. 2013;29(3):160-9.
419. 2024;Pages. Accessed at American Cancer Association at https://www.cancer.org/cancer/types/basal-and-squamous-cell-skin-cancer/about/what-is-basal-and-squamous-cell.html on 5/8/2024 2024.
420. Kim DP, Kus KJB, Ruiz E. Basal Cell Carcinoma Review. Hematol Oncol Clin North Am. 2019;33(1):13-24.
421. 2024;Pages. Accessed at American Cancer Association at https://www.cancer.org/cancer/types/melanoma-skin-cancer/about/key-statistics.html on 5/8/2024 2024.
422. Long GV, Swetter SM, Menzies AM, Gershenwald JE, Scolyer RA. Cutaneous melanoma. Lancet. 2023;402(10400):485-502.
423. Ahmed B, Qadir MI, Ghafoor S. Malignant Melanoma: Skin Cancer-Diagnosis, Prevention, and Treatment. Crit Rev Eukaryot Gene Expr. 2020;30(4):291-7.
424. Christophers AJ. Melanoma is not caused by sunlight. Mutat Res. 1998;422(1):113-7.
425. Elwood JM, Jopson J. Melanoma and sun exposure: an overview of published studies. Int J Cancer. 1997;73(2):198-203.
426. Lindqvist PG, Epstein E, Landin-Olsson M. Sun Exposure - Hazards and Benefits. Anticancer Res. 2022;42(4):1671-7.
427. Peller S, Stephenson CS. Skin irritation and cancer in the United States Navy. Am. J. M. Sc. 1937;194:326-33.
428. Berwick M, Armstrong BK, Ben-Porat L, Fine J, Kricker A, Eberle C, et al. Sun exposure and mortality from melanoma. J Natl Cancer Inst. 2005;97(3):195-9.
429. Gandini S, De Vries E, Tosti G, Botteri E, Spadola G, Maisonneuve P, et al. Sunny holidays before and after melanoma diagnosis are respectively associated with lower Breslow thickness and lower relapse rates in Italy. PLoS One. 2013;8(11):e78820.
430. Westerdahl J, Ingvar C, Måsbäck A, Olsson H. Sunscreen use and malignant melanoma. Int J Cancer. 2000;87(1):145-50.
431. Merrill SJ, Ashrafi S, Subramanian M, Godar DE. Exponentially increasing incidences of cutaneous malignant melanoma in Europe correlate with low personal annual UV doses and suggests 2 major risk factors. Dermatoendocrinol. 2015;7(1):e1004018.

432. Godar DE. Worldwide increasing incidences of cutaneous malignant melanoma. J Skin Cancer. 2011;2011:858425.
433. Bernstein J. MIA In the War on Cancer: Where are the Low-Cost Treatments. https://www.propublica.org/article/where-are-the-low-cost-cancer-treatments: ProPublica; 2014.
434. Anglemyer A, Horvath HT, Bero L. Healthcare outcomes assessed with observational study designs compared with those assessed in randomized trials. Cochrane Database of Syst. Rev. 2014;4:MR000034.
435. Gali-Muhtasib H, Hmadi R, Kareh M, Tohme R, Darwiche N. Cell death mechanisms of plant-derived anticancer drugs: beyond apoptosis. Apoptosis. 2015;20(12):1531-62.
436. Campos-Carrillo A, Weitzel JN, Sahoo P, Rockne R, Mokhnatkin JV, Murtaza M, et al. Circulating tumor DNA as an early cancer detection tool. Pharmacol. Ther. 2020;207:107458.
437. Moding EJ, Nabet BY, Alizadeh AA, Diehn M. Detecting Liquid Remnants of Solid Tumors: Circulating Tumor DNA Minimal Residual Disease. Cancer Discov. 2021;11(12):2968-86.
438. Wang T, Dong Y, Huang Z, Zhang G, Zhao Y, Yao H, et al. Antioxidants stimulate BACH1-dependent tumor angiogenesis. J Clin Invest. 2023.
439. Ambrosone CB, Zirpoli GR, Hutson AD, McCann WE, McCann SE, Barlow WE, et al. Dietary Supplement Use During Chemotherapy and Survival Outcomes of Patients With Breast Cancer Enrolled in a Cooperative Group Clinical Trial (SWOG S0221). J Clin. Oncol. 2020;38(8):804-14.
440. Lawenda BD, Kelly KM, Ladas EJ, Sagar SM, Vickers A, Blumberg JB. Should supplemental antioxidant administration be avoided during chemotherapy and radiation therapy? J Natl. Cancer Inst. 2008;100(11):773-83.
441. Marik PE. Hydrocortisone, Ascorbic Acid and Thiamine (HAT therapy) for the treatment of sepsis. Focus on ascorbic acid. Nutrients. 2018;10:1762.
442. Lee JW, Shahzad MM, Lin YG, Armaiz-Pena G, Mangala LS, Han HD, et al. Surgical stress promotes tumor growth in ovarian carcinoma. Clin Cancer Res. 2009;15(8):2695-702.
443. Hiller JG, Cole SW, Crone EM, Byrne DJ, Shackleford DM, Pang JB, et al. Preoperative β-Blockade with Propranolol Reduces Biomarkers of Metastasis in Breast Cancer: A Phase II Randomized Trial. Clin Cancer Res. 2020;26(8):1803-11.
444. Forget P, Bentin C, Machiels JP, Berliere M, Coulie PG, De Kock M. Intraoperative use of ketorolac or diclofenac is associated with improved disease-free survival and overall survival in conservative breast cancer surgery. Br J Anaesth. 2014;113 Suppl 1:i82-7.
445. Deva S, Jameson M. Histamine type 2 receptor antagonists as adjuvant treatment for resected colorectal cancer. Cochrane Database Syst Rev. 2012(8):Cd007814.
446. Forget P, Vandenhende J, Berliere M, Machiels JP, Nussbaum B, Legrand C, et al. Do intraoperative analgesics influence breast cancer recurrence after mastectomy? A retrospective analysis. Anesth. Analg. 2010;110(6):1630-5.
447. Forget P, Bentin C, Machiels JP, Berliere M, Coulie PG, De KM. Intraoperative use of ketorolac or diclofenac is associated with improved disease-free survival and overall survival in conservative breast cancer surgery. Br. J Anaesth. 2014;113 Suppl 1:i82-i7.
448. Forget P, Bouche G, Duhoux FP, Coulie PG, Decloedt J, Dekleermaker A, et al. Intraoperative ketorolac in high-risk breast cancer patients. A prospective, randomized, placebo-controlled clinical trial. PloS ONE. 2019;14(12):e0225748.
449. Cianchi F, Cortesini C, Schiavone N, Perna F, Magnelli L, Fanti E, et al. The role of cyclooxygenase-2 in mediating the effects of histamine on cell proliferation and vascular endothelial growth factor production in colorectal cancer. Clin. Cancer Res. 2005;11(19 Pt 1):6807-15.

450. Lin CY, Bai DJ, Yuan HY, Wang K, Yang GL, Hu MB, et al. Perioperative cimetidine administration promotes peripheral blood lymphocytes and tumor infiltrating lymphocytes in patients with gastrointestinal cancer: Results of a randomized controlled clinical trial. World J Gastroenterol. 2004;10(1):136-42.
451. Mutschler E, Spahn H, Kirch W. The interaction between H2-receptor antagonists and beta-adrenoceptor blockers. Br J Clin Pharmacol. 1984;17 Suppl 1(Suppl 1):51s-7s.
452. Barron TI, Connolly RM, Sharp L, Bennett K, Visvanathan K. Beta blockers and breast cancer mortality: a population- based study. J Clin Oncol. 2011;29(19):2635-44.
453. Zhang L, Xu L, Zhang F, Vlashi E. Doxycycline inhibits the cancer stem cell phenotype and epithelial-to-mesenchymal transition in breast cancer. Cell Cycle. 2017;16(8):737-45.
454. Tian Y, Song W, Li D, Cai L, Zhao Y. Resveratrol as a natural regulator of autophagy for prevention and treatment of cancer. OncoTargets and Therapy. 2019;12:8601-9.
455. Liu WM, Scott KA, Dennis JL, Kaminska E, Levett AJ, Dalgleish AG. Naltrexone at low doses upregulates a unique gene expression not seen with normal doses: Implications for its use in cancer therapy. Int J Oncol. 2016;49(2):793-802.
456. Kniotek M, Boguska A. Sildenafil can affect innate and adaptive immune system in both experimental animals and patients. Journal of Immunology Research. 2017;2017:4541958.
457. Zulian E, Sartorato P, Benedini S, Baro G, Armanini D, Mantero F, et al. Spironolactone in the treatment of polycystic ovary syndrome: Effects on clinical features, insulin sensitivity and lipid profile. Journal of Endocrinological Investigation. 2005;28(3):49-53.
458. Zou K, Zhao L, Young A, Zhand H-Y, Li B, Zhu W-L, et al. Advances in the study of berberine and its derivatives: a focus on anti-inflammatory and anti-tumor effects in the digestive system. Acta Pharmacologica Sinica. 2017;38:157-67.
459. Zhu Y, Bu S. Curcumin Induces Autophagy, Apoptosis, and Cell Cycle Arrest in Human Pancreatic Cancer Cells. Evidence-Based Complementary and Alternative Medicine. 2017;2017:1-13.
460. Zhao Z, Zeng J, Guo Q, Pu K, Yang Y, Chen N, et al. Berberine Suppresses Stemness and Tumorigenicity of Colorectal Cancer Stem-Like Cells by Inhibiting m(6)A Methylation. Front Oncol. 2021;11:775418.
461. Zhang Y, Fan Y, Huang S, Wang G, Han R, Lei F, et al. Thymoquinone inhibits the metastasis of renal cell cancer cells by inducing autophagy via AMPK/mTOR signaling pathway. Cancer Science. 2018;109(12):3865-73.
462. Zhang J-J, Wang D-W, Cai D, Lu Q, Cheng Y-X. Meroterpenoids From Ganoderma lucidum Mushrooms and Their Biological Roles in Insulin Resistance and Triple-Negative Breast Cancer. Frontiers in Chemistry. 2021;9.
463. Zhang D-W, Fu M, Gao S-H, Liu J-L. Curcumin and Diabetes: A Systematic Review. Evidence-Based Complementary and Alternative Medicine. 2013;2013:1-16.
464. Yu C, Li W-b, Liu J-b, Lu J-w, Feng J-f. Autophagy: Novel applications of nonsteroidal anti-inflammatory drugs for primary cancer. Cancer Medicine. 2017;7.
465. Xing Y, Liqi Z, Jian L, Qinghua Y, Qian Y. Doxycycline Induces Mitophagy and Suppresses Production of Interferon-β in IPEC-J2 Cells. Front Cell Infect Microbiol. 2017;7:21.
466. Wang Y, Lu X, Wang X, Qiu Q, Zhu P, Ma L, et al. atg-7 Based Autophagy Activation Reverses Doxorubicin-Induced Cardiotoxicity. Circulation Research. 2021;129(8):e166-e82.
467. Wang S-F, Hu W-W, Yan H-J, Tan L, Gao J-Q, Tian Y-Y, et al. Modulation of astrocytic glutamine synthetase expression and cell viability by histamine in cultured cortical astrocytes exposed to OGD insults. Neurosciene Letters. 2013;549:69-73.
468. Wang N, Tian X, Chen Y, Tan HQ, Xie PJ, Chen SJ, et al. Low dose doxycycline decreases systemic inflammation and improves glycemic control, lipid profiles, and islet morphology and function in db/db mice. Sci Rep. 2017;7(1):14707.

469. Wang J, Nie D. Modulation of Autophagy by Free Fatty Acids. Cell Death - Autophagy, Apoptosis and Necrosis: InTech; 2015.
470. Szurpnicka A, Kowalczuk A, Szterk A. Biological activity of mistletoe: in vitro and in vivo studies and mechanisms of action. Archives of Pharmacal Research. 2020;43(6):593-629.
471. Sung SJ, Kim H-K, Hong Y-K, Joe YA. Autophagy Is a Potential Target for Enhancing the Anti-Angiogenic Effect of Mebendazole in Endothelial Cells. Biomolecules & Therapeutics. 2019;27(1).
472. Su J, Li D, Chen Q, Li M, Su L, Luo T, et al. Anti-breast Cancer Enhancement of a Polysaccharide From Spore of Ganoderma lucidum With Paclitaxel: Suppression on Tumor Metabolism With Gut Microbiota Reshaping. Frontiers in Microbiology. 2018;9.
473. Shin S, Jing K, Jeong S, Kim N, Song K-S, Heo J-Y, et al. The Omega-3 Polyunsaturated Fatty Acid DHA Induces Simultaneous Apoptosis and Autophagy via Mitochondrial ROS-Mediated Akt-mTOR Signaling in Prostate Cancer Cells Expressing Mutant p53. BioMed Research International. 2013;2013:1-11.
474. Shakya G, Randhi PK, Pajaniradje S, Mohankumar K, Rajagopalan R. Hypoglycaemic role of wheatgrass and its effect on carbohydrate metabolic enzymes in type II diabetic rats. Toxicol Ind Health. 2016;32(6):1026-32.
475. Shakya G, Balasubramanian S, Rajagopalan R. Methanol extract of wheatgrass induces G1 cell cycle arrest in a p53-dependent manner and down regulates the expression of cyclin D1 in human laryngeal cancer cells-an in vitro and in silico approach. Pharmacogn Mag. 2015;11(Suppl 1):S139-47.
476. Sala De Oyanguren FJ, Rainey NE, Moustapha A, Saric A, Sureau F, O'Connor J-E, et al. Highlighting Curcumin-Induced Crosstalk between Autophagy and Apoptosis as Supported by Its Specific Subcellular Localization. Cells. 2020;9(2):361.
477. Rawat SG, Tiwari RK, Jaiswara PK, Gupta VK, Sonker P, Vishvakarma NK, et al. Phosphodiesterase 5 inhibitor sildenafil potentiates the antitumor activity of cisplatin by ROS-mediated apoptosis: a role of deregulated glucose metabolism. Apoptosis. 2022;27(7):606-18.
478. Rainey NE, Moustapha A, Petit PX. Curcumin, a Multifaceted Hormetic Agent, Mediates an Intricate Crosstalk between Mitochondrial Turnover, Autophagy, and Apoptosis. Oxidative Medicine and Cellular Longevity. 2020;2020:1-23.
479. Qin W-M, Wang K, Huang J-R, Mei X-L, Zhi Z. Sildenafil Induces Cell Cycle Arrest and Apoptosis in Human Colorectal Cancer HT-29Cells. Journal of Cancer Research Updates. 2018;7(2):59-63.
480. Propovic KJ, Popvic DJ, Miljkovic D, Popvic JK, Lalosevic D, Posa M, et al. Disulfiram and metformin combination anticancer effect reversible partly by antioxidant nitroglycerin and completely by NF-κB activator mebendazole in hamster fibrosarcoma. Biomedicine & Pharmacotherapy. 2021;143(November).
481. Pantziarka P, Bouche G, Meheus L, Sukhatme V, Sukhatme VP. Repurposing drugs in oncology (ReDO)-cimetidine as an anti-cancer agent. Ecancermedicalscience. 2014;8:485.
482. Nowis D, Malenda A, Furs K, Oleszczak B, Sadowski R, Chlebowska J, et al. Statins impair glucose uptake in human cells. BMJ Open Diabetes Research & Care. 2014;2(1):e000017.
483. Nayeem M, Chauhan K. A comparative study of anti-oxidative potentials of wheat grass, sorghum grass and barley grass juices and its anti-diabetic effectiveness. IJCS. 2019;7(4):2336-41.
484. Nasrollahzadeh A, Momeny M, Fasehee H, Yaghmaie M, Bashash D, Hassani S, et al. Anti-proliferative activity of disulfiram through regulation of the AKT-FOXO axis: A proteomic study of molecular targets. BBA-Molecular Cell Research. 2021;1868(10).
485. Na RS, Ma C, Liu QR, Wu LM, Zheng XL, Liu ZW. Itraconazole attenuates hepatic gluconeogenesis and promotes glucose uptake by regulating AMPK pathway. Exp Ther Med. 2018;15(2):2165-71.

486. Morsi DS, Barnawi IO, Ibrahim HM, El-Morsy AM, El Hassab MA, El Latif HM. Immunomodulatory, apoptotic and anti-proliferative potentials of sildenafil in Ehrlich ascites carcinoma murine model: In vivo and in silico insights. 2023.
487. Mirza-Aghazadeh-Attari M, Ekrami EM, Aghdas SAM, Mihanfar A, Hallaj S, Yousefi B, et al. Targeting PI3K/Akt/mTOR signaling pathway by polyphenols: Implication for cancer therapy. Life Science. 2020;255(15 August).
488. Ming H, Li B, Tian H, Zhou L, Jian J, Zhang T, et al. A minimalist and robust chemo-photothermal nanoplatform capable of augmenting autophagy-modulated immune response against breast cancer. Materials Today Bio. 2022;15.
489. Mhatme MS, Bargade MB, Hiware SK, Motlag MM. Effects of Atorvastatin and Rosuvastatin on the Glycemic Control in Ptients with Type II Diabetes Mellitus: A Comparative, Randomized, Double-Blind Study. Journal of Pharmacognosy and pharmcotherapeutics. 2021;12:54-60.
490. Mengual D, Medrano LE, Villamizar-Villamizar W, Osorio-Llanes E, Mendoza-Torres E, Bolívar S. Novel Effects of Statins on Cancer via Autophagy. Pharmaceuticals (Basel). 2022;15(6).
491. Mei XL, Yang Y, Zhang YJ, Li Y, Zhao JM, Qiu JG, et al. Sildenafil inhibits the growth of human colorectal cancer in vitro and in vivo. Am J Cancer Res. 2015;5(11):3311-24.
492. Marton LT, Pescinini-e-Salzedas LM, Eduarda M, Camargo C, Barbalho SM, dos Santos Haber JF, et al. The Effects of Curcumin on Diabetes Mellitis: A systematic Review. fronteirs in Encocrionology. 2021;12(May).
493. Ma Y, Xu X, Wu H, Li C, Zhong P, Liu Z, et al. Ivermectin contributes to attenuating the severity of acute lung injury in mice. Biomedicine & Pharmacotherapy. 2022;155:113706.
494. Liu Z, Peng Q, Li Y, Gao Y. Resveratrol enhances cisplatin-induced apoptosis in human hepatoma cells via glutamine metabolism inhibition. BMB Rep. 2018;51(9):474-9.
495. Liu Y, Fang S, Sun Q, Liu B. Anthelmintic drug ivermectin inhibits angiogenesis, growth and survival of glioblastoma through inducing mitochondrial dysfunction and oxidative stress. Biochemical and Biophysical Research Communications. 2016;480(3):415-21.
496. Lin M, Heizati M, Wang L, Nurula M, Yang Z, Wang Z, et al. A systematic review and meta-analysis of effects of spironolactone on blood pressure, glucose, lipids, renal function, fibrosis and inflammation in patients with hypertension and diabetes. Blood Pressure. 2021;30(3):145-53.
497. Li Z, Geng YN, Jiang JD, Kong WJ. Antioxidant and anti-inflammatory activities of berberine in the treatment of diabetes mellitus. Evid Based Complement Alternat Med. 2014;2014:289264.
498. Li J, Fan Y, Zhang Y, Liu Y, Yu Y, Ma M. Resveratrol Induces Autophagy and Apoptosis in Non-Small-Cell Lung Cancer Cells by Activating the NGFR-AMPK-mTOR Pathway. Nutrients. 2022;14(12).
499. León D, Uribe E, Zambrano A, Salas M. Implications of Resveratrol on Glucose Uptake and Metabolism. Molecules. 2017;22(3).
500. Kolawole OR, Kashfi K. NSAIDs and Cancer Resolution: New Paradigms beyond Cyclooxygenase. International Journal of Molecular Sciences. 2022;23(3):1432.
501. Khandelwal A, Singh GP, Jamil S. Ivermectin as a multifaceted drug in COVID-19: Current insights. Med J Armed Forces India. 2021;77(Suppl 2):S254-s6.
502. Khadge S, Sharp JG, Mcguire TR, Thiele GM, Black P, Dirusso C, et al. Immune regulation and anti-cancer activity by lipid inflammatory mediators. International Immunopharmacology. 2018;65:580-92.
503. Kapoor S. Emerging clinical and therapeutic applications of Nigella sativa in gastroenterology. World J Gastroenterol. 2009;15(17):2170-1.

504. Jo SB, Sung SJ, Choi HS, Park J-S, Hong Y-K, Joe YA. Modulation of Autophagy is a Potential Strategy for Enhancing the Anti-Tumor Effect of Mebendazole in Glioblastoma Cells. Biomolecules & Therapeutics. 2022;30(6):616-24.
505. Jin F, Xie T, Huang X, Zhao X. Berberine inhibits angiogenesis in glioblastoma xenografts by targeting the VEGFR2/ERK pathway. Pharmaceutical Biology. 2018;56(1):665-71.
506. Gorabi AM, Kiaie N, Aslani S, Sathyapalan T, Jamialahmadi T, Sahebkar A. Implications on the Therapeutic Potential of Statins via Modulation of Autophagy. Oxid Med Cell Longev. 2021;2021:9599608.
507. Fu X, Tan T, Liu P. Regulation of Autophagy by Non-Steroidal Anti-Inflammatory Drugs in Cancer. Cancer Manag Res. 2020;12:4595-604.
508. Ferraresi A, Esposito A, Girone C, Vallino L, Salwa A, Ghezzi I, et al. Resveratrol Contrasts LPA-Induced Ovarian Cancer Cell Migration and Platinum Resistance by Rescuing Hedgehog-Mediated Autophagy. Cells. 2021;10(11).
509. El-Benhawy SA, El-Sheredy HG, Ghanem HB, El-Soud AAA. Berberine can amplify cytotoxic effect of radiotherapy by targeting cancer stem cells. Breast Cancer Management. 2020;9(2):BMT41.
510. De Santi M, Baldelli G, Diotallevi A, Galluzzi L, Schiavano GF, Brandi G. Metformin prevents cell tumorigenesis through autophagy-related cell death. Scientific Reports. 2019;9(1).
511. Das A, Durrant D, Alloum FN, Xi L, Kukreja RC. PDE5 inhibitors as therapeutics for heart disease, diabetes and cancer. Pharmacology & Therapeutics. 2014;147(March):12-21.
512. Cornet-Masana JM, Banús-Mulet A, Carbó JM, Torrente MÁ, Guijarro F, Cuesta-Casanovas L, et al. Dual lysosomal-mitochondrial targeting by antihistamines to eradicate leukaemic cells. eBioMedicine. 2019;47:221-34.
513. Choi YS, Cho HJ, Jung HJ. Atorvastatin inhibits the proliferation of MKN45-derived gastric cancer stem cells in a mevalonate pathway-independent manner. Korean J Physiol Pharmacol. 2022;26(5):367-75.
514. Cao X, Li Y, Wang Y, Yu T, Zhu C, Zhang X, et al. Curcumin suppresses tumorigenesis by ferroptosis in breast cancer. PLOS ONE. 2022;17(1):e0261370.
515. Azadi R, Mousavi SE, Kazemi NM, Yousefi-Manesh H, Rezayat SM, Jaafari MR. Anti-inflammatory efficacy of Berberine Nanomicelle for improvement of cerebral ischemia: formulation, characterization and evaluation in bilateral common carotid artery occlusion rat model. BMC Pharmacology and Toxicology. 2021;22(1):54.
516. Ansary J, Giampieri F, Forbes-Hernandez TY, Regolo L, Quinzi D, Gracia Villar S, et al. Nutritional Value and Preventive Role of Nigella sativa L. and Its Main Component Thymoquinone in Cancer: An Evidenced-Based Review of Preclinical and Clinical Studies. Molecules. 2021;26(8):2108.
517. Andersson CR, Selvin T, Blom K, Rubin J, Berglund M, Jarvius M, et al. Mebendazole is unique among tubulin-active drugs in activating the MEK–ERK pathway. Scientific Reports. 2020;10(1).
518. Alvarez-Jimenez L, Morales-Palomo F, Merno-Cabanas A, Ortega JF, Mora-Rodrigues R. Effects of statin therapy on glycemic control and insulin resistance: A systematic review and meta-analysis. European Journal of Pharmacology. 2023;947(May).
519. AlGhamdi AA, Mohammed MRS, Zamzami MA, Al-Malki AL, Qari MH, Khan MI, et al. Untargeted Metabolomics Identifies Key Metabolic Pathways Altered by Thymoquinone in Leukemic Cancer Cells. Nutrients. 2020;12(6):1792.
520. Adeeyo A, Adefule A, Ofusori D, Aderinola A, Caxton-Martins E. Antihyperglycemic effects of aqueous leaf extracts of mistletoe and Moringa oleifera in streptozotocin-induced diabetes Wistar rats. Diabetologia Croatica. 2013;42(3).
521. Abdel-Hamid NM, Abdel-Ghany MI, Nazmy MH, Amgad SW. Can methanolic extract of Nigella sativa seed affect glyco-regulatory enzymes in experimental hepatocellular carcinoma? Environmental Health and Preventive Medicine. 2013;18(1):49-56.

522. Abbasi F, Lamendola C, Harris CS, Harris V, Tsai M-S, Tripathi P, et al. Statins Are Associated With Increased Insulin Resistance and Secretion. Arteriosclerosis, Thrombosis, and Vascular Biology. 2021;41(11):2786-97.
523. Johnson JR, Lossignol D, Burnell-Nugent M, Fallon MT. An open-label extension study to investigate the long-term safety and tolerability of THC/CBD oromucosal spray and oromucosal THC spray in patients with terminal cancer-related pain refractory to strong opioid analgesics. J Pain Symptom Manage. 2013;46(2):207-18.
524. Johnson JR, Burnell-Nugent M, Lossignol D, Ganae-Motan ED, Potts R, Fallon MT. Multicenter, double-blind, randomized, placebo-controlled, parallel-group study of the efficacy, safety, and tolerability of THC:CBD extract and THC extract in patients with intractable cancer-related pain. J Pain Symptom Manage. 2010;39(2):167-79.
525. Dawson M, Watson TR. The effect of dose form on the bioavailability of mebendazole in man. Br J Clin Pharmacol. 1985;19(1):87-90.
526. Gaziano JM, Brotons C, Coppolecchia R, Cricelli C, Darius H, Gorelick PB, et al. Use of aspirin to reduce risk of initial vascular events in patients at moderate risk of cardiovascular disease (ARRIVE): a randomised, double-blind, placebo-controlled trial. Lancet. 2018;392(10152):1036-46.
527. Burn J, Sheth H, Elliott F, Reed L, Macrae F, Mecklin JP, et al. Cancer prevention with aspirin in hereditary colorectal cancer (Lynch syndrome), 10-year follow-up and registry-based 20-year data in the CAPP2 study: a double-blind, randomised, placebo-controlled trial. Lancet. 2020;395(10240):1855-63.
528. Ko JH, Sethi G, Um JY, Shanmugam MK, Arfuso F, Kumar AP, et al. The Role of Resveratrol in Cancer Therapy. Int. J Mol. Sci. 2017;18(12).
529. Li C, Wang Q, Shen S, Wei X, Li G. HIF-1a/VEGF signaling-mediated epithelial-mesenchymal transition and angiogenesis is critically involved in anti-metastasis effect of luteolin in melanoma cells. Phytother. Res. 2019;33(3):798-807.
530. Greenberg ER, Baron JA, Tosteson TD, Freeman DH, Jr., Beck GJ, Bond JH, et al. A clinical trial of antioxidant vitamins to prevent colorectal adenoma. Polyp Prevention Study Group. New England Journal of Medicine. 1994;331(3):141-7.
531. Wimalawansa SJ. Physiological basis for using Vitamin D to improve health. Biomedicines. 2023;11:1542.
532. Holick MF. Vitamin D deficiency. N. Engl. J. Med. 2002;357:266-81.
533. Brandi ML. Indications on the use of vitamin D and vitamin D metabolites in clinical phenotypes. Clin. Cases. Miner. Bone Metab. 2010;7(3):243-50.
534. Chapuy MC, Preziosi P, Maamer M, Arnaud S, Galan P, Hercberg S, et al. Prevalence of vitamin D insufficiency in an adult normal population. Osteoporos. Int. 1997;7(5):439-43.
535. Vieth R. Why the optimal requirement for Vitamin D3 is probably much higher than what is officially recommended for adults. J Steroid Biochem. Mol. Biol. 2004;89-90(1-5):575-9.
536. Wimalawansa SJ. Rapidly increasing serum 25(OD)D boosts immune system, against infections - Sepsis and COVID-19. Nutrients. 2022;14:2997.
537. Wimalawansa SJ. Effective and practical ways to overcome Vitamin D deficiency. J. Family Med. Community Health. 2021;8:1-8.
538. Reddy P, Edwards LR. Magnesium supplementation in vitamin D deficiency. Am. J. Ther. 2019;26:e124-e32.
539. Schwalfenberg GK. Vitamins K1 and K2: The emerging group of vitamins required for human health. Journal of Nutrition and Metabolism. 2017;2017:6254836.

540. Duan F, Mei C, Yang L, Zheng J, Lu H, Xia Y, et al. Vitamin K2 promotes PI3K/AKT/HIF-1a-mediated glycolysis that leads to AMPK-dependent autophagic cell death in bladder cancer cells. Sci Rep. 2020;10(1):7714.
541. Tokita H, Tsuchida A, Miyazawa K, Ohyashiki K, Katayanagi S, Sudo H, et al. Vitamin K2-induced antitumor effects via cell-cycle arrest and apoptosis in gastric cancer cell lines. Int. J Mol. Med. 2006;17(2):235-43.
542. Welsh J, Bak MJ, Narvaez CJ. New insights into vitamin K biology with relevance to cancer. Trends Mol. Med. 2022;28(10):864-81.
543. Nimptsch K, Rohrmann S, Kaaks R, Linseisen J. Dietary vitamin K intake in relation to cancer incidence and mortality: results from the Heidelberg cohort of the European Prospective Investigation into Cancer and Nutrition (EPIC-Heidelberg). Am. J Clin. Nutr. 2010;91(5):1348-58.
544. Carlberg C, Velleuer E. Vitamin D and the risk for cancer: A molecular analysis. Biochem. Pharmacol. 2022;196:114735.
545. Baeke F, Takiishi T, Korf H, Gysemans C, Mathieu C. Vitamin D: modulator of the immune system. Current Opinion in Pharmacology. 2010;10(4):482-96.
546. Bartley J. Vitamin D: emerging roles in infection and immunity. Expert Review of Antiinfective Therapy. 2010;8(12):1359-69.
547. Chowdhury R, Kunutsor S, Vitezova A, Oliver-Williams C, Chowdhury S, Kiefte-de-Jong JC, et al. Vitamin D and risk of cause specific death: systematic review and meta-analysis of observational cohort and randomised intervention studies. BMJ. 2014;348:g1903.
548. Ng K, Venook AP, Sato K, Yuan C, Hollis BW, Chang IW, et al. Vitamin D status and survival of metastatic colorectal cancer patients: Results form CALGB/SWOG 80405 (Alliance) [Abstract]. J. Clin. Oncol. 2015;33:3503.
549. Sha S, Nguyen TMN, Kuznia S, Niedermaier T, Zhu A, Brenner H, et al. Real-world evidence for the effectiveness of vitamin D supplementation in reduction of total and cause-specific mortality. J Intern Med. 2023;293(3):384-97.
550. Bjelakovic G, Gluud LL, Nikolova D, Whitfield K, Wetterslev J, Simonetti RG, et al. Vitamin D supplementation for prevention of mortality in adults. Cochrane Database Syst. Rev. 2014(1):CD007470.
551. Hossain S, Beydoun MA, Beydoun HA, Chen X, Zonderman AB, Wood RJ. Vitamin D and breast cancer: A systematic review and meta-analysis of observational studies. Clin. Nutr. ESPEN. 2019;30:170-84.
552. Zhang Y, Fang F, Tang J, Jia L, Feng Y, Xu P, et al. Association between vitamin D supplementation and mortality: systematic review and meta-analysis. BMJ. 2019;366:l4673.
553. Manson JE, Cook NR, Lee IM, Christen W, Bassuk SS, Mora S, et al. Vitamin D Supplements and Prevention of Cancer and Cardiovascular Disease. N Engl J Med. 2019;380(1):33-44.
554. Ng K, Nimeiri HS, McCleary NJ, Abrams TA, Yurgelun MB, Cleary JM, et al. Effect of High-Dose vs Standard-Dose Vitamin D3 Supplementation on Progression-Free Survival Among Patients With Advanced or Metastatic Colorectal Cancer: The SUNSHINE Randomized Clinical Trial. JAMA. 2019;321(14):1370-9.
555. Diaz GD, Paraskeva C, Thomas MG, Binderup L, Hague A. Apoptosis is induced by the active metabolite of vitamin D3 and its analogue EB1089 in colorectal adenoma and carcinoma cells: possible implications for prevention and therapy. Cancer Res. 2000;60(8):2304-12.
556. Feldman D, Krishnan AV, Swami S, Giovannucci E, Feldman BJ. The role of vitamin D in reducing cancer risk and progression. Nat. Rev Cancer. 2014;14(5):342-57.
557. Mathieu C, Adorini L. The coming of age of 1,25-dihydroxyvitamin D(3) analogs as immunomodulatory agents. Trends Mol. Med. 2002;8(4):174-9.

558. Zheng W, Cao L, Ouyang L, Zhang Q, Duan B, Zhou W, et al. Anticancer activity of 1,25-(OH)(2)D(3) against human breast cancer cell lines by targeting Ras/MEK/ERK pathway. Onco. Targets Ther. 2019;12:721-32.
559. Abu El Maaty MA, Wolfl S. Effects of 1,25$(OH)_2$ D_3 on Cancer Cells and Potential Applications in Combination with Established and Putative Anti-Cancer Agents. Nutrients. 2017;9(1).
560. Yang ES, Burnstein KL. Vitamin D inhibits G1 to S progression in LNCaP prostate cancer cells through p27Kip1 stabilization and Cdk2 mislocalization to the cytoplasm. J Biol Chem. 2003;278(47):46862-8.
561. Krishnan AV, Swami S, Feldman D. Vitamin D and breast cancer: inhibition of estrogen synthesis and signaling. J Steroid Biochem. Mol. Biol. 2010;121(1-2):343-8.
562. Palmer HG, Sanchez-Carbayo M, Ordonez-Moran P, Larriba MJ, Cordonn-Cardo C, Munoz A. Genetic signatures of differentiation induced by 1alpha,25-dihydroxyvitamin D3 in human colon cancer cells. Cancer Res. 2003;63(22):7799-806.
563. Palmer HG, Gonzalez-Sancho JM, Espada J, Berciano MT, Puig I, Baulida J, et al. Vitamin D(3) promotes the differentiation of colon carcinoma cells by the induction of E-cadherin and the inhibition of beta-catenin signaling. J Cell Biol. 2001;154(2):369-87.
564. Moreno J, Krishnan AV, Swami S, Nonn L, Peehl DM, Feldman D. Regulation of prostaglandin metabolism by calcitriol attenuates growth stimulation in prostate cancer cells. Cancer Res. 2005;65(17):7917-25.
565. Larriba MJ, Garcia de Herreros A, Munoz A. Vitamin D and the Epithelial to Mesenchymal Transition. Stem Cells Int. 2016;2016:6213872.
566. Bernardi RJ, Johnson CS, Modzelewski RA, Trump DL. Antiproliferative effects of 1 alpha,25-dihydroxyvitamin D(3) and vitamin D analogs on tumor-derived endothelial cells. Endocrinology. 2002;143(7):2508-14.
567. Ng K, Meyerhardt JA, Wu K, Feskanich D, Hollis BW, Giovannucci EL, et al. Circulating 25-hydroxyvitamin d levels and survival in patients with colorectal cancer. J Clin. Oncol. 2008;26(18):2984-91.
568. Johansson H, Spadola G, Tosti G, MandalÃ M, Minisini AM, Queirolo P, et al. Vitamin D Supplementation and Disease-Free Survival in Stage II Melanoma: A Randomized Placebo Controlled Trial. Nutrients. 2021;13(6).
569. Yuan C, Sato K, Hollis BW, Zhang S, Niedzwiecki D, Ou FS, et al. Plasma 25-Hydroxyvitamin D Levels and Survival in Patients with Advanced or Metastatic Colorectal Cancer: Findings from CALGB/SWOG 80405 (Alliance). Clin. Cancer Res. 2019;25(24):7497-505.
570. Mezawa H, Sugiura T, Watanabe M, Norizoe C, Takahashi D, Shimojima A, et al. Serum vitamin D levels and survival of patients with colorectal cancer: post-hoc analysis of a prospective cohort study. BMC Cancer. 2010;10:347.
571. Zgaga L, Theodoratou E, Farrington SM, Din FV, Ooi LY, Glodzik D, et al. Plasma vitamin D concentration influences survival outcome after a diagnosis of colorectal cancer. J Clin. Oncol. 2014;32(23):2430-9.
572. Toriola AT, Nguyen N, Scheitler-Ring K, Colditz GA. Circulating 25-hydroxyvitamin D levels and prognosis among cancer patients: a systematic review. Cancer Epidemiol. Biomarkers Prev. 2014;23(6):917-33.
573. Tretli S, Schwartz GG, Torjesen PA, Robsahm TE. Serum levels of 25-hydroxyvitamin D and survival in Norwegian patients with cancer of breast, colon, lung, and lymphoma: a population-based study. Cancer Causes Control. 2012;23(2):363-70.
574. Robsahm TE, Schwartz GG, Tretli S. The Inverse Relationship between 25-Hydroxyvitamin D and Cancer Survival: Discussion of Causation. Cancers (Basel). 2013;5(4):1439-55.

575. Chen QY, Kim S, Lee B, Jeong G, Lee DH, Keum N, et al. Post-Diagnosis Vitamin D Supplement Use and Survival among Cancer Patients: A Meta-Analysis. Nutrients. 2022;14(16).
576. Vaughan-Shaw PG, Buijs LF, Blackmur JP, Theodoratou E, Zgaga L, Din FVN, et al. The effect of vitamin D supplementation on survival in patients with colorectal cancer: systematic review and meta-analysis of randomised controlled trials. Br. J Cancer. 2020;123(11):1705-12.
577. Kuznia S, Zhu A, Akutsu T, Buring JE, Camargo CA, Jr., Cook NR, et al. Efficacy of vitamin D(3) supplementation on cancer mortality: Systematic review and individual patient data meta-analysis of randomised controlled trials. Ageing Res Rev. 2023;87:101923.
578. Wang L, Wang C, Wang J, Huang X, Cheng Y. Longitudinal, observational study on associations between postoperative nutritional vitamin D supplementation and clinical outcomes in esophageal cancer patients undergoing esophagectomy. Sci Rep. 2016;6:38962.
579. Madden JM, Murphy L, Zgaga L, Bennett K. De novo vitamin D supplement use post-diagnosis is associated with breast cancer survival. Breast Cancer Res Treat. 2018;172(1):179-90.
580. Marshall DT, Savage SJ, Garrett-Mayer E, Keane TE, Hollis BW, Horst RL, et al. Vitamin D3 supplementation at 4000 international units per day for one year results in a decrease of positive cores at repeat biopsy in subjects with low-risk prostate cancer under active surveillance. J Clin. Endocrinol. Metab. 2012;97(7):2315-24.
581. Wagner D, Trudel D, Van der Kwast T, Nonn L, Giangreco AA, Li D, et al. Randomized clinical trial of vitamin D3 doses on prostatic vitamin D metabolite levels and ki67 labeling in prostate cancer patients. J Clin. Endocrinol. Metab. 2013;98(4):1498-507.
582. Zeichner SB, Koru-Sengul T, Shah N, Liu Q, Markward NJ, Montero AJ, et al. Improved clinical outcomes associated with vitamin D supplementation during adjuvant chemotherapy in patients with HER2+ nonmetastatic breast cancer. Clin. Breast Cancer. 2015;15(1):e1-11.
583. Cadegiani FA. Remission of severe Myasthenia Gravis after massive-dose vitamin D treatment. Am. J. Case. Rep. 2016;17:51-4.
584. McCullough P, Amend J. Results of daily oral dosing with up to 60,000 international units (iu) of vitamin D3 for 2 to 6 years in 3 adult males. J Steroid Biochem. Mol. Biol. 2017;173:308-12.
585. Amon U, Yaguboglu R, Ennis M, Holick MF, Amon J. Safety Data in Patients with Autoimmune Diseases during Treatment with High Doses of Vitamin D3 According to the "Coimbra Protocol". Nutrients. 2022;14(8).
586. Finamor DC, Sinigaglia-Coimbra R, Neves LC, Gutierrez M, Silva JJ, Torres LD, et al. A pilot study assessing the effect of prolonged administration of high daily doses of vitamin D on the clinical course of vitiligo and psoriasis. Dermatoendocrinol. 2013;5(1):222-34.
587. Kim-Fuchs C, Le CP, Pimentel MA, Shackleford D, Ferrari D, Angst E, et al. Chronic stress accelerates pancreatic cancer growth and invasion: a critical role for beta-adrenergic signaling in the pancreatic microenvironment. Brain Behav Immun. 2014;40:40-7.
588. Yuan A, Wang S, Li Z, Huang C. Psychological aspect of cancer: From stressor to cancer progression. Exp Ther Med. 2010;1(1):13-8.
589. Cole SW, Nagaraja AS, Lutgendorf SK, Green PA, Sood AK. Sympathetic nervous system regulation of the tumour microenvironment. Nat Rev Cancer. 2015;15(9):563-72.
590. Gao G, Sun J, Gao J, Xiong L, Yu L, Gao Y. Chronic stress promoted the growth of ovarian carcinoma via increasing serum levels of norepinephrine and interleukin-10 and altering nm23 and NDRG1 expression in tumor tissues in nude mice. Biosci Trends. 2013;7(1):56-63.
591. Amikishieva AV, Ilnitskaya SI, Nikolin VP, Popova NA, Kaledin VI. Depressive-like psychoemotional state versus acute stresses enhances Lewis lung carcinoma metastasis in C57BL/6J mice. Exp Oncol. 2011;33(4):222-5.

592. Partecke LI, Speerforck S, Käding A, Seubert F, Kühn S, Lorenz E, et al. Chronic stress increases experimental pancreatic cancer growth, reduces survival and can be antagonised by beta-adrenergic receptor blockade. Pancreatology. 2016;16(3):423-33.
593. Pantziarka P, Bouche G, Sukhatme V, Meheus L, Rooman I, Sukhatme VP. Repurposing Drugs in Oncology (ReDO)-Propranolol as an anti-cancer agent. Ecancermedicalscience. 2016;10:680.
594. Lamkin DM, Sloan EK, Patel AJ, Chiang BS, Pimentel MA, Ma JC, et al. Chronic stress enhances progression of acute lymphoblastic leukemia via β-adrenergic signaling. Brain Behav Immun. 2012;26(4):635-41.
595. Sloan EK, Priceman SJ, Cox BF, Yu S, Pimentel MA, Tangkanangnukul V, et al. The sympathetic nervous system induces a metastatic switch in primary breast cancer. Cancer Res. 2010;70(18):7042-52.
596. Rains SL, Amaya CN, Bryan BA. Beta-adrenergic receptors are expressed across diverse cancers. Oncoscience. 2017;4(7-8):95-105.
597. Nissen MD, Sloan EK, Mattarollo SR. β-Adrenergic Signaling Impairs Antitumor CD8(+) T-cell Responses to B-cell Lymphoma Immunotherapy. Cancer Immunol Res. 2018;6(1):98-109.
598. Pundavela J, Roselli S, Faulkner S, Attia J, Scott RJ, Thorne RF, et al. Nerve fibers infiltrate the tumor microenvironment and are associated with nerve growth factor production and lymph node invasion in breast cancer. Mol Oncol. 2015;9(8):1626-35.
599. Osawa H, Printz RL, Whitesell RR, Granner DK. Regulation of hexokinase II gene transcription and glucose phosphorylation by catecholamines, cyclic AMP, and insulin. Diabetes. 1995;44(12):1426-32.
600. Montoya A, Varela-Ramirez A, Dickerson E, Pasquier E, Torabi A, Aguilera R, et al. The beta adrenergic receptor antagonist propranolol alters mitogenic and apoptotic signaling in late stage breast cancer. Biomed J. 2019;42(3):155-65.
601. Wolter JK, Wolter NE, Blanch A, Partridge T, Cheng L, Morgenstern DA, et al. Anti-tumor activity of the beta-adrenergic receptor antagonist propranolol in neuroblastoma. Oncotarget. 2014;5(1):161-72.
602. Pasquier E, Street J, Pouchy C, Carre M, Gifford AJ, Murray J, et al. β-blockers increase response to chemotherapy via direct antitumour and anti-angiogenic mechanisms in neuroblastoma. Br J Cancer. 2013;108(12):2485-94.
603. Entschladen F, Thyssen DA, Drell DW. Re-Use of Established Drugs for Anti-Metastatic Indications. Cells. 2016;5(1).
604. Pantziarka P, Bryan BA, Crispino S, Dickerson EB. Propranolol and breast cancer-a work in progress. Ecancermedicalscience. 2018;12:ed82.
605. Hajighasemi F, Hajighasemi S. Effect of propranolol on angiogenic factors in human hematopoietic cell lines in vitro. Iran Biomed J. 2009;13(4):223-8.
606. Guo K, Ma Q, Wang L, Hu H, Li J, Zhang D, et al. Norepinephrine-induced invasion by pancreatic cancer cells is inhibited by propranolol. Oncol Rep. 2009;22(4):825-30.
607. Xia Y, Wei Y, Li ZY, Cai XY, Zhang LL, Dong XR, et al. Catecholamines contribute to the neovascularization of lung cancer via tumor-associated macrophages. Brain Behav Immun. 2019;81:111-21.
608. Shan T, Ma J, Ma Q, Guo K, Guo J, Li X, et al. β2-AR-HIF-1α: a novel regulatory axis for stress-induced pancreatic tumor growth and angiogenesis. Curr Mol Med. 2013;13(6):1023-34.
609. Park SY, Kang JH, Jeong KJ, Lee J, Han JW, Choi WS, et al. Norepinephrine induces VEGF expression and angiogenesis by a hypoxia-inducible factor-1α protein-dependent mechanism. Int J Cancer. 2011;128(10):2306-16.

610. Rico M, Baglioni M, Bondarenko M, Laluce NC, Rozados V, André N, et al. Metformin and propranolol combination prevents cancer progression and metastasis in different breast cancer models. Oncotarget. 2017;8(2):2874-89.
611. Brohée L, Peulen O, Nusgens B, Castronovo V, Thiry M, Colige AC, et al. Propranolol sensitizes prostate cancer cells to glucose metabolism inhibition and prevents cancer progression. Sci Rep. 2018;8(1):7050.
612. Pasquier E, Ciccolini J, Carre M, Giacometti S, Fanciullino R, Pouchy C, et al. Propranolol potentiates the anti-angiogenic effects and anti-tumor efficacy of chemotherapy agents: implication in breast cancer treatment. Oncotarget. 2011;2(10):797-809.
613. Chang PY, Huang WY, Lin CL, Huang TC, Wu YY, Chen JH, et al. Propranolol Reduces Cancer Risk: A Population-Based Cohort Study. Medicine (Baltimore). 2015;94(27):e1097.
614. Botteri E, Munzone E, Rotmensz N, Cipolla C, De Giorgi V, Santillo B, et al. Therapeutic effect of β-blockers in triple-negative breast cancer postmenopausal women. Breast Cancer Res Treat. 2013;140(3):567-75.
615. Melhem-Bertrandt A, Chavez-Macgregor M, Lei X, Brown EN, Lee RT, Meric-Bernstam F, et al. Beta-blocker use is associated with improved relapse-free survival in patients with triple-negative breast cancer. J Clin Oncol. 2011;29(19):2645-52.
616. Childers WK, Hollenbeak CS, Cheriyath P. β-Blockers Reduce Breast Cancer Recurrence and Breast Cancer Death: A Meta-Analysis. Clin Breast Cancer. 2015;15(6):426-31.
617. Caparica R, Bruzzone M, Agostinetto E, De Angelis C, Fêde Â, Ceppi M, et al. Beta-blockers in early-stage breast cancer: a systematic review and meta-analysis. ESMO Open. 2021;6(2):100066.
618. Powe DG, Voss MJ, Zänker KS, Habashy HO, Green AR, Ellis IO, et al. Beta-blocker drug therapy reduces secondary cancer formation in breast cancer and improves cancer specific survival. Oncotarget. 2010;1(7):628-38.
619. Watkins JL, Thaker PH, Nick AM, Ramondetta LM, Kumar S, Urbauer DL, et al. Clinical impact of selective and nonselective beta-blockers on survival in patients with ovarian cancer. Cancer. 2015;121(19):3444-51.
620. Hwa YL, Shi Q, Kumar SK, Lacy MQ, Gertz MA, Kapoor P, et al. Beta-blockers improve survival outcomes in patients with multiple myeloma: a retrospective evaluation. Am J Hematol. 2017;92(1):50-5.
621. De Giorgi V, Grazzini M, Benemei S, Marchionni N, Botteri E, Pennacchioli E, et al. Propranolol for Off-label Treatment of Patients With Melanoma: Results From a Cohort Study. JAMA Oncol. 2018;4(2):e172908.
622. Léauté-Labrèze C, Hoeger P, Mazereeuw-Hautier J, Guibaud L, Baselga E, Posiunas G, et al. A randomized, controlled trial of oral propranolol in infantile hemangioma. N Engl J Med. 2015;372(8):735-46.
623. Chisholm KM, Chang KW, Truong MT, Kwok S, West RB, Heerema-McKenney AE. β-Adrenergic receptor expression in vascular tumors. Mod Pathol. 2012;25(11):1446-51.
624. Colunga Biancatelli RM, Berrill M, Mohammed YH, Marik PE. Melatonin for the treatment of sepsis: the scientific rationale. J. Thorac. Dis. 2020;12 (Suppl 1):S54-S65.
625. Jung B, Ahmad N. Melatonin in cancer management: Progress and promise. Cancer Res. 2006;66:9789-93.
626. Jockers R, Delagrange P, Dubocovich ML, Markus RP, Renault N, Tosini G, et al. Update on melatonin receptors: IUPHAR Review 20. Br. J Pharmacol. 2016;173(18):2702-25.
627. Yeager RL, Oleske DA, Sanders RA, Eells JT, Henshel DS. Melatonin as a principal component of red light therapy. Medical Hypotheses. 2007;69:372-6.

628. Tan DX, Reiter RJ, Zimmerman S, Hardeland R. Melatonin: Both a messenger of darkness and a participant in cellular actions of non-visible solar radiation of near infrared light. Biology. 2023;12:89.
629. Manouchehri E, Taghipour A, Ghavami V, Ebadi A, Homaei F, Latifnejad RR. Night-shift work duration and breast cancer risk: an updated systematic review and meta-analysis. BMC Womens Health. 2021;21(1):89.
630. Wise J. Danish night shift workers with breast cancer awarded compensation. BMJ. 2009;338:b1152.
631. Mortezaee K, Najafi M, Farhood B, Ahmadi A, Potes Y, Shabeeb D, et al. Modulation of apoptosis by melatonin for improving cancer treatment efficiency: An updated review. Life Sci. 2019;228:228-41.
632. Akbarzadeh M, Movassaghpour AA, Ghanbari H, Kheirandish M, Fathi MN, Rahbarghazi R, et al. The potential therapeutic effect of melatonin on human ovarian cancer by inhibition of invasion and migration of cancer stem cells. Sci Rep. 2017;7(1):17062.
633. Reiter RJ, Sharma R, Ma Q, Rosales-Corral SA, Escames G. Inhibition of mitochondrial pyruvate dehydrogenase kinase: a proposed mechanism by which melatonin causes cancer cells to overcome cytosolic glycolysis, reduce tumor biomass and reverse insensitivity to chemotherapy. Melatonin Res. 2019;2:105-19.
634. Sanchez-Sanchez AM, AAntolin I, Puente-Moncada N, Suarez S, Rodriguez C. Melatonin cytotoxicity is associated to Warburg effect inhibition in Ewing sarcoma cells. PloS ONE. 2015;10:e0135420.
635. Hevia D, Gonzalez-Menendez P, Fernandez-Fernandez M, Cueto S, Rodriguez-Gonzalez P, Garcia-Alonso JI, et al. Melatonin Decreases Glucose Metabolism in Prostate Cancer Cells: A (13)C Stable Isotope-Resolved Metabolomic Study. Int. J Mol. Sci. 2017;18(8).
636. Perfilyeva YV, Ostapchuk YO, Abdolla N, Tleulieva R, Krasnoshtanov VC, Belyaev NN. Exogenous Melatonin Up-Regulates Expression of CD62L by Lymphocytes in Aged Mice under Inflammatory and Non-Inflammatory Conditions. Immunol. Invest. 2019;48(6):632-43.
637. Liu H, Xu L, Wei JE, Xie MR, Wang SE, Zhou RX. Role of CD4+ CD25+ regulatory T cells in melatonin-mediated inhibition of murine gastric cancer cell growth in vivo and in vitro. Anat. Rec. 2011;294(5):781-8.
638. Shiu SY, Law IC, Lau KW, Tam PC, Yip AW, Ng WT. Melatonin slowed the early biochemical progression of hormone-refractory prostate cancer in a patient whose prostate tumor tissue expressed MT1 receptor subtype. J Pineal Res. 2003;35(3):177-82.
639. Tomov B, Popov D, Tomova R, Vladov N, Den Otter W, Krastev Z. Therapeutic response of untreatable hepatocellular carcinoma after application of the immune modulators IL-2, BCG and melatonin. Anticancer Res. 2013;33(10):4531-5.
640. Mills E, Wu P, Seely D, Guyatt G. Melatonin in the treatment of cancer: a systematic review of randomized controlled trials and meta-analysis. J Pineal Res. 2005;39(4):360-6.
641. Seely D, Wu P, Fritz H, Kennedy DA, Tsui T, Seely AJ. Melatonin as adjuvant cancer care with and without chemotherapy: A systematic review and meta-analysis of randomized trials. Integrative Cancer Therapies. 2012;11:293-303.
642. Dowling RJ, Niraula S, Stambolic V, Goodwin PJ. Metformin in cancer: translational challenges. J Mol. Endocrinol. 2012;48(3):R31-R43.
643. Dowling RJ, Zakikhani M, Fantus IG, Pollak M, Sonenberg N. Metformin inhibits mammalian target of rapamycin-dependent translation initiation in breast cancer cells. Cancer Res. 2007;67(22):10804-12.
644. Andrzejewski S, Siegel PM, St-Pierre J. Metabolic profiles associated with metforrmin efficacy in cancer. Front. Endocrinol. 2018;9:372.

645. Barrios-Bernal P, Zatarain-Barron ZL, Hernandez-Pedro N, Orozco-Morales M, Olivera-Ramirez A, Avila-Moreno F, et al. Will we unlock the benefit of metformin for patients with lung cancer? Lessons from current evidence and new hypotheses. Pharmaceuticals. 2022;15:786.
646. Saraei P, Asadi L, Kakar MA, Moradi-Kor N. The beneficial effects of metformin on cancer prevention and therapy: a comprehensive review of recent advances. Cancer Management and Research. 2019;11:3295-313.
647. Shi P, Liu W, Tala, Wang H, Li F, Zhang H, et al. Metformin suppresses triple-negative breast cancer stem cells by targeting KLF5 for degradation. Cell Discov. 2017;3:17010.
648. Lega IC, Shah PS, Margel D, Beyene J, Rochon PA, Lipscombe LL. The effect of metformin on mortality following cancer among patients with diabetes. Cancer Epidemiol. Biomarkers Prev. 2014;23(10):1974-84.
649. Yin M, Zhou J, Gorak EJ, Quddus F. Metformin is associated with survival benefit in cancer patients with concurrent type 2 diabetes: a systematic review and meta-analysis. Oncologist. 2013;18(12):1248-55.
650. Mei ZB, Zhang ZJ, Liu CY, Liu Y, Cui A, Liang ZL, et al. Survival benefits of metformin for colorectal cancer patients with diabetes: a systematic review and meta-analysis. PloS ONE. 2014;9(3):e91818.
651. Coyle C, Cafferty FH, Vale C, Langley RE. Metformin as an adjuvant treatment for cancer: a systematic review and meta-analysis. Annals of Oncolog. 2016;27:2184-95.
652. Eibl G, Rozengurt E. Metformin: Review of epidemiology and mechanisms of action in pancreatic cancer. Cancer Metastasis Rev. 2021;40:865-78.
653. Jimenez-Vacas JM, Herrero-Aguayo V, Montero-Hidalgo AJ, Saez-Martinez P, Gomez-Gomez E. Clinical, cellualr and molecular evidence of the additive antitumor effects of biguanides and statins in prostate cancer. Journal of Clinical Endocrinology & Metabolism. 2012;106:e696-e710.
654. Wang Y, Liu G, Tong D, Parmar H, Hasenmayer D, Yuan W, et al. Metformin represses androgen-dependent and androgen independnet prostrate cancers by targeting androgen receptor. Prostate. 2015;75:1187-96.
655. Buczynska A, Sidorkiewicz I, Kretowski AJ, Zbucka-Kretowska M, Adamska A. Metformin intervention - A panacea for cancer treatment? Cancers. 2022;14:1336.
656. Stopsack KH, Ziehr DR, Rider JR, Giovannucci EL. Metformin and prostate cancer mortality: a meta-analysis. Cancer Causes Control. 2016;27(1):105-13.
657. Giordano A, Tommonaro G. Curcumin and cancer. Nutrients. 2019;11:2376.
658. Pal S, Bhattacharyya S, Choudhuri T, Datta GK, Das T, Sa G. Amelioration of immune cell number depletion and potentiation of depressed detoxification system of tumor-bearing mice by curcumin. Cancer Detect. Prev. 2005;29(5):470-8.
659. Mansouri K, Rasoulpoor S, Daneshkhah A, Abolfathi S, Salari N, Mohammadi M, et al. Clinical effects of curcumin in enhancing cancer therapy: A systematic review. BMC Cancer. 2020;20(1):791.
660. Anand P, Sundaram C, Jhurani S, Kunnumakkara AB, Aggarwal BB. Curcumin and cancer: an "old-age" disease with an "age-old" solution. Cancer Lett. 2008;267(1):133-64.
661. Santosa D, Suharti C, Riwanto I, Dharmana E, Pangarsa EA, Setiawan B, et al. Curcumin as adjuvant therapy to improve remission in myeloma patients: A pilot randomized clinical trial. Caspian. J Intern Med. 2022;13(2):375-84.
662. Cho JW, Lee KS, Kim CW. Curcumin attenuates the expression of IL-1b, IL-6, and TNF-a as well as cyclin E in TNF-a-treated HaCaT cells; NF-kB and MAPKs as potential upstream targets. Int. J Mol. Med. 2007;19(3):469-74.
663. Xiang DB, Zhang KQ, Zeng YL, Yan QZ, Shi Z, Tuo QH, et al. Curcumin: From a controversial "panacea" to effective antineoplastic products. Medicine (Baltimore). 2020;99(2):e18467.

664. Moghaddam SJ, Barta P, Mirabolfathinejad SG, Ammar-Aouchiche Z, Garza NT, Vo TT, et al. Curcumin inhibits COPD-like airway inflammation and lung cancer progression in mice. Carcinogenesis. 2009;30(11):1949-56.
665. Wang JY, Wang X, Wang XJ, Zheng BZ, Wang Y, Wang X, et al. Curcumin inhibits the growth via Wnt/B-catenin pathway in non-small-cell lung cancer cells. Eur Rev Med Pharmacol. Sci. 2018;22(21):7492-9.
666. Alexandrow MG, Song LJ, Altiok S, Gray J, Haura EB, Kumar NB. Curcumin: a novel Stat3 pathway inhibitor for chemoprevention of lung cancer. Eur J Cancer Prev. 2012;21(5):407-12.
667. Ye MX, Li Y, Yin H, Zhang J. Curcumin: updated molecular mechanisms and intervention targets in human lung cancer. Int. J Mol. Sci. 2012;13(3):3959-78.
668. Katta S, Srivastava A, Thangapazham RL, Rosner IL, Cullen J, Li H, et al. Curcumin-Gene Expression Response in Hormone Dependent and Independent Metastatic Prostate Cancer Cells. Int. J Mol. Sci. 2019;20(19).
669. Mach CM, Mathew L, Mosley SA, Kurzrock R, Smith JA. Determination of minimum effective dose and optimal dosing schedule for liposomal curcumin in a xenograft human pancreatic cancer model. Anticancer Res. 2009;29(6):1895-9.
670. Lee JC, Kinniry PA, Arguiri E, Serota M, Kanterakis S, Chatterjee S, et al. Dietary curcumin increases antioxidant defenses in lung, ameliorates radiation-induced pulmonary fibrosis, and improves survival in mice. Radiat. Res. 2010;173(5):590-601.
671. Panahi Y, Darvishi B, Ghanei M, Jowzi N, Beiraghdar F, Varnamkhasti BS. Molecular mechanisms of curcumins suppressing effects on tumorigenesis, angiogenesis and metastasis, focusing on NF-kB pathway. Cytokine Growth Factor Rev. 2016;28:21-9.
672. Dhillon N, Aggarwal BB, Newman RA, Wolff RA, Kunnumakkara AB, Abbruzzese JL, et al. Phase II trial of curcumin in patients with advanced pancreatic cancer. Clin. Cancer Res. 2008;14(14):4491-9.
673. Carroll RE, Benya RV, Turgeon DK, Vareed S, Neuman M, Rodriguez L, et al. Phase IIa clinical trial of curcumin for the prevention of colorectal neoplasia. Cancer Prev. Res (Phila). 2011;4(3):354-64.
674. Li Y, Zhang T. Targeting cancer stem cells by curcumin and clinical applications. Cancer Lett. 2014;346(2):197-205.
675. Zoi V, Galani V, Lianos GD, Voulgaris S, Kyritsis AP, Alexiou GA. The Role of Curcumin in Cancer Treatment. Biomedicines. 2021;9(9).
676. Aggarwal BB, Sethi G, Ahn KS, Sandur SK, Pandey MK, Kunnumakkara AB, et al. Targeting signal-transducer-and-activator-of-transcription-3 for prevention and therapy of cancer: modern target but ancient solution. Ann. N. Y. Acad. Sci. 2006;1091:151-69.
677. Pandey A, Vishnoi K, Mahata S, Tripathi SC, Misra SP, Misra V, et al. Berberine and Curcumin Target Survivin and STAT3 in Gastric Cancer Cells and Synergize Actions of Standard Chemotherapeutic 5-Fluorouracil. Nutr. Cancer. 2015;67(8):1293-304.
678. Yim-im W, Sawatdichaikul O, Semsri S, Horata N, Mokmak W, Tongsima S, et al. Computational analyses of curcuminoid analogs against kinase domain of HER2. BMC Bioinformatics. 2014;15(1):261.
679. Hu S, Xu Y, Meng L, Huang L, Sun H. Curcumin inhibits proliferation and promotes apoptosis of breast cancer cells. Exp Ther. Med. 2018;16(2):1266-72.
680. Wang K, Fan H, Chen Q, Ma G, Zhu M, Zhang X, et al. Curcumin inhibits aerobic glycolysis and induces mitochondrial-mediated apoptosis through hexokinase II in human colorectal cancer cells in vitro. Anticancer Drugs. 2015;26(1):15-24.
681. Starok M, Preira P, Vayssade M, Haupt K, Salome L, Rossi C. EGFR Inhibition by Curcumin in Cancer Cells: A Dual Mode of Action. Biomacromolecules. 2015;16(5):1634-42.

682. Sun XD, Liu XE, Huang DS. Curcumin induces apoptosis of triple-negative breast cancer cells by inhibition of EGFR expression. Mol. Med Rep. 2012;6(6):1267-70.
683. Falconer JS, Fearon KC, Ross JA, Elton R, Wigmore SJ, Garden OJ, et al. Acute-phase protein response and survival duration of patients with pancreatic cancer. Cancer. 1995;75(8):2077-82.
684. James MI, Iwuji C, Irving G, Karmokar A, Higgins JA, Griffin-Teal N, et al. Curcumin inhibits cancer stem cell phenotypes in ex vivo models of colorectal liver metastases, and is clinically safe and tolerable in combination with FOLFOX chemotherapy. Cancer Lett. 2015;364(2):135-41.
685. Kunnumakkara AB, Harsha C, Banik K, Vikkurthi R, Sailo BL, Bordoloi D. Is curcumin bioavailability a problem in humans: Lessons from clinical trials. Expert Opinion on Drug Metabolism & Toxicology. 2019;15:705-33.
686. Bayet-Robert M, Kwiatkowski F, Leheurteur M, Gachon F, Planchat E, Abrial C, et al. Phase I dose escalation trial of docetaxel plus curcumin in patients with advanced and metastatic breast cancer. Cancer Biol Ther. 2010;9(1):8-14.
687. Ghalaut VS, Sangwan L, Dahiya K, Ghalaut PS, Dhankhar R, Saharan R. Effect of imatinib therapy with and without turmeric powder on nitric oxide levels in chronic myeloid leukemia. J Oncol. Pharm Pract. 2012;18(2):186-90.
688. Hejazi J, Rastmanesh R, Taleban FA, Molana SH, Ehtejab G. A pilot clinical trial of radioprotective effects of curcumin supplementation in patients with prostate cancer. J. Cancer. Sci. Ther. 2013;5:320-4.
689. Kanai M, Yoshimura K, Asada M, Imaizumi A, Suzuki C, Matsumoto S, et al. A phase I/II study of gemcitabine-based chemotherapy plus curcumin for patients with gemcitabine-resistant pancreatic cancer. Cancer Chemother. Pharmacol. 2011;68(1):157-64.
690. Mahammedi H, Planchat E, Pouget M, Durando X, CurÃ© H, Guy L, et al. The New Combination Docetaxel, Prednisone and Curcumin in Patients with Castration-Resistant Prostate Cancer: A Pilot Phase II Study. Oncology. 2016;90(2):69-78.
691. Howells LM, Iwuji COO, Irving GRB, Barber S, Walter H, Sidat Z, et al. Curcumin Combined with FOLFOX Chemotherapy Is Safe and Tolerable in Patients with Metastatic Colorectal Cancer in a Randomized Phase IIa Trial. J Nutr. 2019;149(7):1133-9.
692. Pastorelli D, Fabricio ASC, Giovanis P, D'Ippolito S, Fiduccia P, SoldÃ C, et al. Phytosome complex of curcumin as complementary therapy of advanced pancreatic cancer improves safety and efficacy of gemcitabine: Results of a prospective phase II trial. Pharmacol. Res. 2018;132:72-9.
693. Burris HA, III, Moore MJ, Andersen J, Green MR, Rothenberg ML, Modiano MR, et al. Improvements in survival and clinical benefit with gemcitabine as first-line therapy for patients with advanced pancreas cancer: a randomized trial. J Clin. Oncol. 1997;15(6):2403-13.
694. Saghatelyan T, Tananyan A, Janoyan N, Tadevosyan A, Petrosyan H, Hovhannisyan A, et al. Efficacy and safety of curcumin in combination with paclitaxel in patients with advanced, metastatic breast cancer: A comparative, randomized, double-blind, placebo-controlled clinical trial. Phytomedicine. 2020;70:153218.
695. Guorgui J, Wang R, Mattheolabakis G, Mackenzie GG. Curcumin formulated in solid lipid nanoparticles has enhanced efficacy in Hodgkin's lymphoma in mice. Arch Biochem. Biophys. 2018;648:12-9.
696. Moballegh Nasery M, Abadi B, Poormoghadam D, Zarrabi A, Keyhanvar P, Tavakol S, et al. Curcumin delivery mediated by bio-based nanoparticles: A review. Molecules. 2020;25:689.
697. Valizadeh H, Danshina S, Gencer MZ, Ammari A, Sadeghi A, Aslani S. Nano-curcumin therapy, a promising method in modulating inflammatory cytokines in COVID-19 patients. International Immunopharmacology. 2020;89:107088.

698. Ahmadi R, Salari S, Reihani H, Eslami S. Oral nano-curcumin formulation efficacy in the management of mild to moderate outpatient COVID-19: A randomized triple-blind placebo-controlled clinical trial. Food Science & Nutrition. 2021;9:4068-75.
699. Rahimi HR, Nedaeinia R, Shamloo AS, Nikdoust S. Novel delivery system for natural products: Nano-curcumin formulations. AJP. 2016;6:383.
700. Skiba MB, Luis PB, Alfafara C, Billheimer D, Schneider C, Funk JL. Curcuminoid Content and Safety-Related Markers of Quality of Turmeric Dietary Supplements Sold in an Urban Retail Marketplace in the United States. Mol. Nutr. Food Res. 2018;62(14):e1800143.
701. Desai P, Ann D, Wang J, Prabhu S. Pancreatic Cancer: Recent Advances in Nanoformulation-Based Therapies. Crit Rev Ther. Drug Carrier Syst. 2019;36(1):59-91.
702. Nguyen HT, Phung CD, Thapa RK, Pham TT, Tran TH, Jeong JH, et al. Multifunctional nanoparticles as somatostatin receptor-targeting delivery system of polyaniline and methotrexate for combined chemo-photothermal therapy. Acta Biomater. 2018;68:154-67.
703. Tan BL, Norhaizan ME. Curcumin Combination Chemotherapy: The Implication and Efficacy in Cancer. Molecules. 2019;24(14).
704. Notice to US Food and Drug Administraion of the conclusion that the intended use of curcumin is generally recognized as safe. https://www.fda.gov/food/generally-recognized-safe-gras/gras-notice-inventory; 2018.
705. Lao CD, Ruffin MT, Normolle D, Heath DD, Murray SI, Bailey JM, et al. Dose escalation of a curcuminoid formulation. BMC Complement Altern. Med. 2006;6:10.
706. Panahi Y, Saadat A, Beiraghdar F, Nouzari SM, Jalalian HR. Antioxidant effects of bioavailability-enhanced curcuminoids in patients with solid tumors: A randomized double-blind placebo-controlled trial. Journal of Functional Foods. 2014;6:615-22.
707. Halegoua-Demarzio D, Navarro V, Ahmad J, Avula B, Barnhart H, Barritt AS, et al. Liver injury associated with tumeric - A growing problem: Ten cases from the drug-induced liver injury network [DILIN]. Am. J. Med. 2022.
708. Volak LP, Ghirmai S, Cashman JR, MH C. Curcuminoids inhibit multiple human cytochromes P450, UDP-glucuronosyltransferase, and sulfotransferase enzymes, whereas piperine is a relatively selective CYP3A4 inhibitor. Drug Metab Dispos. 2008;36(8):1594-605.
709. Pavithra BH, Prakash N, Jayakumar K. Modification of pharmacokinetics of norfloxacin following oral administration of curcumin in rabbits. J Vet. Sci. 2009;10(4):293-7.
710. Kim DC, Ku SK, Bae JS. Anticoagulant activities of curcumin and its derivative. BMB Rep. 2012;45(4):221-6.
711. Tang M, Hu X, Wang Y, Yao X, Zhang W. Ivermectin, a potential anticancer drug derived from an antiparasitic drug. Pharmacological Research. 2021;163:105207.
712. Juarez M, Schcolnik-Cabrera A, Duenas-Gonzalez A. The multitargeted drug ivermectin: from an antiparasitic agent to a repositioned cancer drug. Am. J. Cancer Res. 2018;8:317-31.
713. Liu J, Zhang K, Cheng L, Zhu H, Xu T. Progress in Understanding the Molecular Mechanisms Underlying the Antitumour Effects of Ivermectin. Drug Des Devel Ther. 2020;14:285-96.
714. Didier A, Loor F. The abamectin derivative ivermectin is a potent P-glycoprotein inhibitor. Anticancer Drugs. 1996;7(7):745-51.
715. Li MY, Zhang J, Lu X, Zhou D, Deng XF, Liu QX, et al. Ivermectin induces nonprotective autophagy by downregulating PAK1 and apoptosis in lung adenocarcinoma cells. Cancer Chemother Pharmacol. 2023.
716. Dou Q, Chen HN, Wang K, Yuan K, Lei Y, Li K, et al. Ivermectin Induces Cytostatic Autophagy by Blocking the PAK1/Akt Axis in Breast Cancer. Cancer Res. 2016;76(15):4457-69.

717. Diao H, Cheng N, Zhao Y, Xu H, Dong H, Thamm DH, et al. Ivermectin inhibits canine mammary tumor growth by regulating cell cycle progression and WNT signaling. BMC Vet. Res. 2019;15(1):276.
718. Melotti A, Mas C, Kuciak M, Lorente-Trigos A, Borges I, Altaba A. The river blindness drug Ivermectin and related macrocyclic lactones inhibit WNT-TCF pathway responses in human cancer. EMBO Mol. Med. 2014;6(10):1263-78.
719. Diana A, Carlino F, Franzese E, Oikonomidou O, Criscitiello C, De VF, et al. Early Triple Negative Breast Cancer: Conventional Treatment and Emerging Therapeutic Landscapes. Cancers (Basel). 2020;12(4).
720. Kwon YJ, Petrie K, Leibovitch BA, Zeng L, Mezei M, Howell L, et al. Selective Inhibition of SIN3 Corepressor with Avermectins as a Novel Therapeutic Strategy in Triple-Negative Breast Cancer. Mol. Cancer Ther. 2015;14(8):1824-36.
721. Chen L, Bi S, Wei Q, Zhao Z, Wang X. Ivermectin suppresses tumour growth and metastasis through degradation of PAK1 in esophageal squamous cell carcinoma. J. Cell. Mol. Med. 2020;24:5387-401.
722. Nappi L, Aguda AH, Nakouzi NA, Lelj-Garolla B, Beraldi E, Lallous N, et al. Ivermectin inhibits HSP27 and potentiates efficacy of oncogene targeting in tumor models. J Clin. Invest. 2020;130(2):699-714.
723. Sharmeen S, Skrtic M, Sukhai MA, Hurren R, Gronda M, Wang X, et al. The antiparasitic agent ivermectin induces chloride-dependent membrane hyperpolarization and cell death in leukemia cells. Blood. 2010;116(18):3593-603.
724. Hu B, Tan H, Yu L, Liao Q, Guo W. Repurposing Ivermectin to augment chemotherapy's efficacy in osteosarcoma. Hum Exp Toxicol. 2022;41:9603271221143693.
725. Draganov D, Han Z, Rana A, Bennett N, Irvine DJ, Lee PP. Ivermectin converts cold tumors hot and synergizes with immune checkpoint blockade for treatment of breast cancer. npj Beast Cancer. 2021;7:22.
726. de Castro CG, Gregianin LJ, Burger JA. Continuous high-dose ivermectin appears to be safe in patients with acute myelogenous leukemia and could inform clinical repurposing for COVID-19 infection. Leuk. Lymphoma. 2020;61:2536-7.
727. Ishiguro T, Ishiguro RH, Ishiguro M, Toki A, Terunuma H. Synergistic Anti-tumor Effect of Dichloroacetate and Ivermectin. Cureus. 2022;14(2):e21884.
728. Pantziarka P, Bouche G, Meheus L, Sukhatme V, Sukhatme VP. Repurposing drugs in oncology (ReDO) - mebendazole as an anti-cancer agent. ecancer. 2014;8:443.
729. Guerini AE, Triggiani L, Maddalo M, Bonu ML, Frassine F, Baiguini A, et al. Mebendazole as a candidate for drug repurposing in oncology: An extensive review of current literature. Cancers. 2019;11:1284.
730. Meco D, Attina G, Mastrangelo S, Navarra P, Ruggiero A. Emerging perspectives on the antiparasitic Mebendazole as a repurposed drug for the treatment of brain cancers. Int. J. Mol. Sci. 2023;24:1334.
731. Nygren P, Larsson R. Drug repositioning from bench to bedside: tumour remission by the antihelmintic drug mebendazole in refractory metastatic colon cancer. Acta Oncol. 2014;53(3):427-8.
732. Dobrosotskaya IY, Hammer GD, Schteingart DE, Maturen KE, Worden FP. Mebendazole monotherapy and long-term disease control in metastatic adrenocortical carcinoma. Endocr. Pract. 2011;17(3):e59-e62.
733. Chiang RS, Syed AB, Wright JL, Montgomery B, Srinivas S. Fenbendazole enhancing anti-tumor effect: A case series. Clin. Oncol. Case Rep. 2021;4:2.

734. Sasaki JI, Ramesh R, Chada S, Gomyo Y, Roth JA, Mukhopadhyay T. The anthelmintic drug mebendazole induces mitotic arrest and apoptosis by depolymerizing tubulin in non-small cell lung cancer cells. Molecular Cancer Therapeutics. 2002;2:1201-9.
735. Bai RY, Staedtke V, Rudin CM, Bunz F, Figgins GJ. Effective treatment of diverse medulloblastoma models with mebendazole and its impact on tumor angiogenesis. Neuro-Oncology. 2015;17:545-54.
736. Doudican NA, Byron AA, Pollock PM, Orlow SJ. XIAP downregulation accompanies mebendazole growth inhibition in melanoma xenografts. Anti-Cancer Drugs. 2013;24:181-8.
737. Simbulan-Rosenthal CM, DDakshanamurthy S, Gaur A, Chen YS, Fang HB, Abdussamad M, et al. The repurposed anthelmintic mebendazole in combination with trametinib suppresses refractory $NRAS^{Q61k}$ melanoma. Oncotarget. 2017;8:12576-95.
738. Walk-Vorderwulbecke V, Pearce K, Brooks T, Hubank M, Zwaan cM, Edwards AD, et al. Targeting acute myeloid leukemia by drug-induced c-MYB degradation. Leukemia. 2018;32:882-9.
739. Tan Z, Chen L, Zhang S. Comprehensive modeling and discovery of mebendazole as a novel TRAF2- and NCK-interacting kinase inhibitor. Scientific Reports. 2016;6:33534.
740. Pinto LC, Soares BM, de Jusus Viana Pinheiro J, Riggins GJ, Assumpcao PP, Burbano RM, et al. The anthelmintic drug mebendazole inhibits growth, migration and invasion in gastric cancer cell model. Toxicology in Vitro. 2015;29:2038-44.
741. Pinto LC, de Fatima Aquino Moreira-Nunes C, Soares BM, Rodriguez Burbano RM, de Lemos JA, Montenegro R. Mebendazole, an antiparasitic drug, inhibits drug transporters expression in preclinical model of gastric peritoneal carcinomatosis. Toxicology in Vitro. 2017;43:87-91.
742. Nygren P, Fryknas M, Agerup B, Larsson R. Repositioning of the anthelmintic drug mebendazole for the treatment for colon cancer. J. Cancer res. Clin. Oncol. 2013;139:2133-40.
743. Gallia GL, Holdhoff M, Brem H, Joshi AD, Hann CL, Bai RY, et al. Mebendazole and temozolomide in patients with newly diagnosed high-grade gliomas: results of a phase 1 clinical trial. Neuro-Oncology Advances. 2021;3:1-8.
744. Caccamo AE, Scaltriti M, Caporali A, D'Arca D, Scorcioni F, Astancolle S, et al. Cell detachment and apoptosis induction of immortalized prostate epithelial cells are associated with early accumulation of a 45 kDa nuclear isoform of clusterin. Biochem. J. 2004;382:157-68.
745. Scaltriti M, Santamaria A, Paciucci R, Bettuzzi S. Intracellular clusterin induces G2-M phase arrest and cell death in PC-3 prostate cancer cells. Cancer Research. 2004;64:6174-82.
746. Liao S, Umekita Y, Guo J, Kokontis JM, Hiipakka RA. Growth inhibition and regression of human prostate and breast tumors in athymic mice by tea epigallocatechin gallate. Cancer Letters. 1995;96:239-43.
747. El-Nashar HA, Aly SH, Ahmadi A, El-Shazly M. The impact of polyphenolics in the management of breast cancer: Mechanistic aspects and recent patents. Recent Patents on Anti-Cancer Drug Discovery. 2022;17:358-79.
748. Kubatka P, Mazurakova A, Samec M, Koklesova L, Zhai K, Kajo K, et al. Flavonoids against non-physiologic inflammation attributed to cancer initiation, development, and progression - 3PM pathways. EPMA Journal. 2021;12:559-87.
749. Katiyar S, Mukhtar H. Tea in chemoprevention. International Journal of Oncology. 1996;8:221-38.
750. Maechler P, Wollheim CB. Mitochondrial glutamate acts as a messenger in glucose-induced insulin exocytosis. Nature. 1999;402:685-9.
751. Rashidi B, Malekzadeh M, Goodarzi M, Masoudifar A, Mirzaei H. Green tea and its anti-angiogenesis effects. Biomed Pharmacother. 2017;89:949-56.

752. Lin CH, Shen YA, Hung PH, Yu YB, Chen YJ. Epigallocathechin gallate, polyphenol present in green tea, inhibits stem-like characteristics and epithelial-mesenchymal transition in nasopharyngeal cancer cell lines. BMC Complement Altern Med. 2012;12:201.
753. Bonuccelli G, Sotgia F, Lisanti MP. Matcha green tea (MGT) inhibits the propagation of cancer stem cells (CSCs), by targeting mitochondrial metabolism, glycolysis and multiple cell signalling pathways. Aging (Albany NY). 2018;10(8):1867-83.
754. Yoon JW, Lee JS, Kim BM, Ahn J, Yang KM. Catechin-7-O-xyloside induces apoptosis via endoplasmic reticulum stress and mitochondrial dysfunction in human non-small cell lung carcinoma H1299 cells. Oncology Reports. 2014;31:314-20.
755. Sun H, Yin M, Hao D, Shen Y. Anti-cancer activity of catechin against A549 lung carcinoma cells by inducion of cyclin kinase inhibitor p21 and suppression of cyclin E1 and p-AKT. Appl. Sci. 2020;10:2065.
756. Song Q, Zhang G, Wang B, Cao G, Li D, Wang Y, et al. Reinforcing the combinational immuno-oncotherapy of switching "cold" tumor to "hot" by responsive penetrating nanogels. ACS Appl. Mater. Interface. 2021;13:36824-38.
757. Menon DR, Li Y, Yamauchi T, Osborne DG, Vaddi PK, wempe MF, et al. EGCG inhibits tumor growth in melanoma by targeting JAK-STAT signaling andits downstream PD-L1/PD-L2-PD1 axis in tumors and enhancing cytotoxic T-cell responses. Pharmaceuticals. 2021;14:1081.
758. McCarty MF, Iloki-Assanga S, Lujany LML. Nutraceutical targeting of TLR4 signaling has potential for prevention of cancer cachexia. Med Hypotheses. 2019;132:109326.
759. Mukherjee S, Hussaini R, White R, Atwi D, Fried A, Sampat S, et al. TriCurin, a synergistic formulation of curcumin, resveratrol, and epicatechin gallate, repolarizes tumor-associated macrophages and triggers an immune response to casue suppression of HPV+ tumors. Cancer Immunology Immunotherapy. 2018;67:761-74.
760. Xu P, Yan F, Zhao Y, Chen X, Sun S, Wang Y, et al. Green tea polyphenol EGCG attenuates MDSCs-mediated immunosuppresion through canonical and non-canoical pathways in a 4T1 murine breast cancer model. Nutrients. 2020;12:1042.
761. Shanafelt TD, Lee YK, Call TG, Nowakowski GS, Dingli D, Zent CS, et al. Clinical effects of oral green tea extracts in four patients with low grade B-cell malignancies. Leuk Res. 2006;30(6):707-12.
762. Michael A, Hedayati B, Dalgleish AG. Disease regression in malignant melanoma: spontaneous resolution or a result of treatment with antioxidants, green tea, and pineapple cores? A case report. Integr Cancer Ther. 2007;6(1):77-9.
763. Lemanne D, Block KI, Kressel BR, Sukhatme VP, White JD. A Case of Complete and Durable Molecular Remission of Chronic Lymphocytic Leukemia Following Treatment with Epigallocatechin-3-gallate, an Extract of Green Tea. Cureus. 2015;7(12):e441.
764. Shanafelt TD, Call TG, Zent CS, LaPlant B, Bowen DA, Roos M, et al. Phase I trial of daily oral Polyphenon E in patients with asymptomatic Rai stage 0 to II chronic lymphocytic leukemia. J Clin Oncol. 2009;27(23):3808-14.
765. Rogovskii VS, Popov SV, Sturov NV, Shimanovski NL. The possibility of preventive and therapeutic use of green tea catechins in prostate cancer. Anti-Cancer Agents in Medicinal Chemistry. 2019;19:1223-31.
766. Mazzanti G, Di Sotto A, Vitalone A. Hepatotoxicity of green tea: an update. Arch. Toxicol. 2015;89:1175-91.
767. Nabavi SF, Bilotto S, Russo GL, Orhan IE, Habtemariam S, Daglia M, et al. Omega-3 polyunsaturated fatty acids and cancer: lessons learned from clinical trials. Cancer Metastasis Rev. 2015;34(3):359-80.

768. Cockbain AJ, Toogood GJ, Hull MA. Omega-3 polyunsaturated fatty acids for the treatment and prevention of colorectal cancer. Gut. 2012;61(1):135-49.
769. Fabian CJ, Kimler BF, Hursting SD. Omega-3 fatty acids for breast cancer prevention and survivorship. Breast Cancer Res. 2015;17(1):62.
770. Xue M, Wang Q, Zhao J, Dong L, Ge Y, Hou L, et al. Docosahexaenoic acid inhibited the Wnt/β-catenin pathway and suppressed breast cancer cells in vitro and in vivo. J Nutr Biochem. 2014;25(2):104-10.
771. Corsetto PA, Montorfano G, Zava S, Jovenitti IE, Cremona A, Berra B, et al. Effects of n-3 PUFAs on breast cancer cells through their incorporation in plasma membrane. Lipids Health Dis. 2011;10:73.
772. Vasudevan A, Yu Y, Banerjee S, Woods J, Farhana L, Rajendra SG, et al. Omega-3 fatty acid is a potential preventive agent for recurrent colon cancer. Cancer Prev Res (Phila). 2014;7(11):1138-48.
773. De Carlo F, Witte TR, Hardman WE, Claudio PP. Omega-3 eicosapentaenoic acid decreases CD133 colon cancer stem-like cell marker expression while increasing sensitivity to chemotherapy. PLoS One. 2013;8(7):e69760.
774. Brasky TM, Lampe JW, Potter JD, Patterson RE, White E. Specialty supplements and breast cancer risk in the VITamins And Lifestyle (VITAL) Cohort. Cancer Epidemiol Biomarkers Prev. 2010;19(7):1696-708.
775. Zheng JS, Hu XJ, Zhao YM, Yang J, Li D. Intake of fish and marine n-3 polyunsaturated fatty acids and risk of breast cancer: meta-analysis of data from 21 independent prospective cohort studies. Bmj. 2013;346:f3706.
776. Kim S, Sandler DP, Galanko J, Martin C, Sandler RS. Intake of polyunsaturated fatty acids and distal large bowel cancer risk in whites and African Americans. Am J Epidemiol. 2010;171(9):969-79.
777. Pot GK, Geelen A, van Heijningen EM, Siezen CL, van Kranen HJ, Kampman E. Opposing associations of serum n-3 and n-6 polyunsaturated fatty acids with colorectal adenoma risk: an endoscopy-based case-control study. Int J Cancer. 2008;123(8):1974-7.
778. Yang B, Ren XL, Fu YQ, Gao JL, Li D. Ratio of n-3/n-6 PUFAs and risk of breast cancer: a meta-analysis of 274135 adult females from 11 independent prospective studies. BMC Cancer. 2014;14:105.
779. West NJ, Clark SK, Phillips RK, Hutchinson JM, Leicester RJ, Belluzzi A, et al. Eicosapentaenoic acid reduces rectal polyp number and size in familial adenomatous polyposis. Gut. 2010;59(7):918-25.
780. Bougnoux P, Hajjaji N, Ferrasson MN, Giraudeau B, Couet C, Le Floch O. Improving outcome of chemotherapy of metastatic breast cancer by docosahexaenoic acid: a phase II trial. Br J Cancer. 2009;101(12):1978-85.
781. Murphy RA, Mourtzakis M, Chu QS, Baracos VE, Reiman T, Mazurak VC. Supplementation with fish oil increases first-line chemotherapy efficacy in patients with advanced nonsmall cell lung cancer. Cancer. 2011;117(16):3774-80.
782. Patterson RE, Flatt SW, Newman VA, Natarajan L, Rock CL, Thomson CA, et al. Marine fatty acid intake is associated with breast cancer prognosis. J Nutr. 2011;141(2):201-6.
783. Aucoin M, Cooley K, Knee C, Fritz H, Balneaves LG, Breau R, et al. Fish-Derived Omega-3 Fatty Acids and Prostate Cancer: A Systematic Review. Integr Cancer Ther. 2017;16(1):32-62.
784. Chagas TR, Borges DS, de Oliveira PF, Mocellin MC, Barbosa AM, Camargo CQ, et al. Oral fish oil positively influences nutritional-inflammatory risk in patients with haematological malignancies during chemotherapy with an impact on long-term survival: a randomised clinical trial. J Hum Nutr Diet. 2017;30(6):681-92.

785. Jin X, Xu XT, Tian MX, Dai Z. Omega-3 polyunsaterated fatty acids improve quality of life and survival, but not body weight in cancer cachexia: A systematic review and meta-analysis of controlled trials. Nutr Res. 2022;107:165-78.
786. Xiong RG, Huang SY, Wu SX, Zhou DD, Yang ZJ, Saimaiti A, et al. Anticancer effects and mechanisms of berberine from medicinal herbs: An update review. Molecules. 2022;27:4523.
787. Yao M, Fan X, Yuan B, Takagi N, Liu S, Han X, et al. Berberine inhibits NLRP3 inflammasone pathway in human triple-negative breast cancer MDA-MB-231 cell. BMC Complementary and Alternative Medicine. 2019;19:216.
788. Pan Y, Zhang F, Zhao Y, Shao D, Zheng X, Chen Y, et al. Berberine enhances chemosensitivity and induces apoptosis through dose-orchestrated AMPK signaling in breast cancer. J. Cancer. 2017;8:1679-89.
789. Shu X, Li M, Cao Y, Li C, Zhou W, Ji G, et al. Berberine alleviates non-alcoholic steatohepatitis through modulating gut microbiota mediated intestinal FXR activation. Front. Pharmacol. 2021;12:750826.
790. Li S, Wang N, Tan HY, Chueng F, Zhang ZJ, Yuen MF, et al. Modulation of gut microbiota mediates berberine-induced expansion of immuno-suppressive cells to against alcoholic liver disease. Clinical and Translational Medicine. 2020;10:e112.
791. Zhu C, Li J, Hua Y, Wang J, Wang K, Sun J. Berberine inhibits the expression of SCT through miR-214-3p stimulation in breast cancer cells. Evidence-Based Complementary and Alternative Medicine. 2020;2020:2817147.
792. Ruan H, Zhan YY, Hou J, Xu B, Chen B, Tian Y, et al. Berberine binds RXRalpha to suppress Beta-catenin signaling in colon cancer cells. Oncogene. 2017;36:6906-18.
793. Samad MA, Saiman MZ, Majid NA, Karsani SA, Yaacob JS. Berberine inhibits telomerase activity and induces cell cycle arrest and telomere erosion in colorectal cancer cell line, HCT 116. Molecules. 2021;26:376.
794. Zhao Z, Zeng J, Guo Q, Pu K, Yang Y, Chen N, et al. Berberine suppresses stemness and tumorigenicity of colorectal cancer stem-like cells by inhibiting m6 A methylation. Front. Oncol. 2021;11:775418.
795. Chen QQ, Shi JM, Ding Z, Xia Q, Zheng TS, Ren YB, et al. Berberine induces apoptosis in non-small-cell lung cancer cells by upregulating miR-19a targeting tissue factor. Cancer Management and Research. 2019;11:9005-15.
796. Kou Y, Tong B, Wu W, Liao X, Zhao M. Berberine improves chemo-sensitivity to cisplatin by enhancing cell apoptosis and repressing PI3K/AKT/mTOR signaling pathway in gastric cancer. Front. Pharmacol. 2020;11:616251.
797. Dai W, Mu L, Cui Y, Li Y, Chen P, Xie H, et al. Berberine promotes apoptosis of colorectal cancer via regulation of the long non-coding RNA (lncRNA) cancer susceptibility candidate 2 (CASC2)/AU-biding factor 1 (AUF1)/Bcell CLL/Lymphoma 2 (Bcl-2) axis. Med. Sci. Monit. 2019;25:730-8.
798. Jeong Y, You D, Kang HG, Yu J, Kim SW, Nam SJ, et al. Berberine suppresses fibronectin expression through inhibition of c-jun phosphorylation in breast cancer cells. J. Breast Cancer. 2018;21:21-7.
799. Chu SC, Yu CC, Hsu LS, Chen KS, Su MY, Chen PN. Berberine reverses epithelial-to-mesenchymal transition and inhibits metastasis and tumor-induced angiogenesis in human cervical cancer cells. Mol. Pharmacol. 2014;86:609-23.
800. Liu CH, Tang WC, Sia P, Huang CC, Yang PM, Wu MH, et al. Berberine inhibits the metastatic ability of prostate cancer cells by suppressing epithelial-to-mesechchymal transition (EMT) associated genes with predictive and prognostic relevance. Int. J. Med. Sci. 2015;12:63-71.

801. Chen Y, Zhang H. Berberine and chemotherapeutic drugs synergistically inhibits cell proliferaion and migration of breast cancer cells. Int. J. Clin. Exp. Med. 2018;11:13243-50.
802. Zhao Y, Jing Z, Li Y, Mao W. Berberine in combination with cisplatin suppresses breast cancer cell growth through induction of DNA breaks and caspase-3-dependent apoptosis. Oncology Reports. 2016;36:567-72.
803. Chen P, Dai CH, Shi ZH, Wang Y, Wu JN, Chen K, et al. Synergistic inhibitory effect of berberine and icotinib on non-small cell lung cancer cells via inducing autophagic cell death and apoptosis. Apoptosis. 2021;26:639-56.
804. You HY, Xie XM, Zhang WJ, Zhu HL, Jiang FZ. Berberine modulates cisplatin sensitivity of human gastric cancer cells by upregulation of miR-203. In Vitro Cellular & Developmental Biology - Animal. 2016;52:857-63.
805. Chen YX, Gao QY, Zou TH, Wang BM, Liu SD, Sheng JQ, et al. Berberine versus placebo for the prevention of recurrence of colorectal adenoma: a multicentre, double-blinded, randomised controlled study. Lancet Gastroenterol. Hepatol. 2020;5(3):267-75.
806. Zhang Q, Wang X, Cao S, Sun Y, He X, Jiang B, et al. Berberine represses human gastric cancer cell growth in vitro and in vivo by inducing cytostatic autophagy via inhibition of MAPK/mTOR/p70S6K and Akt signaling pathways. Biomedicine and Pharmacotherapy. 2020;128:110245.
807. Parrales A, Thoenen E, Iwakuma T. The interplay between mutant p53 and the mevalonate pathway. Cell Death & Differentiation. 2017;25:460-70.
808. Cruz PM, Mo H, McConathy WJ, Sabnis N, Lacko AG. The role of cholestrol metabolism and cholestrol transport in carcinogenesis: a review of scientific findings, relevant to future cancer therapeutics. Front. Pharmacol. 2013;4:119.
809. Borgquist S, Bjarnadottir O, Kimbung S, Ahern TP. Statins: a role in breast cancer therapy? J. Intern. Med. 2018;284:346-57.
810. Farwell WR, D'Avolio LW, Scranton RE, Lawler EV, Gaziano JM. Statins and prostate cancer diagnosis and grade in a veterans population. J Natl. Cancer Inst. 2011;103(11):885-92.
811. Nelson JE, Harris RE. Inverse association of prostate cancer and non-steroidal anti-inflammatory drugs (NSAIDs): results of a case-control study. Oncol. Rep. 2000;7(1):169-70.
812. Nielsen SF, Nordestgaard BG, Bojesen SE. Statin use and reduced cancer-related mortality. N. Engl. J Med. 2012;367(19):1792-802.
813. Zhong S, Zhang X, Chen L, Ma T, Tang J, Zhao J. Statin use and mortality in cancer patients: Systematic review and meta-analysis of observational studies. Cancer Treat. Rev. 2015;41(6):554-67.
814. Yu O, Eberg M, Benayoun S, Aprikian A, Batist G, Suissa S, et al. Use of statins and the risk of death in patients with prostate cancer. J Clin. Oncol. 2014;32(1):5-11.
815. Manthravadi S, Shrestha A, Madhusudhana S. Impact of statin use on cancer recurrence and mortality in breast cancer: A systematic review and meta-analysis. Int. J Cancer. 2016;139(6):1281-8.
816. Ahern TP, Pedersen L, Tarp M, Cronin-Fenton DP, Garne JP, Silliman RA, et al. Statin prescriptions and breast cancer recurrence risk: a Danish nationwide prospective cohort study. J Natl. Cancer Inst. 2011;103(19):1461-8.
817. Lash TL, Riis AH, Ostenfeld EB, Erichsen R, Vyberg M, Ahern TP, et al. Associations of Statin Use With Colorectal Cancer Recurrence and Mortality in a Danish Cohort. Am. J Epidemiol. 2017;186(6):679-87.
818. Shao JY, Lee FP, Chang CL, Wu SY. Statin-Based Palliative Therapy for Hepatocellular Carcinoma. Medicine (Baltimore). 2015;94(42):e1801.

819. Gray RT, Coleman HG, Hughes C, Murray LJ, Cardwell CR. Statin use and survival in colorectal cancer: Results from a population-based cohort study and an updated systematic review and meta-analysis. Cancer Epidemiol. 2016;45:71-81.

820. Lin JJ, Ezer N, Sigel K, Mhango G, Wisnivesky JP. The effect of statins on survival in patients with stage IV lung cancer. Lung Cancer. 2016;99:137-42.

821. Li L, Cui N, Hao T, Zou J, Wu J, Yi K, et al. Statins use and the prognosis of colorectal cancer: a meta-analysis. Clinics and Research in Hepatology and Gastroenterology. 2021;45:101588.

822. Lu C, Li X, Ren Y, Zhang X. Disulfiram: a novel repurposed drug for cancer therapy. Cancer Chemother Pharmacol. 2021;87(2):159-72.

823. Liu P, Kumar IS, Brown S, Kannappan V, Tawari PE, Tang JZ, et al. Disulfiram targets cancer stem-like cells and reverses resistance and cross-resistance in acquired paclitaxel-resistant triple-negative breast cancer cells. Br J Cancer. 2013;109(7):1876-85.

824. Kang X, Jadhav S, Annaji M, Huang CH, Amin R, Shen J, et al. Advancing Cancer Therapy with Copper/Disulfiram Nanomedicines and Drug Delivery Systems. Pharmaceutics. 2023;15(6).

825. Denoyer D, Masaldan S, La Fontaine S, Cater MA. Targeting copper in cancer therapy: 'Copper That Cancer'. Metallomics. 2015;7(11):1459-76.

826. Liu P, Wang Z, Brown S, Kannappan V, Tawari PE, Jiang W, et al. Liposome encapsulated Disulfiram inhibits NFκB pathway and targets breast cancer stem cells in vitro and in vivo. Oncotarget. 2014;5(17):7471-85.

827. Zha J, Chen F, Dong H, Shi P, Yao Y, Zhang Y, et al. Disulfiram targeting lymphoid malignant cell lines via ROS-JNK activation as well as Nrf2 and NF-kB pathway inhibition. J Transl Med. 2014;12:163.

828. Yip NC, Fombon IS, Liu P, Brown S, Kannappan V, Armesilla AL, et al. Disulfiram modulated ROS-MAPK and NFκB pathways and targeted breast cancer cells with cancer stem cell-like properties. Br J Cancer. 2011;104(10):1564-74.

829. Park YM, Go YY, Shin SH, Cho JG, Woo JS, Song JJ. Anti-cancer effects of disulfiram in head and neck squamous cell carcinoma via autophagic cell death. PLoS One. 2018;13(9):e0203069.

830. Triscott J, Lee C, Hu K, Fotovati A, Berns R, Pambid M, et al. Disulfiram, a drug widely used to control alcoholism, suppresses the self-renewal of glioblastoma and over-rides resistance to temozolomide. Oncotarget. 2012;3(10):1112-23.

831. Liu P, Brown S, Goktug T, Channathodiyil P, Kannappan V, Hugnot JP, et al. Cytotoxic effect of disulfiram/copper on human glioblastoma cell lines and ALDH-positive cancer-stem-like cells. Br J Cancer. 2012;107(9):1488-97.

832. Terashima Y, Toda E, Itakura M, Otsuji M, Yoshinaga S, Okumura K, et al. Targeting FROUNT with disulfiram suppresses macrophage accumulation and its tumor-promoting properties. Nat Commun. 2020;11(1):609.

833. Dufour P, Lang JM, Giron C, Duclos B, Haehnel P, Jaeck D, et al. Sodium dithiocarb as adjuvant immunotherapy for high risk breast cancer: a randomized study. Biotherapy. 1993;6(1):9-12.

834. Nechushtan H, Hamamreh Y, Nidal S, Gotfried M, Baron A, Shalev YI, et al. A phase IIb trial assessing the addition of disulfiram to chemotherapy for the treatment of metastatic non-small cell lung cancer. Oncologist. 2015;20(4):366-7.

835. Huang J, Campian JL, Gujar AD, Tran DD, Lockhart AC, DeWees TA, et al. A phase I study to repurpose disulfiram in combination with temozolomide to treat newly diagnosed glioblastoma after chemoradiotherapy. J Neurooncol. 2016;128(2):259-66.

836. Huang J, Campian JL, Gujar AD, Tsien C, Ansstas G, Tran DD, et al. Final results of a phase I dose-escalation, dose-expansion study of adding disulfiram with or without copper to adjuvant temozolomide for newly diagnosed glioblastoma. J Neurooncol. 2018;138(1):105-11.

837. Huang J, Chaudhary R, Cohen AL, Fink K, Goldlust S, Boockvar J, et al. A multicenter phase II study of temozolomide plus disulfiram and copper for recurrent temozolomide-resistant glioblastoma. J Neurooncol. 2019;142(3):537-44.
838. Pantziarka P, Bouche G, Meheus L, Sukhatme S. Repurposing drugs in oncology (ReDO) - cimetidine as an anti-cancer agent. ecancer. 2014;8:485.
839. Aponte-Lopez A, Fuentes-PananÃ¡ EM, Cortes-MuÃ±oz D, Munoz-Cruz S. Mast Cell, the Neglected Member of the Tumor Microenvironment: Role in Breast Cancer. J Immunol. Res. 2018;2018:2584243.
840. Ibrahim SSA, El-Aal SAA, Reda AM, Achy SE, Shahine Y. Anti-neoplastic action of Cimetidine/Vitamin C on histamine and the PI3K/AKT/mTOR pathway in Ehrlich breast cancer. Sci Rep. 2022;12(1):11514.
841. Liu FR, Jiang CG, Li YS, Li JB, Li F. Cimetidine inhibits the adhesion of gastric cancer cells expressing high levels of sialyl Lewis x in human vascular endothelial cells by blocking E-selectin expression. Int. J Mol. Med. 2011;27(4):537-44.
842. Kennedy L, Hodges K, Meng F, Alpini G, Francis H. Histamine and histamine receptor regulation of gastrointestinal cancers. Transl. Gastrointest. Cancer. 2012;1(3):215-27.
843. O'Mahony L, Akdis M, Akdis CA. Regulation of the immune response and inflammation by histamine and histamine receptors. J Allergy Clin. Immunol. 2011;128(6):1153-62.
844. Martin RK, Saleem SJ, Folgosa L, Zellner HB, Damle SR, Nguyen GK, et al. Mast cell histamine promotes the immunoregulatory activity of myeloid-derived suppressor cells. J Leukoc. Biol. 2014;96(1):151-9.
845. Katoh J, Tsuchiya K, Osawa H, Sato W, Matsumura G, Iida Y, et al. Cimetidine reduces impairment of cellular immunity after cardiac operations with cardiopulmonary bypass. J Thorac. Cardiovasc. Surg. 1998;116(2):312-8.
846. TC vdPK, Snijders A, Boeije LC, De Groot ER, Alewijnse AE, Leurs R, et al. Histamine inhibits the production of interleukin-12 through interaction with H2 receptors. J Clin. Invest. 1998;102(10):1866-73.
847. Caron G, Delneste Y, Roelandts E, Duez C, Bonnefoy JY, Pestel J, et al. Histamine polarizes human dendritic cells into Th2 cell-promoting effector dendritic cells. J Immunol. 2001;167(7):3682-6.
848. Elenkov IJ, Webster E, Papanicolaou DA, Fleisher TA, Chrousos GP, Wilder RL. Histamine potently suppresses human IL-12 and stimulates IL-10 production via H2 receptors. J Immunol. 1998;161(5):2586-93.
849. Ghosh AK, Hirasawa N, Ohuchi K. Enhancement by histamine of vascular endothelial growth factor production in granulation tissue via H(2) receptors. Br. J Pharmacol. 2001;134(7):1419-28.
850. Chihara Y, Fujimoto K, Miyake M, Hiasa Y, Hirao Y. Anti-tumor effect of cimetidine via inhibiting angiogenesis factors in N-butyl-N-(4-hydroxybutyl) nitrosamine-induced mouse and rat bladder carcinogenesis. Oncol. Rep. 2009;22(1):23-8.
851. Deva S, Jameson M. Histamine type 2 receptor antagonists as adjuvant treatment for resected colorectal cancer. Cochrane Database Syst. Rev. 2012(8):CD007814.
852. Borgstrom S, von Eyben FE, Flodgren P, Axelsson B, Sjogren HO. Human leukocyte interferon and cimetidine for metastatic melanoma. N. Engl. J Med. 1982;307(17):1080-1.
853. Flodgren P, Borgstrom S, Jonsson PE, Lindstrom C, Sjogren HO. Metastatic malignant melanoma: regression induced by combined treatment with interferon [HuIFN-alpha(Le)] and cimetidine. Int. J Cancer. 1983;32(6):657-65.
854. Tonnesen H, Knigge U, Bulow S, Damm P, Fischerman K, Hesselfeldt P, et al. Effect of cimetidine on survival after gastric cancer. Lancet. 1988;2(8618):990-2.

855. Matsumoto S, Imaeda Y, Umemoto S, Kobayashi K, Suzuki H, Okamoto T. Cimetidine increases survival of colorectal cancer patients with high levels of sialyl Lewis-X and sialyl Lewis-A epitope expression on tumour cells. Br. J Cancer. 2002;86(2):161-7.
856. Adams WJ, Lawson JA, Morris DL. Cimetidine inhibits in vivo growth of human colon cancer and reverses histamine stimulated in vitro and in vivo growth. Gut. 1994;35(11):1632-6.
857. Kubota T, Fujiwara H, Ueda Y, Itoh T, Yamashita T, Yoshimura T, et al. Cimetidine modulates the antigen presenting capacity of dendritic cells from colorectal cancer patients. Br. J Cancer. 2002;86(8):1257-61.
858. Sarasola MP, TÃ¡quez Delgado MA, Nicoud MB, Medina VA. Histamine in cancer immunology and immunotherapy. Current status and new perspectives. Pharmacol. Res Perspect. 2021;9(5):e00778.
859. Breuer S, Maimon O, Appelbaum L, Peretz T, Hubert A. TL-118-anti-angiogenic treatment in pancreatic cancer: a case report. Med Oncol. 2013;30(2):585.
860. Niwa K, Onogi K, Wu Y, Mori H, Inoue Y, Tamaya T. Prognostic implications of cimetidine on advanced serous ovarian carcinoma related to cyclooxygenase-2 expression. Mol. Med Rep. 2008;1(1):119-22.
861. Fukuda M, Kusama K, Sakashita H. Cimetidine inhibits salivary gland tumor cell adhesion to neural cells and induces apoptosis by blocking NCAM expression. BMC Cancer. 2008;8:376.
862. Kinouchi T, Saiki S, Maeda O, Kuroda M, Usami M, Kotake T. Treatment of advanced renal cell carcinoma with a combination of human lymphoblastoid interfereon-alpha and cimetidine. J. Urol. 1997;157:1604-7.
863. Tatokoro M, Fujii Y, Kawakami S, Saito K, Koga F, Matsuoka Y, et al. Phase-II trial of combination treatment of interferon-alpha, cimetidine, cyclooxygenase-2 inhibitor and renin-angiotensin-system inhibitor (I-CCA therapy) for advanced renal cell carcinoma. Cancer Sci. 2011;102(1):137-43.
864. Bobek V, Boubelik M, KovarÃ-k J, Taltynov O. Inhibition of adhesion breast cancer cells by anticoagulant drugs and cimetidine. Neoplasma. 2003;50(2):148-51.
865. Lefranc F, James S, Camby I, Gaussin JF, Darro F, Brotchi J, et al. Combined cimetidine and temozolomide, compared with temozolomide alone: significant increases in survival in nude mice bearing U373 human glioblastoma multiforme orthotopic xenografts. J Neurosurg. 2005;102(4):706-14.
866. Thronicke A, Schad F, Debus M, Grabowski J, Soldner G. Viscum album L. Therapy in Oncology: An Update on Current Evidence. Complement Med Res. 2022;29(4):362-8.
867. Loef M, Walach H. Quality of life in cancer patients treated with mistletoe: a systematic review and meta-analysis. BMC Complement Med Ther. 2020;20(1):227.
868. Huber R, Rostock M, Goedl R, Lüdtke R, Urech K, Buck S, et al. Mistletoe treatment induces GM-CSF- and IL-5 production by PBMC and increases blood granulocyte- and eosinophil counts: a placebo controlled randomized study in healthy subjects. Eur J Med Res. 2005;10(10):411-8.
869. Oei SL, Thronicke A, Schad F. Mistletoe and Immunomodulation: Insights and Implications for Anticancer Therapies. Evid Based Complement Alternat Med. 2019;2019:5893017.
870. Harmsma M, Grommé M, Ummelen M, Dignef W, Tusenius KJ, Ramaekers FC. Differential effects of Viscum album extract IscadorQu on cell cycle progression and apoptosis in cancer cells. Int J Oncol. 2004;25(6):1521-9.
871. Kwon YS, Chun SY, Kim MK, Nan HY, Lee C, Kim S. Mistletoe Extract Targets the STAT3-FOXM1 Pathway to Induce Apoptosis and Inhibits Metastasis in Breast Cancer Cells. Am J Chin Med. 2021;49(2):487-504.

872. Ben-Arye E, Lavie O, Samuels N, Khamaisie H, Schiff E, Raz OG, et al. Safety of herbal medicine use during chemotherapy in patients with ovarian cancer: a "bedside-to-bench" approach. Med Oncol. 2017;34(4):54.
873. Horneber MA, Bueschel G, Huber R, Linde K, Rostock M. Mistletoe therapy in oncology. Cochrane Database Syst Rev. 2008;2008(2):Cd003297.
874. Kienle GS, Kiene H. Review article: Influence of Viscum album L (European mistletoe) extracts on quality of life in cancer patients: a systematic review of controlled clinical studies. Integr Cancer Ther. 2010;9(2):142-57.
875. Loef M, Walach H. Survival of Cancer Patients Treated with Non-Fermented Mistletoe Extract: A Systematic Review and Meta-Analysis. Integr Cancer Ther. 2022;21:15347354221133561.
876. Pelzer F, Loef M, Martin DD, Baumgartner S. Cancer-related fatigue in patients treated with mistletoe extracts: a systematic review and meta-analysis. Support Care Cancer. 2022;30(8):6405-18.
877. Paller CJ, Wang L, Fu W, Kumar R, Durham JN, Azad NS, et al. Phase I Trial of Intravenous Mistletoe Extract in Advanced Cancer. Cancer Res Commun. 2023;3(2):338-46.
878. Kienle GS, Mussler M, Fuchs D, Kiene H. Intravenous Mistletoe Treatment in Integrative Cancer Care: A Qualitative Study Exploring the Procedures, Concepts, and Observations of Expert Doctors. Evid Based Complement Alternat Med. 2016;2016:4628287.
879. Dutta R, Khalil R, Green R, Mohapatra SS, Mohapatra S. Withania Somnifera (Ashwagandha) and Withaferin A: Potential in Integrative Oncology. Int J Mol Sci. 2019;20(21).
880. Mikulska P, Malinowska M, Ignacyk M, Szustowski P, Nowak J, Pesta K, et al. Ashwagandha (Withania somnifera)-Current Research on the Health-Promoting Activities: A Narrative Review. Pharmaceutics. 2023;15(4).
881. Nagy Z, Cheung BB, Tsang W, Tan O, Herath M, Ciampa OC, et al. Withaferin A activates TRIM16 for its anti-cancer activity in melanoma. Sci Rep. 2020;10(1):19724.
882. Jawarneh S, Talib WH. Combination of Ashwagandha Water Extract and Intermittent Fasting as a Therapy to Overcome Cisplatin Resistance in Breast Cancer: An in vitro and in vivo Study. Front Nutr. 2022;9:863619.
883. Tang Q, Ren L, Liu J, Li W, Zheng X, Wang J, et al. Withaferin A triggers G2/M arrest and intrinsic apoptosis in glioblastoma cells via ATF4-ATF3-CHOP axis. Cell Prolif. 2020;53(1):e12706.
884. Lee HE, Shin JA, Jeong JH, Jeon JG, Lee MH, Cho SD. Anticancer activity of Ashwagandha against human head and neck cancer cell lines. J Oral Pathol Med. 2016;45(3):193-201.
885. Widodo N, Priyandoko D, Shah N, Wadhwa R, Kaul SC. Selective killing of cancer cells by Ashwagandha leaf extract and its component Withanone involves ROS signaling. PLoS One. 2010;5(10):e13536.
886. Choi BY, Kim BW. Withaferin-A Inhibits Colon Cancer Cell Growth by Blocking STAT3 Transcriptional Activity. J Cancer Prev. 2015;20(3):185-92.
887. Sikandan A, Shinomiya T, Nagahara Y. Ashwagandha root extract exerts anti-inflammatory effects in HaCaT cells by inhibiting the MAPK/NF-κB pathways and by regulating cytokines. Int J Mol Med. 2018;42(1):425-34.
888. Chen L, Liu Y, Becher A, Diepold K, Schmid E, Fehn A, et al. Sildenafil triggers tumor lethality through altered expression of HSP90 and degradation of PKD2. Carcinogenesis. 2020;41(10):1421-31.
889. Chhonker SK, Rawat D, Koiri RK. Repurposing PDE5 inhibitor tadalafil and sildenafil as anticancer agent against hepatocellular carcinoma via targeting key events of glucose metabolism and multidrug resistance. J Biochem. Mol. Toxicol. 2022;36(8):e23100.
890. Islam BN, Sharman SK, Hou Y, Bridges AE, Singh N, Kim S, et al. Sildenafil Suppresses Inflammation-Driven Colorectal Cancer in Mice. Cancer Prev. Res (Phila). 2017;10(7):377-88.

891. Booth L, Roberts JL, Cruickshanks N, Conley A, Durrant DE, Das A, et al. Phosphodiesterase 5 inhibitors enhance chemotherapy killing in gastrointestinal/genitourinary cancer cells. Mol. Pharmacol. 2014;85(3):408-19.
892. Booth L, Roberts JL, Cruickshanks N, Tavallai S, Webb T, Samuel P, et al. PDE5 inhibitors enhance celecoxib killing in multiple tumor types. J Cell Physiol. 2015;230(5):1115-27.
893. Domvri K, Zarogoulidis K, Zogas N, Zarogoulidis P, Petanidis S, Porpodis K, et al. Potential synergistic effect of phosphodiesterase inhibitors with chemotherapy in lung cancer. J Cancer. 2017;8(18):3648-56.
894. Dent P, Booth L, Roberts JL, Poklepovic A, Hancock JF. (Curcumin+sildenafil) enhances the efficacy of 5FU and anti-PD1 therapies in vivo. J Cell Physiol. 2020;235(10):6862-74.
895. Tai LH, Alkayyal AA, Leslie AL, Sahi S, Bennett S, Tanese de SC, et al. Phosphodiesterase-5 inhibition reduces postoperative metastatic disease by targeting surgery-induced myeloid derived suppressor cell-dependent inhibition of Natural Killer cell cytotoxicity. Oncoimmunology. 2018;7(6):e1431082.
896. Cruz-Burgos M, Losada-Garcia A, Cruz-Hernandez CD, Cortes-Ramirez SA, Camacho-Arroyo I, Gonzalez-Covarrubias V, et al. New Approaches in Oncology for Repositioning Drugs: The Case of PDE5 Inhibitor Sildenafil. Front Oncol. 2021;11:627229.
897. Serafini P, Meckel K, Kelso M, Noonan K, Califano J, Koch W, et al. Phosphodiesterase-5 inhibition augments endogenous antitumor immunity by reducing myeloid-derived suppressor cell function. J Exp Med. 2006;203(12):2691-702.
898. Klutzny S, Anurin A, Nicke B, Regan JL, Lange M, Schulze L, et al. PDE5 inhibition eliminates cancer stem cells via induction of PKA signaling. Cell Death Dis. 2018;9(2):192.
899. Sutton SS, Magagnoli J, Cummings TH, Hardin JW. The Association Between Phosphodiesterase-5 Inhibitors and Colorectal Cancer in a National Cohort of Patients. Clin. Transl. Gastroenterol. 2020;11(6):e00173.
900. Weed DT, Vella JL, Reis IM, De la Fuente AC, Gomez C, Sargi Z, et al. Tadalafil reduces myeloid-derived suppressor cells and regulatory T cells and promotes tumor immunity in patients with head and neck squamous cell carcinoma. Clin. Cancer Res. 2015;21(1):39-48.
901. Califano JA, Khan Z, Noonan KA, Rudraraju L, Zhang Z, Wang H, et al. Tadalafil augments tumor specific immunity in patients with head and neck squamous cell carcinoma. Clin. Cancer Res. 2015;21(1):30-8.
902. Huang W, Sundquist J, Sundquist K, Ji J. Phosphodiesterase-5 inhibitors use and risk for mortality and metastases among male patients with colorectal cancer. Nat. Commun. 2020;11(1):3191.
903. Danley KT, Tan A, Catalona WJ, Leikin R, Helenowski I, Jovanovic B, et al. The association of phosphodiesterase-5 inhibitors with the biochemical recurrence-free and overall survival of patients with prostate cancer following radical prostatectomy. Urol. Oncol. 2022;40(2):57-.
904. Tsubamoto H, Ueda T, Inoue K, Sakata K, Shibahara H, Sonoda T. Repurposing itraconazole as an anticancer agent. Oncology Letters. 2017;14(2):1240-6.
905. Ali T, Rahman SU, Hao Q, Li W, Liu Z, Ali Shah F, et al. Melatonin prevents neuroinflammation and relieves depression by attenuating autophagy impairment through FOXO3a regulation. J Pineal Res. 2020;69(2):e12667.
906. Pounds R, Leonard S, Dawson C, Kehoe S. Repurposing itraconazole for the treatment of cancer. Oncology Letters. 2017;14(3):2587-97.
907. Kim DJ, Kim J, Spaunhurst K, Montoya J, Khodosh R, Chandra K, et al. Open-Label, Exploratory Phase II Trial of Oral Itraconazole for the Treatment of Basal Cell Carcinoma. Journal of Clinical Oncology. 2014;32(8).

908. Kim J, Tang JY, Gong R, Kim J, Lee JJ, Clemons KV, et al. Itraconazole, a Commonly Used Antifungal that Inhibits Hedgehog Pathway Activity and Cancer Growth. Cancerer Cell. 2010;17:388-99.
909. Wang W, Dong X, Liu Y, Ni B, Sai N, You L, et al. Itraconazole exerts anti-liver cancer potential through the Wnt, PI3K/AKT/mTOR, and ROS pathways. Biomedicine & Pharmacotherapy. 2020;131.
910. Antonarakis ES, Heath EI, Smith DC, Rathkopf D, Blackford AL, Danila DC, et al. Repurposing Itraconazole as a Treatment for Advanced Prostate Cancer: A Noncomparative Randomized Phase II Trial in Men With Metastatic Castration-Resistant Prostate Cancer. Oncologist. 2013;18:163-73.
911. Chen C, Zhang W. Itraconazole Alters the Stem Cell Characteristics of A549 and NCI-H460 Human Lung Cancer Cells by Suppressing Wnt Signaling. Medical Science Monitor. 2019;25:9509-16.
912. Chong CR, Xu J, Lu J, Bhat S, Sullivan DJ, Liu JO. Inhibition of Angiogenesis by the Antigungal Drug Itraconazole. ACS Chem. Biol. 2007;2(4):263-70.
913. Mamtani R, Yang Y-X, Scott FI, Lewis JD, Boursi B. Association of Itraconazole, a Hedgehog Inhibitor, and Bladder Cancer. Journal of Urology. 2016;196(2):343-8.
914. Marastoni S, Madariaga A, Pesic A, Nair SN, Li ZJ, Salev Z, et al. Repurposing Itraconazole and Hydroxychloroquine to Target Lysosomal Homeostasis in Epithelial Ovarian Cancer. cancer Research Communications. 2022;4(2 (5)):293-306.
915. Nacev BA, Grassi P, Dell A, Haslam SM, Liu JO. The Antifungal Drug Itraconazole Inhibits Vascular Endothelial Growth Factor Receptor 2 (VEGFR2) Glycosylation, Trafficking, and Signaling in Endothelial Cells. Journal of Biological Chemistry. 2011;286(51):44045-56.
916. Chen S, Zhuang K, Sun K, Yang Q, Ran X, Xu X, et al. Itraconazole Induces Regression of Infantile Hemangioma via Downregulation of the Platelet-Derived Growth Factor–D/PI3K/Akt/mTOR Pathway. Journal of Investigative Dermatology. 2019;139(7):1574-82.
917. Head SA, Shi WQ, Yang EJ, Nacev BA, Hong SY, Pasunooti KK, et al. Simultaneous Targeting of NPC1 and VDAC1 by Itraconazole Leads to Synergistic Inhibition of mTOR Signaling and Angiogenesis. ACS Chemical Biology. 2017;12(1):174-82.
918. Zhang W, Bhagwath A, Ramzan Z, Williams TA, Subramaniyan I, Edpuganti V, et al. Itraconazole Exerts Its Antitumor Effect in Esophageal Cancer By Suppressing the HER2/AKT Signaling Pathway. Molecular Cancer Therapeutics. 2021;20(101904-1915).
919. Gerber DD, Putnam WC, Fattah FJ, Kernstine KH, Brekken R, A. , Pedrosa I, et al. Concentration-dependent Early Antivascular and Antitumor Effects of Itraconazole in Non-Small Cell Lung Cancer. Clinical Cancer Research. 2021.
920. Hiroshi T, Takashi S, Yamasaki M, Inoue K. Impact of Combination Chemotherapy with Itraconazole on Survival of Patients with Refractory Ovarian Cancer. Anticancer Research. 2014;34(5):2481-7.
921. Lan K, Yan R, Zhu K, Li W, Xu Z, Dang C, et al. Itraconazole inhibits the proliferation of gastric cancer cells in vitro and improves patient survival. Oncology Letters. 2018.
922. Rudin CM, Brahmer JR, Juergens RA, Hann CL, Ettinger DS, Sebree R, et al. Phase 2 Study of Pemetrexed and Itraconazole as Second-Line Therapy for Metastatic Nonsquamous Non–Small-Cell Lung Cancer. Journal of Thoracic Oncology. 2013;8(5):619-23.
923. Shen P-W, Chou Y-M, Li C-L, Liao E-C, Huang H-S, Yin C-H, et al. Itraconazole improves survival outcomes in patients with colon cancer by inducing autophagic cell death and inhibiting transketolase expression. Oncology Letters. 2021;22(5).
924. Tsubamoto H, Sonoda T, Ikuta S, Tani S, Inoue K, Yamanaka K. Combination Chemotherapy with Itraconazole for Treating Metastatic pancreatic Cancer in the Second-line or Additional Setting. Anticancer Research. 2015;35:4191-6.

925. Tsubamoto H, Sonoda T, Inoue K. Impact of Itraconazole on the Survival of Heavily Pre-treated Patients with Triple-Negative Breast Cancer. Anticancer Research. 2014;34:3839-44.
926. Tsubamoto H, Sonoda T, Yamasaki M, Inoue K. Impact of combination chemotherapy with itraconazole on survival for patients with recurrent or persistent ovarian clear cell carcinoma. Anticancer Res. 2014;34(4):2007-14.
927. Tsubamoto H, Sonoda T, Ikuta S, Tani S, Inoue K, Yamanaka N. Impact of Itraconazole After First-line Chemotherapy on Survival of Patients with Metastatic Biliary Tract Cancer. Anticancer Res. 2015;35(9):4923-7.
928. Rinshausen I, Feuerstacke Y, Krainz P, Hollander JD, Hermann K, Buck A, et al. Antifungal Therapy with Itraconazole Impairs the Anti-Lymphoma Effects of Rituximab by Inhibiting Recruitment of CD20 to Cell Surface Lipid Rafts. Caner Research. 2010;70:4292-6.
929. Yang BR, Seong J-M, Choi N-K, Shin J-Y, Lee J, Kim Y-J, et al. Co-Medication of Statins with Contraindicated Drugs. PLOS ONE. 2015;10(5):e0125180.
930. Liu WM, Dalgleish AG. Naltrexone at low doses (LDN) and its relevance to cancer therapy. Expert Rev Anticancer Ther. 2022;22(3):269-74.
931. Zagon IS, McLaughlin PJ. Naltrexone modulates tumor response in mice with neuroblastoma. Science. 1983;221(4611):671-3.
932. Parkitny L, Younger J. Reduced Pro-Inflammatory Cytokines after Eight Weeks of Low-Dose Naltrexone for Fibromyalgia. Biomedicines. 2017;5(2).
933. Cant R, Dalgleish AG, Allen RL. Naltrexone Inhibits IL-6 and TNFα Production in Human Immune Cell Subsets following Stimulation with Ligands for Intracellular Toll-Like Receptors. Front Immunol. 2017;8:809.
934. Meng J, Meng Y, Plotnikoff NP, Youkilis G, Griffin N, Shan F. Low dose naltrexone (LDN) enhances maturation of bone marrow dendritic cells (BMDCs). Int Immunopharmacol. 2013;17(4):1084-9.
935. Lennon FE, Mirzapoiazova T, Mambetsariev B, Salgia R, Moss J, Singleton PA. Overexpression of the μ-opioid receptor in human non-small cell lung cancer promotes Akt and mTOR activation, tumor growth, and metastasis. Anesthesiology. 2012;116(4):857-67.
936. Liu N, Yan L, Shan F, Wang X, Qu N, Handley MK, et al. Low-dose naltrexone plays antineoplastic role in cervical cancer progression through suppressing PI3K/AKT/mTOR pathway. Transl Oncol. 2021;14(4):101028.
937. Tripolt S, Neubauer HA, Knab VM, Elmer DP, Aberger F, Moriggl R, et al. Opioids drive breast cancer metastasis through the δ-opioid receptor and oncogenic STAT3. Neoplasia. 2021;23(2):270-9.
938. Ma M, Wang X, Liu N, Shan F, Feng Y. Low-dose naltrexone inhibits colorectal cancer progression and promotes apoptosis by increasing M1-type macrophages and activating the Bax/Bcl-2/caspase-3/PARP pathway. Int. Immunopharmacol. 2020;83:106388.
939. Couto RD, Fernandes BJD. Low Doses Naltrexone: The Potential Benefit Effects for its Use in Patients with Cancer. Curr. Drug Res Rev. 2021;13(2):86-9.
940. Miskoff JA, Chaudhri M. Low Dose Naltrexone and Lung Cancer: A Case Report and Discussion. Cureus. 2018;10(7):e2924.
941. Berkson BM, Calvo Riera F. The Long-Term Survival of a Patient With Stage IV Renal Cell Carcinoma Following an Integrative Treatment Approach Including the Intravenous α-Lipoic Acid/Low-Dose Naltrexone Protocol. Integr Cancer Ther. 2018;17(3):986-93.
942. Berkson BM, Rubin DM, Berkson AJ. The long-term survival of a patient with pancreatic cancer with metastases to the liver after treatment with the intravenous alpha-lipoic acid/low-dose naltrexone protocol. Integr Cancer Ther. 2006;5(1):83-9.

943. Berkson BM, Rubin DM, Berkson AJ. Reversal of signs and symptoms of a B-cell lymphoma in a patient using only low-dose naltrexone. Integr Cancer Ther. 2007;6(3):293-6.
944. Berkson BM, Rubin DM, Berkson AJ. Revisiting the ALA/N (alpha-lipoic acid/low-dose naltrexone) protocol for people with metastatic and nonmetastatic pancreatic cancer: a report of 3 new cases. Integr Cancer Ther. 2009;8(4):416-22.
945. Khan A. Long-term remission of adenoid cystic tongue carcinoma with low dose naltrexone and vitamin D3--a case report. Oral Health Dent Manag. 2014;13(3):721-4.
946. Lissoni P, Malugani F, Bordin V, Conti A, Maestroni G, Tancini G. A new neuroimmunotherapeutic strategy of subcutaneous low-dose interleukin-2 plus the long-acting opioid antagonist naltrexone in metastatic cancer patients progressing on interleukin-2 alone. Neuro Endocrinol Lett. 2002;23(3):255-8.
947. Rok J, Rzepka Z, Kowalska J, Banach K, Beberok A, Wrzesniok D. The Anticancer Potential of Doxycycline and Minocycline-A Comparative Study on Amelanotic Melanoma Cell Lines. Int. J Mol. Sci. 2022;23(2).
948. Garrido-Mesa N, Zarzuelo A, Galvez J. Minocycline: far beyond an antibiotic. Br. J Pharmacol. 2013;169(2):337-52.
949. Rok J, Rzepka Z, Beberok A, Pawlik J, Wrzesniok D. Cellular and Molecular Aspects of Anti-Melanoma Effect of Minocycline-A Study of Cytotoxicity and Apoptosis on Human Melanotic Melanoma Cells. Int. J Mol. Sci. 2020;21(18).
950. Rok J, Karkoszka M, Rzepka Z, Respondek M, Banach K, Beberok A, et al. Cytotoxic and proapoptotic effect of doxycycline - An in vitro study on the human skin melanoma cells. Toxicol. In Vitro. 2020;65:104790.
951. Weiler J, Dittmar T. Minocycline impairs TNF-a induced cell fusion of M13SV1-Cre cells with MDA-MB-435-pFDR1 cells by suppressing NF-kB transcriptional activity and its induction of target-gene expression of fusion-relevant factors. Cell Commun. Signal. 2019;17(1):71.
952. Lokeshwar BL. Chemically modified non-antimicrobial tetracyclines are multifunctional drugs against advanced cancers. Pharmacol. Res. 2011;63(2):146-50.
953. Niu G, Liao Z, Cai L, Wei R, Sun L. The combined effects of celecoxib and minocycline hydrochloride on inhibiting the osseous metastasis of breast cancer in nude mice. Cancer Biother. Radiopharm. 2008;23(4):469-76.
954. Gilbertson-Beadling S, Powers EA, Stamp-Cole M, Scott PS, Wallace TL, Copeland J, et al. The tetracycline analogs minocycline and doxycycline inhibit angiogenesis in vitro by a non-metalloproteinase-dependent mechanism. Cancer Chemother. Pharmacol. 1995;36(5):418-24.
955. Liu FY, Wu YH, Zhou SJ, Deng YL, Zhang ZY, Zhang EL, et al. Minocycline and cisplatin exert synergistic growth suppression on hepatocellular carcinoma by inducing S phase arrest and apoptosis. Oncol. Rep. 2014;32(2):835-44.
956. Masumori N, Tsukamoto T, Miyao N, Kumamoto Y, Saiki I, Yoneda J. Inhibitory effect of minocycline on in vitro invasion and experimental metastasis of mouse renal adenocarcinoma. J Urol. 1994;151(5):1400-4.
957. Markovic DS, Vinnakota K, van RN, Kiwit J, Synowitz M, Glass R, et al. Minocycline reduces glioma expansion and invasion by attenuating microglial MT1-MMP expression. Brain Behav. Immun. 2011;25(4):624-8.
958. Carlos-Escalante JA, de Jesús-Sánchez M, Rivas-Castro A, Pichardo-Rojas PS, Arce C, Wegman-Ostrosky T. The Use of Antihypertensive Drugs as Coadjuvant Therapy in Cancer. Front Oncol. 2021;11:660943.
959. Shahar OD, Kalousi A, Eini L, Fisher B, Weiss A, Darr J, et al. A high-throughput chemical screen with FDA approved drugs reveals that the antihypertensive drug Spironolactone impairs cancer cell survival by inhibiting homology directed repair. Nucleic Acids Res. 2014;42(9):5689-701.

960. Ueda M, Matsuura K, Kawai H, Wakasugi M, Matsunaga T. Spironolactone-induced XPB degradation depends on CDK7 kinase and SCF(FBXL18) E3 ligase. Genes Cells. 2019;24(4):284-96.
961. Mohammadi Z, Mostakhdem Hashemi M, Saghaeian Jazi M. Spironolactone Induces Apoptotic Cell Death in Human Glioblastoma U87-MG Cancer Cells. International Journal of Cancer Management. 2022;15(10).
962. Chauhan AK, Li P, Sun Y, Wani G, Zhu Q, Wani AA. Spironolactone-induced XPB degradation requires TFIIH integrity and ubiquitin-selective segregase VCP/p97. Cell Cycle. 2021;20(1):81-95.
963. Gabbard RD, Hoopes RR, Kemp MG. Spironolactone and XPB: An Old Drug with a New Molecular Target. Biomolecules. 2020;10(5).
964. Leung W-H, Vong QP, Lin W, Janke L, Chen T, Leung W. Modulation of NKG2D ligand expression and metastasis in tumors by spironolactone via RXRγ activation. Journal of Experimental Medicine. 2013;210(12):2675-92.
965. Vela D, Vela-Gaxha Z. Differential regulation of hepcidin in cancer and non-cancer tissues and its clinical implications. Experimental & Molecular Medicine. 2018;50(2):e436-e.
966. Mleczko-Sanecka K, Da Silva AR, Call D, Neves J, Schmeer N, Damm G, et al. Imatinib and spironolactone suppress hepcidin expression. Haematologica. 2017;102(7):1173-84.
967. Areloegbe SE, Peter MU, Oyeleke MB, Olaniyi KS. Low-dose spironolactone ameliorates adipose tissue inflammation and apoptosis in letrozole-induced PCOS rat model. BMC Endocrine Disorders. 2022;22(1).
968. Sanomachi T, Suzuki S, Togashi K, Sugai A, Seino S, Okada M, et al. Spironolactone, a Classic Potassium-Sparing Diuretic, Reduces Survivin Expression and Chemosensitizes Cancer Cells to Non-DNA-Damaging Anticancer Drugs. Cancers. 2019;11(10):1550.
969. Hiebert BM, Janzen BW, Sanjanwala RM, Ong AD, Feldman RD, Kim JO. Impact of spironolactone exposure on prostate cancer incidence amongst men with heart failure: A Pharmacoepidemiological study. British Journal of Clinical Pharmacology. 2021;87(4):1801-13.
970. Mackenzie IS, Morant SV, Wei L, Thompson AM, Macdonald TM. Spironolactone use and risk of incident cancers: a retrospective, matched cohort study. British Journal of Clinical Pharmacology. 2017;83(3):653-63.
971. Bommareddy K, Hamade H, Lopez-Olivo MA, Wehner M, Tosh T, Barbieri JS. Association of Spironolactone Use With Risk of Cancer: A Systematic Review and Meta-analysis. JAMA Dermatol. 2022;158(3):275-82.
972. Schemiedek P, Sadee W, Baethmann A. Cerebral uptake of a 3H-labelled spirolactone compound in the dog. Eur J Pharmacol. 1973;21.
973. Achterberg C, Astrup A, Bier DM, King JC, Krauss RM, Teicholz N. An analysis of the recent US dietary guidelines process in light of its federal mandate and a National Academies report. PNAS Nexus. 2022;1:1-12.
974. Jazi SMH, Tayebi F, Teimouri-Jervekani Z, Mokarian F, Mehrzad V, Sadeghi A. Comparative Evaluation of Captopril, Spironolactone, and Carvedilol Effect on Endothelial Function in Breast Cancer Women Undergoing Chemotherapy. Adv Biomed Res. 2023;15(12):116.
975. Tome-Carneiro J, Larrosa M, Gonzalez-Sarrias A, Tomas-Barberan FA, Garcia-Conesa MT, Espin JC. Resveratrol and clinical trials: the crossroad from in vitro studies to human evidence. Curr. Pharm Des. 2013;19(34):6064-93.
976. Kundu JK, Surh YJ. Cancer chemopreventive and therapeutic potential of resveratrol: mechanistic perspectives. Cancer Lett. 2008;269(2):243-61.
977. Harikumar KB, Kunnumakkara AB, Sethi G, Diagaradjane P, Anand P, Pandey MK, et al. Resveratrol, a multitargeted agent, can enhance antitumor activity of gemcitabine in vitro and in orthotopic mouse model of human pancreatic cancer. Int. J Cancer. 2010;127(2):257-68.

978. Benitez DA, Pozo-Guisado E, Alvarez-Barrientos A, Fernandez-Salguero PM, Castellon EA. Mechanisms involved in resveratrol-induced apoptosis and cell cycle arrest in prostate cancer-derived cell lines. J Androl. 2007;28(2):282-93.
979. Hsieh TC, Wong C, John BD, Wu JM. Regulation of p53 and cell proliferation by resveratrol and its derivatives in breast cancer cells: an in silico and biochemical approach targeting integrin avB3. Int. J Cancer. 2011;129(11):2732-43.
980. Aziz MH, Nihal M, Fu VX, Jarrard DF, Ahmad N. Resveratrol-caused apoptosis of human prostate carcinoma LNCaP cells is mediated via modulation of phosphatidylinositol 3'-kinase/Akt pathway and Bcl-2 family proteins. Mol. Cancer Ther. 2006;5(5):1335-41.
981. Bhardwaj A, Sethi G, Vadhan-Raj S, Bueso-Ramos C, Takada Y, Gaur U, et al. Resveratrol inhibits proliferation, induces apoptosis, and overcomes chemoresistance through down-regulation of STAT3 and nuclear factor-kappaB-regulated antiapoptotic and cell survival gene products in human multiple myeloma cells. Blood. 2007;109(6):2293-302.
982. Zhang L, Wen X, Li M, Li S, Zhao H. Targeting cancer stem cells and signaling pathways by resveratrol and pterostilbene. Biofactors. 2018;44(1):61-8.
983. Vergara D, Valente CM, Tinelli A, Siciliano C, Lorusso V, Acierno R, et al. Resveratrol inhibits the epidermal growth factor-induced epithelial mesenchymal transition in MCF-7 cells. Cancer Lett. 2011;310(1):1-8.
984. Li K, Dias SJ, Rimando AM, Dhar S, Mizuno CS, Penman AD, et al. Pterostilbene acts through metastasis-associated protein 1 to inhibit tumor growth, progression and metastasis in prostate cancer. PLoS One. 2013;8(3):e57542.
985. Chen RJ, Kuo HC, Cheng LH, Lee YH, Chang WT, Wang BJ, et al. Apoptotic and Nonapoptotic Activities of Pterostilbene against Cancer. Int J Mol Sci. 2018;19(1).
986. Lee YH, Chen YY, Yeh YL, Wang YJ, Chen RJ. Stilbene Compounds Inhibit Tumor Growth by the Induction of Cellular Senescence and the Inhibition of Telomerase Activity. Int J Mol Sci. 2019;20(11).
987. Wang D, Guo H, Yang H, Wang D, Gao P, Wei W. Pterostilbene, An Active Constituent of Blueberries, Suppresses Proliferation Potential of Human Cholangiocarcinoma via Enhancing the Autophagic Flux. Front Pharmacol. 2019;10:1238.
988. Gore RD, Palaskar SJ, Bartake AR. Wheatgrass: Green Blood can Help to Fight Cancer. J Clin Diagn Res. 2017;11(6):Zc40-zc2.
989. Bar-Sela G, Cohen M, Ben-Arye E, Epelbaum R. The Medical Use of Wheatgrass: Review of the Gap Between Basic and Clinical Applications. Mini Rev Med Chem. 2015;15(12):1002-10.
990. Jakab F, Shoenfeld Y, Balogh A, Nichelatti M, Hoffmann A, Kahán Z, et al. A medical nutriment has supportive value in the treatment of colorectal cancer. Br J Cancer. 2003;89(3):465-9.
991. Avisar A, Cohen M, Katz R, Shentzer Kutiel T, Aharon A, Bar-Sela G. Wheatgrass Juice Administration and Immune Measures during Adjuvant Chemotherapy in Colon Cancer Patients: Preliminary Results. Pharmaceuticals (Basel). 2020;13(6).
992. Bar-Sela G, Tsalic M, Fried G, Goldberg H. Wheat grass juice may improve hematological toxicity related to chemotherapy in breast cancer patients: a pilot study. Nutr Cancer. 2007;58(1):43-8.
993. Attoub S, Gaben AM, Al-Salam S, Al Sultan MA, John A, Nicholls MG, et al. Captopril as a potential inhibitor of lung tumor growth and metastasis. Ann N Y Acad Sci. 2008;1138:65-72.
994. Radin DP, Krebs A, Maqsudlu A, Patel P. Our ACE in the HOLE: Justifying the Use of Angiotensin-converting Enzyme Inhibitors as Adjuvants to Standard Chemotherapy. Anticancer Res. 2018;38(1):45-9.
995. Ronquist G, Rodríguez LA, Ruigómez A, Johansson S, Wallander MA, Frithz G, et al. Association between captopril, other antihypertensive drugs and risk of prostate cancer. Prostate. 2004;58(1):50-6.

996. Liu H, Naxerova K, Pinter M, Incio J, Lee H, Shigeta K, et al. Use of Angiotensin System Inhibitors Is Associated with Immune Activation and Longer Survival in Nonmetastatic Pancreatic Ductal Adenocarcinoma. Clin Cancer Res. 2017;23(19):5959-69.
997. Riddiough GE, Fifis T, Walsh KA, Muralidharan V, Christophi C, Tran BM, et al. Captopril, a Renin-Angiotensin System Inhibitor, Attenuates Features of Tumor Invasion and Down-Regulates C-Myc Expression in a Mouse Model of Colorectal Cancer Liver Metastasis. Cancers (Basel). 2021;13(11).
998. Pinheiro L, Perdomo-Pantoja A, Casaos J, Huq S, Paldor I, Vigilar V, et al. Captopril inhibits Matrix Metalloproteinase-2 and extends survival as a temozolomide adjuvant in an intracranial gliosarcoma model. Clin Neurol Neurosurg. 2021;207:106771.
999. Kast RE, Halatsch ME. Matrix metalloproteinase-2 and -9 in glioblastoma: a trio of old drugs-captopril, disulfiram and nelfinavir-are inhibitors with potential as adjunctive treatments in glioblastoma. Arch Med Res. 2012;43(3):243-7.
1000. Crouchet E, Li S, Sojoodi M, Bandiera S, Fujiwara N, El Saghire H, et al. Hepatocellular carcinoma chemoprevention by targeting the angiotensin-converting enzyme and EGFR transactivation. JCI Insight. 2022;7(13).
1001. Fisher M, Knappertz V. The dose of aspirin for the prevention of cardiovascular and cerebrovascular events. Curr. Med Res Opin. 2006;22(7):1239-48.
1002. Tao DL, Tassi YS, Williams CD, McCarty OJT. Aspirin and antiplatelet treatments in cancer. Blood. 2021;137(23):3201-11.
1003. Negi RR, Rana SV, Gupta V, Gupta R, Chadha VD, Prasad KK, et al. Over-Expression of Cyclooxygenase-2 in Colorectal Cancer Patients. Asian Pac. J Cancer Prev. 2019;20(6):1675-81.
1004. Wilson AJ, Fadare O, Beeghly-Fadiel A, Son DS, Liu Q, Zhao S, et al. Aberrant over-expression of COX-1 intersects multiple pro-tumorigenic pathways in high-grade serous ovarian cancer. Oncotarget. 2015;6(25):21353-68.
1005. Chan TA, Morin PJ, Vogelstein B, Kinzler KW. Mechanisms underlying nonsteroidal antiinflammatory drug-mediated apoptosis. Proc. Natl. Acad. Sci U. S. A. 1998;95(2):681-6.
1006. McCarty MF, Block KI. Preadministration of high-dose salicylates, suppressors of NF-kappa B activation, may increase the chemosensitivity of many cancers: an example of proapoptotic signal modulation therapy. Integr Cancer Ther. 2006;5(3):252-68.
1007. Pan MR, Chang HC, Hung WC. Non-steroidal anti-inflammatory drugs suppress the ERK signaling pathway via block of Ras/c-Raf interaction and activation of MAP kinase phosphatases. Cell Signal. 2008;20(6):1134-41.
1008. Thun MJ, Namboodiri MM, Heath CW, Jr. Aspirin use and reduced risk of fatal colon cancer. N. Engl. J Med. 1991;325(23):1593-6.
1009. Baron JA, Cole BF, Sandler RS, Haile RW, Ahnen D, Bresalier R, et al. A randomized trial of aspirin to prevent colorectal adenomas. N. Engl. J Med. 2003;348(10):891-9.
1010. Sandler RS, Halabi S, Baron JA, Budinger S, Paskett E, Keresztes R, et al. A randomized trial of aspirin to prevent colorectal adenomas in patients with previous colorectal cancer. N. Engl. J Med. 2003;348(10):883-90.
1011. Gann PH, Manson JE, Glynn RJ, Buring JE, Hennekens CH. Low-dose aspirin and incidence of colorectal tumors in a randomized trial. J Natl. Cancer Inst. 1993;85(15):1220-4.
1012. Cook NR, Lee IM, Gaziano JM, Gordon D, Ridker PM, Manson JE, et al. Low-dose aspirin in the primary prevention of cancer: the Women's Health Study: a randomized controlled trial. JAMA. 2005;294(1):47-55.
1013. Routine aspirin or nonsteroidal anti-inflammatory drugs for the primary prevention of colorectal cancer: U.S. Preventive Services Task Force recommendation statement. Ann. Intern Med. 2007;146(5):361-4.

1014. Rothwell PM, Wilson M, Elwin CE, Norrving B, Algra A, Warlow CP, et al. Long-term effect of aspirin on colorectal cancer incidence and mortality: 20-year follow-up of five randomised trials. Lancet. 2010;376(9754):1741-50.
1015. Chubak J, Whitlock EP, Williams SB, Kamineni A, Burda BU, Buist DS, et al. Aspirin for the Prevention of Cancer Incidence and Mortality: Systematic Evidence Reviews for the U.S. Preventive Services Task Force. Ann. Intern Med. 2016;164(12):814-25.
1016. Chan AT, Ladabaum U. Where Do We Stand With Aspirin for the Prevention of Colorectal Cancer? The USPSTF Recommendations. Gastroenterology. 2016;150(1):14-8.
1017. McNeil JJ, Nelson MR, Woods RL, Lockery JE, Wolfe R, Reid CM, et al. Effect of Aspirin on All-Cause Mortality in the Healthy Elderly. N. Engl. J Med. 2018;379(16):1519-28.
1018. McNeil JJ, Woods RL, Nelson MR, Reid CM, Kirpach B, Wolfe R, et al. Effect of Aspirin on Disability-free Survival in the Healthy Elderly. N. Engl. J Med. 2018;379(16):1499-508.
1019. Guirguis-Blake JM, Evans CV, Perdue LA, Bean SI, Senger CA. Aspirin Use to Prevent Cardiovascular Disease and Colorectal Cancer: Updated Evidence Report and Systematic Review for the US Preventive Services Task Force. JAMA. 2022;327(16):1585-97.
1020. Simon TG, Duberg AS, Aleman S, Chung RT, Chan AT, Ludvigsson JF. Association of Aspirin with Hepatocellular Carcinoma and Liver-Related Mortality. N. Engl. J Med. 2020;382(11):1018-28.
1021. Risch HA, Lu L, Streicher SA, Wang J, Zhang W, Ni Q, et al. Aspirin Use and Reduced Risk of Pancreatic Cancer. Cancer Epidemiol. Biomarkers Prev. 2017;26(1):68-74.
1022. Wu D, Zhou B, Yang J, Qiu FB, Hu SY, Zhan HX. Can aspirin use reduce the risk of pancreatic cancer: an updated systematic review and meta-analysis. Journal of Pancreatology. 2020;3:201-10.
1023. Elwood PC, Morgan G, Delon C, Protty M, Galante J, Pickering J, et al. Aspirin and cancer survival: a systematic review and meta-analyses of 118 observational studies of aspirin and 18 cancers. Ecancermedicalscience. 2021;15:1258.
1024. Wang X, Luo Y, Chen T, Zhang K. Low-dose aspirin use and cancer-specific mortality: a meta-analysis of cohort studies. J Public Health (Oxf). 2021;43(2):308-15.
1025. Lebeau B, Chastang C, Muir JF, Vincent J, Massin F, Fabre C. No effect of an antiaggregant treatment with aspirin in small cell lung cancer treated with CCAVP16 chemotherapy. Results from a randomized clinical trial of 303 patients. The "Petites Cellules" Group. Cancer. 1993;71(5):1741-5.
1026. Chen WY, Winder EP, Ballman KV, Winer EP, Openshaw TH, Hahn OM, et al. A randomized phase III, double-blinded, placebo-controlled trial of aspirin as adjuvent therapy for breast cancer (A011502): The aspirin after breast cancer (ABC) trial [abstract]. J. Clin. Oncol. 2022;40 (suppl):360922.
1027. Chen WY, Ballman KV, Partridge AH, Hahn OM, Briccetti FM, Irvin WJ, et al. Aspirin vs Placebo as Adjuvant Therapy for Breast Cancer: The Alliance A011502 Randomized Trial. Jama. 2024.
1028. Pantziarka P, Sukhatme V, Bouche G, Meheus L, Sukhatme VP. Repurposing drugs in oncology (reDO)- diclofenac as an anti-cancer agent. ecancer. 2023;10:610.
1029. Giuliano F, Warner TD. Ex vivo assay to determine the cyclooxygenase selectivity of non-steroidal anti-inflammatory drugs. Br. J Pharmacol. 1999;126(8):1824-30.
1030. Nakanishi M, Rosenberg DW. Multifaceted roles of PGE2 in inflammation and cancer. Semin. Immunopathol. 2013;35(2):123-37.
1031. Tinsley HN, Gary BD, Keeton AB, Lu W, Li Y, Piazza GA. Inhibition of PDE5 by sulindac sulfide selectively induces apoptosis and attenuates oncogenic Wnt/B-catenin-mediated transcription in human breast tumor cells. Cancer Prev. Res (Phila). 2011;4(8):1275-84.

1032. Seed MP, Brown JR, Freemantle CN, Papworth JL, Colville-Nash PR, Willis D, et al. The inhibition of colon-26 adenocarcinoma development and angiogenesis by topical diclofenac in 2.5% hyaluronan. Cancer Res. 1997;57(9):1625-9.
1033. Amano H, Hayashi I, Endo H, Kitasato H, Yamashina S, Maruyama T, et al. Host prostaglandin E(2)-EP3 signaling regulates tumor-associated angiogenesis and tumor growth. J Exp Med. 2003;197(2):221-32.
1034. Kalinski P. Regulation of immune responses by prostaglandin E2. J Immunol. 2012;188(1):21-8.
1035. Obermajer N, Muthuswamy R, Odunsi K, Edwards RP, Kalinski P. PGE(2)-induced CXCL12 production and CXCR4 expression controls the accumulation of human MDSCs in ovarian cancer environment. Cancer Res. 2011;71(24):7463-70.
1036. Talmadge JE, Hood KC, Zobel LC, Shafer LR, Coles M, Toth B. Chemoprevention by cyclooxygenase-2 inhibition reduces immature myeloid suppressor cell expansion. Int. Immunopharmacol. 2007;7(2):140-51.
1037. Chesney JA, Mitchell RA, Yaddanapudi K. Myeloid-derived suppressor cells-a new therapeutic target to overcome resistance to cancer immunotherapy. J Leukoc. Biol. 2017;102(3):727-40.
1038. Fujita M, Kohanbash G, Fellows-Mayle W, Hamilton RL, Komohara Y, Decker SA, et al. COX-2 blockade suppresses gliomagenesis by inhibiting myeloid-derived suppressor cells. Cancer Res. 2011;71(7):2664-74.
1039. Yaqub S, Henjum K, Mahic M, Jahnsen FL, Aandahl EM, BjÃ¸rnbeth BA, et al. Regulatory T cells in colorectal cancer patients suppress anti-tumor immune activity in a COX-2 dependent manner. Cancer Immunol. Immunother. 2008;57(6):813-21.
1040. Chirasani SR, Leukel P, Gottfried E, Hochrein J, Stadler K, Neumann B, et al. Diclofenac inhibits lactate formation and efficiently counteracts local immune suppression in a murine glioma model. Int. J Cancer. 2013;132(4):843-53.
1041. Inoue A, Muranaka S, Fujita H, Kanno T, Tamai H, Utsumi K. Molecular mechanism of diclofenac-induced apoptosis of promyelocytic leukemia: dependency on reactive oxygen species, Akt, Bid, cytochrome and caspase pathway. Free Radic. Biol Med. 2004;37(8):1290-9.
1042. Gottfried E, Lang SA, Renner K, Bosserhoff A, Gronwald W, Rehli M, et al. New aspects of an old drug--diclofenac targets MYC and glucose metabolism in tumor cells. PloS ONE. 2013;8(7):e66987.
1043. Sareddy GR, Kesanakurti D, Kirti PB, Babu PP. Nonsteroidal anti-inflammatory drugs diclofenac and celecoxib attenuates Wntb-catenin/Tcf signaling pathway in human glioblastoma cells. Neurochem. Res. 2013;38(11):2313-22.
1044. Gerthofer V, Kreutz M, Renner K, Jachnik B, Dettmer K, Oefner P, et al. Combined Modulation of Tumor Metabolism by Metformin and Diclofenac in Glioma. Int. J Mol. Sci. 2018;19(9).
1045. Yi T, Cho SG, Yi Z, Pang X, Rodriguez M, Wang Y, et al. Thymoquinone inhibits tumor angiogenesis and tumor growth through suppressing AKT and ERK signaling pathways. Mol. Cancer Ther. 2008;7:1789-96.
1046. Kundu J, Chun KS, Aruoma OI, Kundu JK. Mechanistic perpsectives on cancer chemoprevention/chemotherapeutic effects of thymoquinone. Mutation Research/Fundamental and Molecular Mechanisms of Mutagenesis. 2014;768:22-34.
1047. Rahim MA, Shoukat A, Khalid W, Ejaz A, Itrat N, Majeed I, et al. A narrative review on various oil extraction methods, encapsulation processes, fatty acid profiles, oxidative stability, and medicinal properties of black seed (Nigella sativa). Foods. 2022;11:2826.
1048. Mostofa AG, Hossain K, Basak D, Sayeed MS. Thymoquinone as a potential adjuvant therapy for cancer treatment: Evidence from preclinical studies. Front. Pharmacol. 2017;8:295.
1049. Darakhshan S, Pou AB, Colagar AH, Sisakhtnezhad S. Thymoquinone and its therapeutic potentials. Pharmacological Research. 2015;95:138-58.

1050. Wei J, Wang B, Chen V, Wang Q, Ahmed AF, Zhang Y, et al. The immunomodulatory effects of active ingredients from Nigella sativa in RAW264.7 cells through NF-KB/MAPK signaling pathways. Front. Nutr. 2022;9:899797.
1051. Majdalawich AF, Fayyad MW, Nasrallah GK. Anti-cancer properties and mechanisms of action of thymoquinone, the major active ingredient of Nigella sativa. Critical Reviews in Food Science and Nutrition. 2017;57:3911-28.
1052. Zhao Z, Liu L, Li S, Hou X, Yang J. Advances in research on the relationship between thymoquinone and pancreatic cancer. Front. Oncol. 2023;12:1092020.
1053. Majdalawieh AF, Fayyad MW. Recent advances on the anti-cancer properties of Nigella sativa, a widely used food additive. Journal of Ayurevda and Integrative Medicine. 2016;7:173-80.
1054. Johnson-Ajinwo OR, Ullah I, Mbye H, Richardson A, Horrocks P, Li WW. The synthesis and evaluation of thymoquinone analogues as anti-ovarian cancer and antimalarial agents. Biorganic & Medicinal Chemistry Letters. 2018;28:1219-22.
1055. Ha JH, ayaraman M, adhakrishnan R, omathinayagam R, an M, ong YS. Differential effects of thymoquinone on lysophosphatidic acid-induced oncogenic pathways in ovarian cells. Journal of Traditional and Complementary Medicine. 2020;10:207-18.
1056. El-Mahdy MA, Zhu Q, Wang QE, Wani G, Wani AA. Thymoquinone induces apoptosis through activation of caspase-8 and mitochondrial events in p53-null myeloblastic leukemia HL-60 cells. Int. J. Cancer. 2005;117:409-17.
1057. Shariare MH, Khan A, Al-Masum A, Khan JH, Uddin J, Kazi M. Development of stable liposomal drug delivery system of thymoquinone and its In Vitro anticancer studies using breast cancer and cervical cancer cell lines. Molecules. 2022;27:6744.
1058. Ng WK, Yazan LS, Ismail M. Thymoquinone from Nigella sativa was more potent than cisplatin in eliminating of SiHa cells via apoptosis with down-regulaiopn of Bcl-2 protein. Toxicology in Vitro. 2011;25:1392-8.
1059. Alsanosi S, Sheikh RA, Sonbul S, Altayb HN, Batubara AS, Hosawani S, et al. The potential role of Nigella sativa seed oil as epigenetic therapy of cancer. Molecules. 2022;27:2779.
1060. Elkady AI, Hussein RA, El-Assouli SM. Mechanism of action of Nigella sativa on human colon cancer cells: the suppression of AP-1 and NF-kB transcription factors and the inducion of cytoprotective genes. Asian Pac. J. Cancer. Prev. 2015;16:7943-57.
1061. El-Far AH, Godugu K, Noreldin AE, Saddiq AA, Almaghrabi OA, Al Jaouni SK, et al. Thymoquinone and Costunolide induce apoptosis of both proliferative and doxorubin-induced-senescent colon and breast cancer cells. Integrative Cancer Therapies. 2021;30:1-20.
1062. Abdualmjid RJ, Sergi CM. Mitochonfrial dysfunction and induction of apoptosis in hepatocellular carcinoma and cholangiocarcinoma cell lines by thymoquinone. Int. J. Mol. Sci. 2022;23:14669.
1063. Thabrew MI, Mitry RR, Morsy MA, Hughes RD. Cytotoxic effects of a decoction of Nigella sativa, Hemidesmus indicus and Smalax glabra on human hepatoma HepG2 cells. Life Sci. 2005;77:1319-30.
1064. Mbarek LA, Mouse HA, Elabbadi N, Bensalah M, Gamouh A, Aboufatima R, et al. Anti-tumor properties of blackseed (Nigella sativa L.) extracts. Brazilian Journal of Medical and Biological Research. 2007;40:839-47.
1065. Khader M, Bresgen N, Eckl PM. Antimutagenic effects of ethanolic extracts from selected Palestinian medicinal plants. Journal of Ethnopharmacology. 2010;127:319-24.
1066. Kaseb AO, Chinnakannu K, Chen D, Sivanandam A, Tejwani S, Menon M, et al. Androgen receptor- and E2F-1-targeted thymoquinone therapy for hormone-refractory prostate cancer. Cancer Res. 2007;67:7782-8.

1067. Shahraki S, Mohebbati R, Shafei MN, Mahmoudi M, Hosseinian S, Parhizgar S, et al. Induction of apoptosis and growth-inhibition by thymoquinone in ACHN and GP-293 cell lines in comparable with Cis-Platinum. Journal of Pharmacopuncture. 2019;22:176-83.
1068. Chehi N, Chipitsyna G, Gong Q, Yeo CJ, Arafat HA. Anti-inflammatory effectsof the Nigella Sativa seed extract, thymoquinone, in pancreatic cancer cells. HPB. 2009;11:373-81.
1069. Al-Sheddi ES, Farshori NN, Al-Oqail MM, Musarrat J, Al-Khedhairy AA, Siddiqui MA. Cytotoxicity of Nigella Sativa seed oil and extractt against human lung cancer cell line. Asian Pac. J. Cancer. Prev. 2023;15:983-7.
1070. Kia ZA, Bizaki ST, Tapeh EA, Harijani SM, Katal N, Baziary RG. Recovering the angiogenic/angiostatic balance in NNK-induced lung carcinoma via 12 weeks of submaximal swimming and Nigella sativa nanocapsule. Toxicology Reports. 2022;9:1452-60.
1071. Ayeka PA. Potential of Mushroom Compounds as Immunomodulators in Cancer Immunotherapy: A Review. Evid. Based Complement Alternat. Med. 2018;2018:7271509.
1072. Park HJ. Current Uses of Mushrooms in Cancer Treatment and Their Anticancer Mechanisms. Int. J Mol. Sci. 2022;23(18).
1073. Dixon A, Elyaguov J, Choudhury M, Konno S. Anticancer effect of medicinal mushroom extract on renal cell carsinoma: Alternative therapeutic implication. World J. Nephrol. Urol. 2022;11:1-9.
1074. Liu MM, Liu T, Yeung S, Wang Z, Andresen B, Parsa C, et al. Inhibitory activity of medicinal mushroom Ganoderma lucidum on colorectal cancer by attenuating inflammation. Precis. Clin. Med. 2021;4(4):231-45.
1075. Cao Y, Xu X, Liu S, Huang L, Gu J. Ganoderma: A Cancer Immunotherapy Review. Front Pharmacol. 2018;9:1217.
1076. Placido AI, roque F, Morgado M. The promising role of mushrooms as a therapeutic adjuvant of conventional cancer therapies. Biologics. 2022;2:58-68.
1077. Jin X, Ruiz Beguerie J, Size D, Chan GC. *Ganoderma lucidum* (Reishi mushroom) for cancer treatment (Review). Cochrane Database of Syst. Rev. 2016;4:CD007731.
1078. Zhong C, Li Y, Li W, Lian S, Li Y, Wu C, et al. Ganoderma lucidum extract promotes tumor cell pyroptosis and inhibits metastasis in breast cancer. Food Chem Toxicol. 2023;174:113654.
1079. Kumagai Y, Akira S. Identification and functions of pattern-recognition receptors. J Allergy Clin. Immunol. 2010;125(5):985-92.
1080. Wasser SP. Medicinal mushroom science: Current perspectives, advances, evidences, and challenges. Biomed J. 2014;37(6):345-56.
1081. Yu P, Zhang X, Liu N, Tang L, Peng C, Chen X. Pyroptosis: mechanisms and diseases. Signal Transduct. Target Ther. 2021;6(1):128.
1082. Oka S, Tanaka S, Yoshida S, Hiyama T, Ueno Y, Ito M, et al. A water-soluble extract from culture medium of Ganoderma lucidum mycelia suppresses the development of colorectal adenomas. Hiroshima J Med Sci. 2010;59(1):1-6.
1083. Chen X, Hu ZP, Yang XX, Huang M, Gao Y, Tang W, et al. Monitoring of immune responses to a herbal immuno-modulator in patients with advanced colorectal cancer. Int. Immunopharmacol. 2006;6(3):499-508.
1084. Gao Y, Zhou S, Jiang W, Huang M, Dai X. Effects of ganopoly (a Ganoderma lucidum polysaccharide extract) on the immune functions in advanced-stage cancer patients. Immunol. Invest. 2003;32(3):201-15.
1085. Jeitler M, Michalsen A, Frings D, HÃ¼bner M, Fischer M, Koppold-Liebscher DA, et al. Significance of Medicinal Mushrooms in Integrative Oncology: A Narrative Review. Front Pharmacol. 2020;11:580656.

1086. Nowakowski P, Markiewicz-Å»ukowska R, Bielecka J, Mielcarek K, Grabia M, Socha K. Treasures from the forest: Evaluation of mushroom extracts as anti-cancer agents. Biomed Pharmacother. 2021;143:112106.
1087. Klupp NL, Chang D, Hawke F, Kiat H, Cao H, Grant SJ, et al. Ganoderma lucidum mushroom for the treatment of cardiovascular risk factors. Cochrane Database Syst. Rev. 2015;2015(2):CD007259.
1088. Spano D, Marshall JC, Marino N, De MD, Romano A, Scoppettuolo MN, et al. Dipyridamole prevents triple-negative breast-cancer progression. Clin. Exp Metastasis. 2013;30(1):47-68.
1089. Gresele P, Momi S, Malvestiti M, Sebastiano M. Platelet-targeted pharmacologic treatments as anti-cancer therapy. Cancer Metastasis Rev. 2017;36(2):331-55.
1090. Tsuruo T, Fujita N. Platelet aggregation in the formation of tumor metastasis. Proc. Jpn. Acad. Ser. B Phys. Biol Sci. 2008;84(6):189-98.
1091. Gao J, Zhou C, Zhong Y, Shi L, Luo X, Su H, et al. Dipyridamole interacts with the N-terminal domain of HSP90 and antagonizes the function of the chaperone in multiple cancer cell lines. Biochem. Pharmacol. 2023;207:115376.
1092. Budd GT, Herzog P, Bukowski RM. Phase I/II trial of dipyridamole, 5-fluorouracil, leukovorin, and mitoxantrone in metastatic breast cancer. Invest New Drugs. 1994;12(4):283-7.
1093. Kohnoe S, Maehara Y, Takahashi I, Emi Y, Baba H, Sugimachi K. Treatment of advanced gastric cancer with 5-fluorouracil and cisplatin in combination with dipyridamole. Int. J Oncol. 1998;13(6):1203-6.
1094. Raschko JW, Synold TW, Chow W, Coluzzi P, Hamasaki V, Leong LA, et al. A phase I study of carboplatin and etoposide administered in conjunction with dipyridamole, prochlorperazine and cyclosporine A. Cancer Chemother. Pharmacol. 2000;46(5):403-10.
1095. Fleming RA, Capizzi RL, Muss HB, Smith S, Fernandes DJ, Homesley H, et al. Phase I study of N-(phosphonacetyl)-L-aspartate with fluorouracil and with or without dipyridamole in patients with advanced cancer. Clin. Cancer Res. 1996;2(7):1107-14.
1096. Zasowska-Nowak A, Nowak PJ, Cialkowska-Rysz A. High-Dose Vitamin C in Advanced-Stage Cancer Patients. Nutrients. 2021;13(3).
1097. Cameron E, Pauling L. Ascorbic acid and the glycosaminoglycans. An orthomolecular approach to cancer and other diseases. Oncology. 1973;27(2):181-92.
1098. Cameron E, Pauling L. Supplemental ascorbate in the supportive treatment of cancer: Prolongation of survival times in terminal human cancer. Proceedings of the National Academy of Sciences of the United States of America. 1976;73(10):3685-9.
1099. Creagan ET, Moertel C, O'Fallon JR, Schuitt AJ, Rubin J, Frytak S. Failure of high-dose vitamin C (ascorbic acid) therapy to benefit patients with advanced cancer. A controlled trial. New England Journal of Medicine. 1979;301(13):687-90.
1100. Moertel CG, Fleming TR, Creagan ET, Rubin J, O'Connel MJ, Ames MM. High-dose vitamin C versus placebo in the treatment of patients with advanced cancer who have had no prior chemotherapy. A randomized double-blind comparison. New England Journal of Medicine. 1985;312(3):137-41.
1101. Padayatty SJ, Sun H, Wang Y, Riordan HD, Hewitt SM, Katz A, et al. Vitamin C pharmacokinetics: implications for oral and intravenous use. Annals of Internal Medicine. 2004;140(7):533-7.
1102. Padayatty SJ, Levine M. Reevaluation of ascorbate in cancer treatment: emerging evidence, open minds and serendipity. J Am. Coll. Nutr. 2000;19(4):423-5.
1103. Leung PY, Miyashita K, Young M, Tsao CS. Cytotoxic effect of ascorbate and its derivatives on cultured malignant and nonmalignant cell lines. Anticancer Res. 1993;13(2):475-80.
1104. Makino Y, Sakagami H, Takeda M. Induction of cell death by ascorbic acid derivatives in human renal carcinoma and glioblastoma cell lines. Anticancer Res. 1999;19(4B):3125-32.

1105. Maramag C, Menon M, Balaji KC, Reddy PG, Laxmanan S. Effect of vitamin C on prostate cancer cells in vitro: effect on cell number, viability, and DNA synthesis. Prostate. 1997;32(3):188-95.
1106. Davis JL, Paris HL, Beals JW, Binns SE, Giordano GR, Scalzo RL, et al. Liposomal-encapsulated Ascorbic Acid: Influence on Vitamin C bioavailability and capacity to protect against ischemia-reperfusion injury. Nutrition and Metabolic Insights. 2016;9:25-30.
1107. Hickey S, Roberts HJ, Miller NJ. Pharmacokinetics of oral vitamin C. Journal of Nutritional & Environmental Medicine. 2008;17:169-77.
1108. Mikirova N, Levy T, Hunningshake R. The levels of ascorbic acid in blood and mononuclear blood cells after oral liposome-encapsulated and oral non-encapsulated vitamin C supplementation, taken without and with IV hydrocortisone. J. Orthomol. Med. 2019;34.
1109. Mikirova NA. Ascorbic Acid and Dehydroascorbic Acid Concentrations in Plasma and Peripheral Blood Mononuclear Cells after Oral Liposomal-Encapsulated or Intravenous Ascorbic Acid Delivery. J. Orthomol. Med. 2017;32:1-9.
1110. Lee B, Oh SW, Myung SK. Efficacy of Vitamin C Supplements in Prevention of Cancer: A Meta-Analysis of Randomized Controlled Trials. Korean J Fam Med. 2015;36(6):278-85.
1111. Benade L, Howard T, Burk D. Synergistic killing of Ehrlich ascites carcinoma cells by ascorbate and 3-amino-1,2,4,-triazole. Oncology. 1969;23(1):33-43.
1112. Yun J, Mullarky E, Lu C, Bosch KN, Kavalier A, Rivera K, et al. Vitamin C selectively kills KRAS and BRAF mutant colorectal cancer cells by targeting GAPDH. Science. 2015;350(6266):1391-6.
1113. Riordan HD, Riordan NH, Jackson JA, Casciari JJ, Hunninghake R, Gonzalez MJ, et al. Intravenous vitamin C as a chemotherapy agent: a report on clinical cases. P. R. Health Sci J. 2004;23(2):115-8.
1114. Gonzalez MJ, Berdiel MJ, Cintron AV. High dose IV vitamin C and metastatic breast cancer: A case report. J. Orthomol. Med. 2017;32:1.
1115. Garcia KM, De Jesus C, Berdiel MJ, Miranda-Massari JR, Gonzalez MJ. Intravenous vitamin C and metabolic correction as adjuvant therapy for prostate cancer: a case report. J. Cancer Prev. Curr. Res. 2016;5:00164.
1116. Nielsen TK, Hojgaard M, Andersen JT, Jorgensen NR, Zerahn B, Kristensen B, et al. Weekly ascorbic acid infusion in castration-resistant prostate cancer patients: a single-arm phase II trial. Transl. Androl Urol. 2017;6(3):517-28.
1117. Wilson MK, Baguley BC, Wall C, Jameson MB, Findlay MP. Review of high-dose intravenous vitamin C as an anticancer agent. Asia Pac. J Clin. Oncol. 2014;10(1):22-37.
1118. Carr AC, Cook J. Intravenous Vitamin C for Cancer Therapy - Identifying the Current Gaps in Our Knowledge. Front Physiol. 2018;9:1182.
1119. Jacobs C, Hutton B, Ng T, Shorr R, Clemons M. Is there a role for oral or intravenous ascorbate (vitamin C) in treating patients with cancer? A systematic review. Oncologist. 2015;20(2):210-23.
1120. Hoffer LJ, Robitaille L, Zakarian R, Meinychuk D, Kavan P, Agulnik J, et al. High-dose intravenous vitamin C combined with cytotoxic chemotherapy in patients with advanced cancer: a phase I-II clinical trial. PloS ONE. 2015;10(4):e0120228.
1121. Wang F, He MM, Xiao J, Zhang YQ, Yuan XL, Fang WJ, et al. A Randomized, Open-Label, Multicenter, Phase 3 Study of High-Dose Vitamin C Plus FOLFOX ± Bevacizumab versus FOLFOX ± Bevacizumab in Unresectable Untreated Metastatic Colorectal Cancer (VITALITY Study). Clin. Cancer Res. 2022;28(19):4232-9.
1122. Stacpoole PW. Therapeutic Targeting of the Pyruvate Dehydrogenase Complex/Pyruvate Dehydrogenase Kinase (PDC/PDK) Axis in Cancer. J Natl. Cancer Inst. 2017;109(11).
1123. Abdel-Wahab AF, Mahmoud W, Al-Harizy RM. Targeting glucose metabolism to suppress cancer progression: prospective of anti-glycolytic cancer therapy. Pharmacol. Res. 2019;150:104511.

1124. Albayrak G, Konac E, Dere UA, Emmez H. Targeting Cancer Cell Metabolism with Metformin, Dichloroacetate and Memantine in Glioblastoma (GBM). Turk. Neurosurg. 2021;31(2):233-7.
1125. Powell SF, Mazurczak M, Dib EG, Bleeker JS, Geeraerts LH, Tinguely M, et al. Phase II study of dichloroacetate, an inhibitor of pyruvate dehydrogenase, in combination with chemoradiotherapy for unresected, locally advanced head and neck squamous cell carcinoma. Invest New Drugs. 2022;40(3):622-33.
1126. Strum SB, Adalsteinsson O, Black RR, Segal D, Peress NL, Waldenfels J. Case report: Sodium dichloroacetate (DCA) inhibition of the "Warburg Effect" in a human cancer patient: complete response in non-Hodgkin's lymphoma after disease progression with rituximab-CHOP. J Bioenerg. Biomembr. 2013;45(3):307-15.
1127. Khan A, Andrews D, Blackburn AC. Long-term stabilization of stage 4 colon cancer using sodium dichloroacetate therapy. World J Clin. Cases. 2016;4(10):336-43.
1128. Khan A, Andrews D, Shainhouse J, Blackburn AC. Long-term stabilization of metastatic melanoma with sodium dichloroacetate. World J Clin. Oncol. 2017;8(4):371-7.
1129. Brandsma D, Dorlo TP, Haanen JH, Beijnen JH, Boogerd W. Severe encephalopathy and polyneuropathy induced by dichloroacetate. J Neurol. 2010;257(12):2099-100.
1130. Bayat Mokhtari R, Baluch N, Homayouni TS, Morgatskaya E, Kumar S, Kazemi P, et al. The role of Sulforaphane in cancer chemoprevention and health benefits: a mini-review. J Cell Commun Signal. 2018;12(1):91-101.
1131. Clarke JD, Dashwood RH, Ho E. Multi-targeted prevention of cancer by sulforaphane. Cancer Lett. 2008;269(2):291-304.
1132. Li Y, Zhang T. Targeting cancer stem cells with sulforaphane, a dietary component from broccoli and broccoli sprouts. Future Oncol. 2013;9(8):1097-103.
1133. Li Y, Zhang T, Korkaya H, Liu S, Lee HF, Newman B, et al. Sulforaphane, a dietary component of broccoli/broccoli sprouts, inhibits breast cancer stem cells. Clin Cancer Res. 2010;16(9):2580-90.
1134. Rodova M, Fu J, Watkins DN, Srivastava RK, Shankar S. Sonic hedgehog signaling inhibition provides opportunities for targeted therapy by sulforaphane in regulating pancreatic cancer stem cell self-renewal. PLoS One. 2012;7(9):e46083.
1135. Ge M, Zhang L, Cao L, Xie C, Li X, Li Y, et al. Sulforaphane inhibits gastric cancer stem cells via suppressing sonic hedgehog pathway. Int J Food Sci Nutr. 2019;70(5):570-8.
1136. Burnett JP, Lim G, Li Y, Shah RB, Lim R, Paholak HJ, et al. Sulforaphane enhances the anticancer activity of taxanes against triple negative breast cancer by killing cancer stem cells. Cancer Lett. 2017;394:52-64.
1137. Castro NP, Rangel MC, Merchant AS, MacKinnon G, Cuttitta F, Salomon DS, et al. Sulforaphane Suppresses the Growth of Triple-negative Breast Cancer Stem-like Cells In vitro and In vivo. Cancer Prev Res (Phila). 2019;12(3):147-58.
1138. Srivastava RK, Tang SN, Zhu W, Meeker D, Shankar S. Sulforaphane synergizes with quercetin to inhibit self-renewal capacity of pancreatic cancer stem cells. Front Biosci (Elite Ed). 2011;3(2):515-28.
1139. Chen H, Landen CN, Li Y, Alvarez RD, Tollefsbol TO. Epigallocatechin gallate and sulforaphane combination treatment induce apoptosis in paclitaxel-resistant ovarian cancer cells through hTERT and Bcl-2 down-regulation. Exp Cell Res. 2013;319(5):697-706.
1140. Cipolla BG, Mandron E, Lefort JM, Coadou Y, Della Negra E, Corbel L, et al. Effect of Sulforaphane in Men with Biochemical Recurrence after Radical Prostatectomy. Cancer Prev Res (Phila). 2015;8(8):712-9.
1141. Alumkal JJ, Slottke R, Schwartzman J, Cherala G, Munar M, Graff JN, et al. A phase II study of sulforaphane-rich broccoli sprout extracts in men with recurrent prostate cancer. Invest New Drugs. 2015;33(2):480-9.

1142. Clarke JD, Hsu A, Riedl K, Bella D, Stevens JF, Ho E. Bioavailability and inter-conversion of sulforaphane and erucin in human subjects consuming broccoli sprouts or broccoli supplement in a cross-over study design. Pharmacol. Res. 2011;64:456-63.
1143. Khandouzi N, Shidfar F, Rajab A, Rahideh T, Hosseini P, Taheri MM. The effects of Ginger on fasting blood sugar, hemoglobin A1C, Apolipoprotein B, Apolipoprotein A-1 and malondialdehyde in type 2 diabetic patients. Iranian Journal of Pharmaceutical Research. 2015;14:131-40.
1144. Das AK. Anticancer Effect of AntiMalarial Artemisinin Compounds. Ann Med Health Sci Res. 2015;5(2):93-102.
1145. Li P, Yang S, Dou M, Chen Y, Zhang J, Zhao X. Synergic effects of artemisinin and resveratrol in cancer cells. J Cancer Res Clin Oncol. 2014;140(12):2065-75.
1146. Nandakumar DN, Nagaraj VA, Vathsala PG, Rangarajan P, Padmanaban G. Curcumin-artemisinin combination therapy for malaria. Antimicrob Agents Chemother. 2006;50(5):1859-60.
1147. Gerhardt T, Jones R, Park J, Lu R, Chan HW, Fang Q, et al. Effects of antioxidants and pro-oxidants on cytotoxicity of dihydroartemisinin to Molt-4 human leukemia cells. Anticancer Res. 2015;35(4):1867-71.
1148. Kwok JC, Richardson DR. The iron metabolism of neoplastic cells: alterations that facilitate proliferation? Crit Rev Oncol Hematol. 2002;42(1):65-78.
1149. Obrador-Hevia A, Fernández de Mattos S, Villalonga P, Rodríguez J. Molecular biology of mantle cell lymphoma: from profiling studies to new therapeutic strategies. Blood Rev. 2009;23(5):205-16.
1150. Yang ND, Tan SH, Ng S, Shi Y, Zhou J, Tan KS, et al. Artesunate induces cell death in human cancer cells via enhancing lysosomal function and lysosomal degradation of ferritin. J Biol Chem. 2014;289(48):33425-41.
1151. Strik H, Efferth T, Kaina B. Artesunate in glioblastoma therapy: Case reports and review of clinical studies. Phytomedicine. 2024;123:155274.
1152. von Hagens C, Walter-Sack I, Goeckenjan M, Storch-Hagenlocher B, Sertel S, Elsässer M, et al. Long-term add-on therapy (compassionate use) with oral artesunate in patients with metastatic breast cancer after participating in a phase I study (ARTIC M33/2). Phytomedicine. 2019;54:140-8.
1153. von Hagens C, Walter-Sack I, Goeckenjan M, Osburg J, Storch-Hagenlocher B, Sertel S, et al. Prospective open uncontrolled phase I study to define a well-tolerated dose of oral artesunate as add-on therapy in patients with metastatic breast cancer (ARTIC M33/2). Breast Cancer Res Treat. 2017;164(2):359-69.
1154. Deeken JF, Wang H, Hartley M, Cheema AK, Smaglo B, Hwang JJ, et al. A phase I study of intravenous artesunate in patients with advanced solid tumor malignancies. Cancer Chemother Pharmacol. 2018;81(3):587-96.
1155. Berger TG, Dieckmann D, Efferth T, Schultz ES, Funk JO, Baur A, et al. Artesunate in the treatment of metastatic uveal melanoma--first experiences. Oncol Rep. 2005;14(6):1599-603.
1156. Krishna S, Ganapathi S, Ster IC, Saeed ME, Cowan M, Finlayson C, et al. A Randomised, Double Blind, Placebo-Controlled Pilot Study of Oral Artesunate Therapy for Colorectal Cancer. EBioMedicine. 2015;2(1):82-90.
1157. Abrams DI. Cannabis, Cannabinoids and Cannabis-Based Medicines in Cancer Care. Integr Cancer Ther. 2022;21:15347354221081772.
1158. Abu-Amna M, Salti T, Khoury M, Cohen I, Bar-Sela G. Medical Cannabis in Oncology: a Valuable Unappreciated Remedy or an Undesirable Risk? Curr Treat Options Oncol. 2021;22(2):16.
1159. Abrahamov A, Abrahamov A, Mechoulam R. An efficient new cannabinoid antiemetic in pediatric oncology. Life Sci. 1995;56(23-24):2097-102.

1160. Smith LA, Azariah F, Lavender VT, Stoner NS, Bettiol S. Cannabinoids for nausea and vomiting in adults with cancer receiving chemotherapy. Cochrane Database Syst Rev. 2015;2015(11):Cd009464.

1161. Hesketh PJ, Kris MG, Basch E, Bohlke K, Barbour SY, Clark-Snow RA, et al. Antiemetics: ASCO Guideline Update. J Clin Oncol. 2020;38(24):2782-97.

1162. Portenoy RK, Ganae-Motan ED, Allende S, Yanagihara R, Shaiova L, Weinstein S, et al. Nabiximols for opioid-treated cancer patients with poorly-controlled chronic pain: a randomized, placebo-controlled, graded-dose trial. J Pain. 2012;13(5):438-49.

1163. Fallon MT, Albert Lux E, McQuade R, Rossetti S, Sanchez R, Sun W, et al. Sativex oromucosal spray as adjunctive therapy in advanced cancer patients with chronic pain unalleviated by optimized opioid therapy: two double-blind, randomized, placebo-controlled phase 3 studies. Br J Pain. 2017;11(3):119-33.

1164. Guggisberg J, Schumacher M, Gilmore G, Zylla DM. Cannabis as an Anticancer Agent: A Review of Clinical Data and Assessment of Case Reports. Cannabis Cannabinoid Res. 2022;7(1):24-33.

1165. Likar R, Koestenberger M, Stultschnig M, Nahler G. Concomitant Treatment of Malignant Brain Tumours With CBD - A Case Series and Review of the Literature. Anticancer Res. 2019;39(10):5797-801.

1166. Guzmán M, Duarte MJ, Blázquez C, Ravina J, Rosa MC, Galve-Roperh I, et al. A pilot clinical study of Delta9-tetrahydrocannabinol in patients with recurrent glioblastoma multiforme. Br J Cancer. 2006;95(2):197-203.

1167. Twelves C, Sabel M, Checketts D, Miller S, Tayo B, Jove M, et al. A phase 1b randomised, placebo-controlled trial of nabiximols cannabinoid oromucosal spray with temozolomide in patients with recurrent glioblastoma. Br J Cancer. 2021;124(8):1379-87.

1168. Lian X, Wang G, Zhou H, Zheng Z, Fu Y, Cai L. Anticancer Properties of Fenofibrate: A Repurposing Use. J Cancer. 2018;9(9):1527-37.

1169. Li T, Zhang Q, Zhang J, Yang G, Shao Z, Luo J, et al. Fenofibrate induces apoptosis of triple-negative breast cancer cells via activation of NF-κB pathway. BMC Cancer. 2014;14:96.

1170. Jiao HL, Zhao BL. Cytotoxic effect of peroxisome proliferator fenofibrate on human HepG2 hepatoma cell line and relevant mechanisms. Toxicol Appl Pharmacol. 2002;185(3):172-9.

1171. Binello E, Mormone E, Emdad L, Kothari H, Germano IM. Characterization of fenofibrate-mediated anti-proliferative pro-apoptotic effects on high-grade gliomas and anti-invasive effects on glioma stem cells. J Neurooncol. 2014;117(2):225-34.

1172. Han DF, Zhang JX, Wei WJ, Tao T, Hu Q, Wang YY, et al. Fenofibrate induces G0/G1 phase arrest by modulating the PPARα/FoxO1/p27 kip pathway in human glioblastoma cells. Tumour Biol. 2015;36(5):3823-9.

1173. Zhao H, Zhu C, Qin C, Tao T, Li J, Cheng G, et al. Fenofibrate down-regulates the expressions of androgen receptor (AR) and AR target genes and induces oxidative stress in the prostate cancer cell line LNCaP. Biochem Biophys Res Commun. 2013;432(2):320-5.

1174. Chen W, Mook RA, Jr., Premont RT, Wang J. Niclosamide: Beyond an antihelminthic drug. Cell Signal. 2018;41:89-96.

1175. Figarola JL, Singhal J, Singhal S, Kusari J, Riggs A. Bioenergetic modulation with the mitochondria uncouplers SR4 and niclosamide prevents proliferation and growth of treatment-naïve and vemurafenib-resistant melanomas. Oncotarget. 2018;9(97):36945-65.

1176. Kumar R, Coronel L, Somalanka B, Raju A, Aning OA, An O, et al. Mitochondrial uncoupling reveals a novel therapeutic opportunity for p53-defective cancers. Nat Commun. 2018;9(1):3931.

1177. Wang J, Ren XR, Piao H, Zhao S, Osada T, Premont RT, et al. Niclosamide-induced Wnt signaling inhibition in colorectal cancer is mediated by autophagy. Biochem J. 2019;476(3):535-46.

1178. Park SY, Kim JY, Choi JH, Kim JH, Lee CJ, Singh P, et al. Inhibition of LEF1-Mediated DCLK1 by Niclosamide Attenuates Colorectal Cancer Stemness. Clin Cancer Res. 2019;25(4):1415-29.
1179. Li Y, Li PK, Roberts MJ, Arend RC, Samant RS, Buchsbaum DJ. Multi-targeted therapy of cancer by niclosamide: A new application for an old drug. Cancer Lett. 2014;349(1):8-14.
1180. Chen M, Wang J, Lu J, Bond MC, Ren XR, Lyerly HK, et al. The anti-helminthic niclosamide inhibits Wnt/Frizzled1 signaling. Biochemistry. 2009;48(43):10267-74.
1181. Deng Y, Wang Z, Zhang F, Qiao M, Yan Z, Wei Q, et al. A Blockade of IGF Signaling Sensitizes Human Ovarian Cancer Cells to the Anthelmintic Niclosamide-Induced Anti-Proliferative and Anticancer Activities. Cell Physiol Biochem. 2016;39(3):871-88.
1182. Yo YT, Lin YW, Wang YC, Balch C, Huang RL, Chan MW, et al. Growth inhibition of ovarian tumor-initiating cells by niclosamide. Mol Cancer Ther. 2012;11(8):1703-12.
1183. Pu J, Guardia CM, Keren-Kaplan T, Bonifacino JS. Mechanisms and functions of lysosome positioning. J Cell Sci. 2016;129(23):4329-39.
1184. Circu ML, Dykes SS, Carroll J, Kelly K, Galiano F, Greer A, et al. A Novel High Content Imaging-Based Screen Identifies the Anti-Helminthic Niclosamide as an Inhibitor of Lysosome Anterograde Trafficking and Prostate Cancer Cell Invasion. PLoS One. 2016;11(1):e0146931.
1185. Beljanski M, Crochet S. The selective anticancer agents PB-100 and BG-8 are active against human melanoma cells, but do not affect non malignant fibroblasts. Int J Oncol. 1996;8(6):1143-8.
1186. Beljanski M, Crochet S. The selective anticancer agent pb-100 inhibits interleukin-6 induced enhancement of glioblastoma cell-proliferation in-vitro. Int J Oncol. 1994;5(4):873-9.
1187. Chang C, Zhao W, Xie B, Deng Y, Han T, Cui Y, et al. Pao Pereira Extract Suppresses Castration-Resistant Prostate Cancer Cell Growth, Survival, and Invasion Through Inhibition of NFκB Signaling. Integr Cancer Ther. 2014;13(3):249-58.
1188. Chen P, Dong R, Chen Q. Extracts of the Medicinal Plants Pao Pereira and Rauwolfia vomitoria Inhibit Ovarian Cancer Stem Cells In Vitro. Integr Cancer Ther. 2022;21:15347354221123019.
1189. Dong R, Chen P, Chen Q. Extract of the Medicinal Plant Pao Pereira Inhibits Pancreatic Cancer Stem-Like Cell In Vitro and In Vivo. Integr Cancer Ther. 2018;17(4):1204-15.
1190. Bemis DL, Capodice JL, Desai M, Katz AE, Buttyan R. beta-carboline alkaloid-enriched extract from the amazonian rain forest tree pao pereira suppresses prostate cancer cells. J Soc Integr Oncol. 2009;7(2):59-65.
1191. Yu J, Chen Q. The plant extract of Pao pereira potentiates carboplatin effects against ovarian cancer. Pharm Biol. 2014;52(1):36-43.
1192. Yu J, Drisko J, Chen Q. Inhibition of pancreatic cancer and potentiation of gemcitabine effects by the extract of Pao Pereira. Oncol Rep. 2013;30(1):149-56.
1193. Fan M, Zhang X, Song H, Zhang Y. Dandelion (Taraxacum Genus): A Review of Chemical Constituents and Pharmacological Effects. Molecules. 2023;28(13).
1194. Li Y, Deng Y, Zhang X, Fu H, Han X, Guo W, et al. Dandelion Seed Extract Affects Tumor Progression and Enhances the Sensitivity of Cisplatin in Esophageal Squamous Cell Carcinoma. Front Pharmacol. 2022;13:897465.
1195. Ovadje P, Ammar S, Guerro JA, Arnason JT, Pandey S. Dandelion root extract affects colorectal cancer proliferation and survival through the activation of multiple death signalling pathways. Oncotarget. 2016;45:73080-100.
1196. Zhu H, Zhao H, Zhang L, Xu J, Zhu C, Zhao H. Dandelion root extract suppressed gastric cancer cells proliferaion and migraion through targeting lncRNA-CCAT1. Biomedicine & Pharmacotherapy. 2017;93:1010-7.
1197. Deng XX, Jiao YN, Hao HF, Xue D, Bai CC, Han SY. Taraxacum mongolicum extract inhibited malignant phenotype of triple-negative breast cancer cells in tumor-associated macrophages

microenvironment through suppressing IL-10 / STAT3 / PD-L1 signaling pathways. J Ethnopharmacol. 2021;274:113978.

1198. Wang S, Hao HF, Fu JL, Guo ZW, Guo Y, Yuan Y, et al. Dandelion extract inhibits triple-negative breast cancer cell proliferaion by interfering with glycerophospholipids and unsaturated fatty acids metabolism. Front. Pharmacol. 2022;13:942996.

1199. Lin CJ, Chen JT, Yeh LJ, Yang RC, Huang SM, Chen TW. Characteristics of the Cytotoxicity of Taraxacum mongolicum and Taraxacum formosanum in Human Breast Cancer Cells. Int J Mol Sci. 2022;23(19).

1200. Lonn E, Yusuf S, Arnold MJ, Sheridan P, Pogue J, Micks M, et al. Homocysteine lowering with folic acid and B vitamins in vascular disease. N Engl J Med. 2006;354(15):1567-77.

1201. Cole BF, Baron JA, Sandler RS, Haile RW, Ahnen DJ, Bresalier RS, et al. Folic acid for the prevention of colorectal adenomas: a randomized clinical trial. Jama. 2007;297(21):2351-9.

1202. Ebbing M, Bleie Ø, Ueland PM, Nordrehaug JE, Nilsen DW, Vollset SE, et al. Mortality and cardiovascular events in patients treated with homocysteine-lowering B vitamins after coronary angiography: a randomized controlled trial. Jama. 2008;300(7):795-804.

1203. Bønaa KH, Njølstad I, Ueland PM, Schirmer H, Tverdal A, Steigen T, et al. Homocysteine lowering and cardiovascular events after acute myocardial infarction. N Engl J Med. 2006;354(15):1578-88.

1204. Ebbing M, Bønaa KH, Nygård O, Arnesen E, Ueland PM, Nordrehaug JE, et al. Cancer incidence and mortality after treatment with folic acid and vitamin B12. Jama. 2009;302(19):2119-26.

1205. Klein EA, Thompson IM, Jr., Tangen CM, Crowley JJ, Lucia MS, Goodman PJ, et al. Vitamin E and the risk of prostate cancer: the Selenium and Vitamin E Cancer Prevention Trial (SELECT). Jama. 2011;306(14):1549-56.

1206. Dhyani P, Quispe C, Sharma E, Bahukhandi A, Sati P, Attri DC, et al. Anticancer potential of alkaloids: a key emphasis to colchicine, vinblastine, vincristine, vindesine, vinorelbine and vincamine. Cancer Cell International. 2022;22(1).

1207. Kumar A, Sharma PR, Mondhe DM. Potential anticancer role of colchicine-based derivatives: an overview. Anticancer Drugs. 2017;28(3):250-62.

1208. Angelidis C, Kotsialou Z, Kossyvakis C, Vrettou AR, Zacharoulis A, Kolokathis F, et al. Colchicine Pharmacokinetics and Mechanism of Action. Curr Pharm Des. 2018;24(6):659-63.

1209. Marzo-Mas A, Conesa-Milián L, Noppen S, Liekens S, Falomir E, Murga J, et al. N-alpha-Aminoacyl Colchicines as Promising Anticancer Agents. Med Chem. 2021;17(1):21-32.

1210. Cheng Z, Lu X, Feng B. A review of research progress of antitumor drugs based on tubulin targets. Translational Cancer Research. 2020;9(6):4020-7.

1211. Jordan MA. Mechanism of Action of Antitumor Drugs that Interact with Microtubules and Tubulin. Curr. Med. Chem- Anti-Cancer Agents. 2002;2:1-17.

1212. Karahalil B, Yardim-Akaydin S, Baytas SN. An overview of microtubule targeting agents for cancer therapy. Arh Hig Rada Toksikol. 2019;70(3):160-72.

1213. Leung YY, Yao Hui LL, Kraus VB. Colchicine—Update on mechanisms of action and therapeutic uses. Seminars in Arthritis and Rheumatism. 2015;45(3):341-50.

1214. Charpentier MS, Whipple RA, Vitolo MI, Boggs AE, Slovic J, Thompson KN, et al. Curcumin targets breast cancer stem–like cells with microtentacles that persist in mammospheres and promote reattachment. Cancer Res. 2014;74(4):1250-60.

1215. Ganguly A, Yang H, Zhang H, Cabral F, Patel KD. Microtubule Dynamics Control Tail Retraction in Migrating Vascular Endothelial Cells. Molecular Cancer Therapeutics. 2013;12(12):2837-46.

1216. Chen X-m, Liu J, Wang T, Shang J. Colchicine-induced apoptosis in human normal liver L-02 cells by mitochondrial mediated pathways. Toxicology in Vitro. 2012;26:649-55.

1217. Acuna-Castroviejo D. Melatonin, clock genes and mitochondria in sepsis. Cellular & Molecular Life Sciences. 2017;74(21):3965-87.
1218. Huang Z, Xu Y, Peng W. Colchicine induces apoptosis in HT-29 human colon cancer cells via the AKT and c-Jun N-terminal kinase signaling pathways. Molecular Medicine Reports. 2015;12(4):5939-44.
1219. Zhang T, Chen W, Jiang X, Liu L, Wei K, Du H, et al. Anticancer effects and underlying mechanism of Colchicine on human gastric cancer cell lines in vitro and in vivo. Bioscience Reports. 2019;39.
1220. Singh B, Kumar A, Joshi P, Guru S, Kumar S, Wani Z, et al. Colchicine derivatives with potent anticancer activity and reduced P-glycoprotein induction liability. Org Biomol Chem. 2015;13(20):5674-89.
1221. Abouaitah K, Hassan HA, Swiderska-Sroda A, Gohar L, Shaker OG, Wojnarowicz J, et al. Targeted Nano-Drug Delivery of Colchicine against Colon Cancer Cells by Means of Mesoporous Silica Nanoparticles. Cancers. 2020;12(1):144.
1222. Bakar-Ateş F, Özmen N, Kaya-Sezginer E, Kurt E. Effects of colchicine on cell cycle arrest and MMP-2 mRNA expression in MCF-7 breast adenocarcinoma cells. 2018(75):239-44.
1223. Larocque K, Ovadje P, Djurdjevic S, Mehdi M, Green J, Pandey S. Novel Analogue of Colchicine Induces Selective Pro-Death Autophagy and Necrosis in Human Cancer Cells. PLoS ONE. 2014;9(1):e87064.
1224. Lin Z-Y, Kuo C-H, Wu D-C, Chuang W-L. Anticancer effects of clinically acceptable colchicine concentrations on human gastric cancer cell lines. The Kaohsiung Journal of Medical Sciences. 2016;32(2):68-73.
1225. Kuo M-C, Chang S-J, Hsieh M-C. Colchicine Significantly Reduces Incident Cancer in Gout Male Patients. Medicine. 2015;94(50).
1226. Finkelstein Y, Aks SE, Hutson JR, Juurlink DN, Nguyen P, Dubnov-Raz G, et al. Colchicine poisoning: the dark side of an ancient drug. Clin Toxicol (Phila). 2010;48(5):407-14.
1227. Vatansever G, Karadeniz C, Kendirli T. An Insidious Danger in Children With Familial Mediterranean Fever: Colchicine Intoxication. Pediatr Emerg Care. 2015;31(9):652-3.
1228. Ernst E. Shark cartilage for cancer? Lancet. 1998;351(9098):298.
1229. Ostrander GK, Cheng KC, Wolf JC, Wolfe MJ. Shark cartilage, cancer and the growing threat of pseudoscience. Cancer Res. 2004;64(23):8485-91.
1230. González RP, Leyva A, Moraes MO. Shark cartilage as source of antiangiogenic compounds: from basic to clinical research. Biol Pharm Bull. 2001;24(10):1097-101.
1231. Miller DR, Anderson GT, Stark JJ, Granick JL, Richardson D. Phase I/II trial of the safety and efficacy of shark cartilage in the treatment of advanced cancer. J Clin Oncol. 1998;16(11):3649-55.
1232. Loprinzi CL, Levitt R, Barton DL, Sloan JA, Atherton PJ, Smith DJ, et al. Evaluation of shark cartilage in patients with advanced cancer: a North Central Cancer Treatment Group trial. Cancer. 2005;104(1):176-82.
1233. Jaszczak-Wilke E, Polkowska Ż, Koprowski M, Owsianik K, Mitchell AE, Bałczewski P. Amygdalin: Toxicity, Anticancer Activity and Analytical Procedures for Its Determination in Plant Seeds. Molecules. 2021;26(8).
1234. Shi J, Chen Q, Xu M, Xia Q, Zheng T, Teng J, et al. Recent updates and future perspectives about amygdalin as a potential anticancer agent: A review. Cancer Med. 2019;8(6):3004-11.
1235. Song Z, Xu X. Advanced research on anti-tumor effects of amygdalin. J Cancer Res Ther. 2014;10 Suppl 1:3-7.
1236. Chang HK, Shin MS, Yang HY, Lee JW, Kim YS, Lee MH, et al. Amygdalin induces apoptosis through regulation of Bax and Bcl-2 expressions in human DU145 and LNCaP prostate cancer cells. Biol Pharm Bull. 2006;29(8):1597-602.

1237. Milazzo S, Lejeune S, Ernst E. Laetrile for cancer: a systematic review of the clinical evidence. Support Care Cancer. 2007;15(6):583-95.
1238. Chen Y, Ma J, Wang F, Hu J, Cui A, Wei C, et al. Amygdalin induces apoptosis in human cervical cancer cell line HeLa cells. Immunopharmacol Immunotoxicol. 2013;35(1):43-51.
1239. Stock CC, Martin DS, Sugiura K, Fugmann RA, Mountain IM, Stockert E, et al. Antitumor tests of amygdalin in spontaneous animal tumor systems. J Surg Oncol. 1978;10(2):89-123.
1240. Dorr RT, Paxinos J. The current status of laetrile. Ann Intern Med. 1978;89(3):389-97.
1241. Ellison NM, Byar DP, Newell GR. Special report on Laetrile: the NCI Laetrile Review. Results of the National Cancer Institute's retrospective Laetrile analysis. N Engl J Med. 1978;299(10):549-52.
1242. Moertel CG, Fleming TR, Rubin J, Kvols LK, Sarna G, Koch R, et al. A clinical trial of amygdalin (Laetrile) in the treatment of human cancer. N Engl J Med. 1982;306(4):201-6.
1243. Milazzo S, Horneber M. Laetrile treatment for cancer. Cochrane Database Syst Rev. 2015;2015(4):Cd005476.
1244. Kinzel A, Ambrogi M, Varshaver M, Kirson ED. Tumor Treating Fields for Glioblastoma Treatment: Patient Satisfaction and Compliance With the Second-Generation Optune(Â®) System. Clin. Med Insights Oncol. 2019;13:1179554918825449.
1245. Moser JC, Salvador E, Deniz K, Swanson K, Tuszynski J, Carlson KW, et al. The Mechanisms of Action of Tumor Treating Fields. Cancer Res. 2022;82(20):3650-8.
1246. Stupp R, Taillibert S, Kanner A, Read W, Steinberg D, Lhermitte B, et al. Effect of Tumor-Treating Fields Plus Maintenance Temozolomide vs Maintenance Temozolomide Alone on Survival in Patients With Glioblastoma: A Randomized Clinical Trial. JAMA. 2017;318(23):2306-16.
1247. Kim CY, Paek SH, Nam DH, Chang JH, Hong YK, Kim JH, et al. Tumor treating fields plus temozolomide for newly diagnosed glioblastoma: a sub-group analysis of Korean patients in the EF-14 phase 3 trial. J Neurooncol. 2020;146(3):399-406.
1248. NCCN clinical practice guidelines in oncology, Central nervous systems cancer, Version 1. https://www.nccn.org/login?returnURL=https://www.nccn.org/professionals/physician_gls/pdf/cns.pdf; 2018.
1249. Ghiaseddin AP, Shin D, Melnick K, Tran DD. Tumor Treating Fields in the Management of Patients with Malignant Gliomas. Curr. Treat. Options Oncol. 2020;21(9):76.
1250. Yanovsky RL, Bartenstein DW, Rogers GS, Isakoff SJ, Chen ST. Photodynamic therapy for solid tumors: A review of the literature. Photodermatol. Photoimmunol. Photomed. 2019;35(5):295-303.
1251. Dos Santos AF, de Almeida DR, Terra LF, Baptista M, Labriola L. Photodynamic therapy in cancer treatment - an update review. J. Cancer Metastasis Treat. 2019;5:25.
1252. Reiter RJ, Ma Q, Sharma R. Melatonin in mitochondria: Mitigating clear and present dangers. Physiology. 2020;35:86-95.
1253. Zimmerman S, Reiter RJ. Melatonin and the optics of the human body. Melatonin Res. 2019;2:138-60.
1254. Moore CM, Nathan TR, Lees WR, Mosse CA, Freeman A, Emberton M, et al. Photodynamic therapy using meso tetra hydroxy phenyl chlorin (mTHPC) in early prostate cancer. Lasers Surg. Med. 2006;38(5):356-63.
1255. Dos Santos AF, Terra LF, Wailemann RA, Oliveira TC, Gomes VM, Mineiro MF, et al. Methylene blue photodynamic therapy induces selective and massive cell death in human breast cancer cells. BMC Cancer. 2017;17(1):194.
1256. Kostron H. Photodynamic diagnosis and therapy and the brain. In: Gomer CJ, ed. Photodynamic Therapy. Methods and Protocols: Humana Press; 2010:261-80.

1257. Windahl T, Andersson SO, Lofgren L. Photodynamic therapy of localised prostatic cancer. Lancet. 1990;336(8723):1139.
1258. Bredell MG, Besic E, Maake C, Walt H. The application and challenges of clinical PD-PDT in the head and neck region: a short review. J Photochem. Photobiol. B. 2010;101(3):185-90.
1259. Moen I, Stuhr LE. Hyperbaric oxygen therapy and cancer--a review. Target Oncol. 2012;7(4):233-42.
1260. Raa A, Stansberg C, Steen VM, Bjerkvig R, Reed RK, Stuhr LE. Hyperoxia retards growth and induces apoptosis and loss of glands and blood vessels in DMBA-induced rat mammary tumors. BMC Cancer. 2007;7:23.
1261. Stuhr LE, Raa A, Oyan AM, Kalland KH, Sakariassen PO, Petersen K, et al. Hyperoxia retards growth and induces apoptosis, changes in vascular density and gene expression in transplanted gliomas in nude rats. J Neurooncol. 2007;85(2):191-202.
1262. Gore A, Muralidhar M, Espey MG, Degenhardt K, Mantell LL. Hyperoxia sensing: from molecular mechanisms to significance in disease. J Immunotoxicol. 2010;7(4):239-54.
1263. Moen I, Oyan AM, Kalland KH, Tronstad KJ, Akslen LA, Chekenya M, et al. Hyperoxic treatment induces mesenchymal-to-epithelial transition in a rat adenocarcinoma model. PloS ONE. 2009;4(7):e6381.
1264. Poff AM, Ari C, Seyfried TN, D'Agostino DP. The ketogenic diet and hyperbaric oxygen therapy prolong survival in mice with systemic metastatic cancer. PloS ONE. 2013;8(6):e65522.
1265. Bennett MH, Feldmeier J, Smee R, Milross C. Hyperbaric oxygenation for tumour sensitisation to radiotherapy. Cochrane Database Syst. Rev. 2018;4(4):CD005007.
1266. Cazzaniga ME, Cordani N, Capici S, Cogliati V, Riva F, Cerrito MG. Metronomic Chemotherapy. Cancers (Basel). 2021;13(9).
1267. Wichmann V, Eigeliene N, Saarenheimo J, Jekunen A. Recent clinical evidence on metronomic dosing in controlled clinical trials: a systematic literature review. Acta Oncol. 2020;59(7):775-85.
1268. Liu Y, Gu F, Liang J, Dai X, Wan C, Hong X, et al. The efficacy and toxicity profile of metronomic chemotherapy for metastatic breast cancer: A meta-analysis. PloS ONE. 2017;12(3):e0173693.
1269. DeVita VT, Jr., Chu E. A history of cancer chemotherapy. Cancer Res. 2008;68(21):8643-53.
1270. Bukowski K, Kciuk M, Kontek R. Mechanisms of Multidrug Resistance in Cancer Chemotherapy. Int J Mol Sci. 2020;21(9).
1271. Nussbaumer S, Bonnabry P, Veuthey JL, Fleury-Souverain S. Analysis of anticancer drugs: a review. Talanta. 2011;85(5):2265-89.
1272. Jones R. Cytotoxic chemotherapy: clinical aspects. Medicine. 2015;44:25-9.
1273. Fernando J, Jones R. The Principles of cancer treatment by chemotherapy. Surgery. 2015;33:131-5.
1274. McDivitt RW, Stone KR, Craig RB, Palmer JO, Meyer JS, Bauer WC. A proposed classification of breast cancer based on kinetic information: derived from a comparison of risk factors in 168 primary operable breast cancers. Cancer. 1986;57(2):269-76.
1275. Savage P. Chemotherapy curable malignancies and cancer stem cells: a biological review and hypothesis. BMC Cancer. 2016;16(1):906.
1276. Savage P, Stebbing J, Bower M, Crook T. Why does cytotoxic chemotherapy cure only some cancers? Nat Clin Pract Oncol. 2009;6(1):43-52.
1277. Goldberg GS, Airley R. Cancer Chemotherapy. Basic Science to the Clinic. 2nd ed. Hoboken, NJ: Wiley Blackwell; 2020.
1278. Arai T, Kuroishi T, Saito Y, Kurita Y, Naruke T, Kaneko M. Tumor doubling time and prognosis in lung cancer patients: evaluation from chest films and clinical follow-up study. Japanese Lung Cancer Screening Research Group. Jpn J Clin Oncol. 1994;24(4):199-204.

1279. Harris K, Khachaturova I, Azab B, Maniatis T, Murukutla S, Chalhoub M, et al. Small cell lung cancer doubling time and its effect on clinical presentation: a concise review. Clin Med Insights Oncol. 2012;6:199-203.
1280. Wang JC, Sone S, Feng L, Yang ZG, Takashima S, Maruyama Y, et al. Rapidly growing small peripheral lung cancers detected by screening CT: correlation between radiological appearance and pathological features. Br J Radiol. 2000;73(873):930-7.
1281. Dahan M, Hequet D, Bonneau C, Paoletti X, Rouzier R. Has tumor doubling time in breast cancer changed over the past 80 years? A systematic review. Cancer Med. 2021;10(15):5203-17.
1282. Baharvand M, Jafari S, Mortazavi H. Herbs in Oral Mucositis. J Clin Diagn Res. 2017;11(3):Ze05-ze11.
1283. Nagi R, Patil DJ, Rakesh N, Jain S, Sahu S. Natural agents in the management of oral mucositis in cancer patients-systematic review. J Oral Biol Craniofac Res. 2018;8(3):245-54.
1284. Motallebnejad M, Akram S, Moghadamnia A, Moulana Z, Omidi S. The effect of topical application of pure honey on radiation-induced mucositis: a randomized clinical trial. J Contemp Dent Pract. 2008;9(3):40-7.
1285. Hawley P, Hovan A, McGahan CE, Saunders D. A randomized placebo-controlled trial of manuka honey for radiation-induced oral mucositis. Support Care Cancer. 2014;22(3):751-61.
1286. Su CK, Mehta V, Ravikumar L, Shah R, Pinto H, Halpern J, et al. Phase II double-blind randomized study comparing oral aloe vera versus placebo to prevent radiation-related mucositis in patients with head-and-neck neoplasms. Int J Radiat Oncol Biol Phys. 2004;60(1):171-7.
1287. Alkhouli M, Laflouf M, Alhaddad M. Efficacy of Aloe-Vera Use for Prevention of Chemotherapy-Induced Oral Mucositis in Children with Acute Lymphoblastic Leukemia: A Randomized Controlled Clinical Trial. Compr Child Adolesc Nurs. 2021;44(1):49-62.
1288. Ahmadi A. Potential prevention: Aloe vera mouthwash may reduce radiation-induced oral mucositis in head and neck cancer patients. Chin J Integr Med. 2012;18(8):635-40.
1289. Elhadad MA, El-Negoumy E, Taalab MR, Ibrahim RS, Elsaka RO. The effect of topical chamomile in the prevention of chemotherapy-induced oral mucositis: A randomized clinical trial. Oral Dis. 2022;28(1):164-72.
1290. Maleki M, Mardani A, Manouchehri M, Ashghali Farahani M, Vaismoradi M, Glarcher M. Effect of Chamomile on the Complications of Cancer: A Systematic Review. Integr Cancer Ther. 2023;22:15347354231164600.
1291. Rao S, Dinkar C, Vaishnav LK, Rao P, Rai MP, Fayad R, et al. The Indian Spice Turmeric Delays and Mitigates Radiation-Induced Oral Mucositis in Patients Undergoing Treatment for Head and Neck Cancer: An Investigational Study. Integr Cancer Ther. 2014;13(3):201-10.
1292. Francis M, Williams S. Effectiveness of Indian Turmeric Powder with Honey as Complementary Therapy on Oral Mucositis : A Nursing Perspective among Cancer Patients in Mysore. Nurs J India. 2014;105(6):258-60.
1293. Steinmann D, Babadağ Savaş B, Felber S, Joy S, Mertens I, Cramer H, et al. Nursing Procedures for the Prevention and Treatment of Mucositis Induced by Cancer Therapies: Clinical Practice Guideline Based on an Interdisciplinary Consensus Process and a Systematic Literature Search. Integr Cancer Ther. 2021;20:1534735420940412.
1294. Schönknecht K, Surdacka A, Rudenko L. Effectiveness of composed herbal extract in the treatment of gingivitis and oral and pharyngeal mucosa - Review of studies. Wiad Lek. 2021;74(7):1737-49.
1295. Eita AAB. Milk thistle (Silybum marianum (L.)Gaertn.): An overview about its pharmacology and medicinal uses with an emphasis on oral diseases. J Oral Biosci. 2022;64(1):71-6.

1296. Mutluay Yayla E, Izgu N, Ozdemir L, Aslan Erdem S, Kartal M. Sage tea-thyme-peppermint hydrosol oral rinse reduces chemotherapy-induced oral mucositis: A randomized controlled pilot study. Complement Ther Med. 2016;27:58-64.
1297. Marucci L, Farneti A, Di Ridolfi P, Pinnaro P, Pellini R, Giannarelli D, et al. Double-blind randomized phase III study comparing a mixture of natural agents versus placebo in the prevention of acute mucositis during chemoradiotherapy for head and neck cancer. Head Neck. 2017;39(9):1761-9.
1298. Borges DO, Freitas K, Minicucci EM, Popim RC. Benefits of ginger in the control of chemotherapy-induced nausea and vomiting. Rev Bras Enferm. 2020;73(2):e20180903.
1299. Marx W, Ried K, McCarthy AL, Vitetta L, Sali A, McKavanagh D, et al. Ginger-Mechanism of action in chemotherapy-induced nausea and vomiting: A review. Crit Rev Food Sci Nutr. 2017;57(1):141-6.
1300. Saneei Totmaj A, Emamat H, Jarrahi F, Zarrati M. The effect of ginger (Zingiber officinale) on chemotherapy-induced nausea and vomiting in breast cancer patients: A systematic literature review of randomized controlled trials. Phytother Res. 2019;33(8):1957-65.
1301. Kim SD, Kwag EB, Yang MX, Yoo HS. Efficacy and Safety of Ginger on the Side Effects of Chemotherapy in Breast Cancer Patients: Systematic Review and Meta-Analysis. Int J Mol Sci. 2022;23(19).
1302. Sanaati F, Najafi S, Kashaninia Z, Sadeghi M. Effect of Ginger and Chamomile on Nausea and Vomiting Caused by Chemotherapy in Iranian Women with Breast Cancer. Asian Pac J Cancer Prev. 2016;17(8):4125-9.
1303. Molassiotis A, Zhao IY, Crichton M, Olver I, Fleury M, Giusti R, et al. Effects of food-based interventions in the management of chemoradiotherapy-induced nausea and vomiting: a systematic review. Support Care Cancer. 2023;31(7):413.
1304. Chow R, Valdez C, Chow N, Zhang D, Im J, Sodhi E, et al. Oral cannabinoid for the prophylaxis of chemotherapy-induced nausea and vomiting-a systematic review and meta-analysis. Support Care Cancer. 2020;28(5):2095-103.
1305. Machado Rocha FC, Stéfano SC, De Cássia Haiek R, Rosa Oliveira LM, Da Silveira DX. Therapeutic use of Cannabis sativa on chemotherapy-induced nausea and vomiting among cancer patients: systematic review and meta-analysis. Eur J Cancer Care (Engl). 2008;17(5):431-43.
1306. Arring NM, Millstine D, Marks LA, Nail LM. Ginseng as a Treatment for Fatigue: A Systematic Review. J Altern Complement Med. 2018;24(7):624-33.
1307. Sadeghian M, Rahmani S, Zendehdel M, Hosseini SA, Zare Javid A. Ginseng and Cancer-Related Fatigue: A Systematic Review of Clinical Trials. Nutr Cancer. 2021;73(8):1270-81.
1308. Valdés-González JA, Sánchez M, Moratilla-Rivera I, Iglesias I, Gómez-Serranillos MP. Immunomodulatory, Anti-Inflammatory, and Anti-Cancer Properties of Ginseng: A Pharmacological Update. Molecules. 2023;28(9).
1309. Wang CZ, Anderson S, Du W, He TC, Yuan CS. Red ginseng and cancer treatment. Chin J Nat Med. 2016;14(1):7-16.
1310. Remenapp A, Coyle K, Orange T, Lynch T, Hooper D, Hooper S, et al. Efficacy of Withania somnifera supplementation on adult's cognition and mood. J Ayurveda Integr Med. 2022;13(2):100510.
1311. Speers AB, Cabey KA, Soumyanath A, Wright KM. Effects of Withania somnifera (Ashwagandha) on Stress and the Stress- Related Neuropsychiatric Disorders Anxiety, Depression, and Insomnia. Curr Neuropharmacol. 2021;19(9):1468-95.
1312. Piao BK, Wang YX, Xie GR, Mansmann U, Matthes H, Beuth J, et al. Impact of complementary mistletoe extract treatment on quality of life in breast, ovarian and non-small cell lung cancer patients. A prospective randomized controlled clinical trial. Anticancer Res. 2004;24(1):303-9.

1313. Schnell-Inderst P, Steigenberger C, Mertz M, Otto I, Flatscher-Thöni M, Siebert U. Additional treatment with mistletoe extracts for patients with breast cancer compared to conventional cancer therapy alone - efficacy and safety, costs and cost-effectiveness, patients and social aspects, and ethical assessment. Ger Med Sci. 2022;20:Doc10.
1314. Donelli D, Antonelli M, Bellinazzi C, Gensini GF, Firenzuoli F. Effects of lavender on anxiety: A systematic review and meta-analysis. Phytomedicine. 2019;65:153099.

Made in the United States
[illegible]
November 2020

Made in United States
Orlando, FL
11 November 2026

90609399R00129